HEMATOLOGY FOR INTERNISTS

This book is based on an American College of Physicians Course on Hematology for Internists, with Emphasis on Recent Advances, given at The University of Rochester School of Medicine and Dentistry, Rochester, New York

HEMATOLOGY

BY 26 AUTHORS

EDITOR

ROBERT I. WEED, M.D.

Professor of Medicine and of Radiation Biology and Biophysics and Head, Hematology Unit, The University of Rochester School of Medicine and Dentistry, Rochester

FOR INTERNISTS

ASSOCIATE EDITORS

RICHARD F. BAKEMEIER, M.D.

Associate Professor of Medicine, The University of Rochester School of Medicine and Dentistry, Rochester

LEON W. HOYER, M.D.

Associate Professor of Medicine, University of Connecticut School of Medicine, Hartford

STANLEY B. TROUP, M.D.

Professor of Medicine, The University of Rochester School of Medicine and Dentistry, Rochester

LITTLE, BROWN AND COMPANY, BOSTON

Library of Congress catalog card No. 73-146341

First Edition

ISBN 0-316-92773

4337-21D2-M09/71

Published in Great Britain by Churchill/Livingstone, Edinburgh and London

Printed in the United States of America

PREFACE

Several elementary hematology texts are currently available, as are recent revisions of inclusive advanced texts and new comprehensive works of value to those with an extensive background in hematology. This book has been written for practicing physicians with a special interest in hematology; the complexity and coverage of individual topics are oriented toward a general medical audience. Like the American College of Physicians Course on Hematology for Internists, with Emphasis on Recent Advances, given at The University of Rochester, the book is intended for practicing internists as well as residents and fellows in training; but it is hoped that much of the content will be of interest also to pediatricians, general practitioners, and clinical pathologists.

Selection of topics for the book was based in large part on the interests of the various chapters were all members of the faculty of The University given in Rochester, although much of the material has been updated and several new subjects have been added. With the important exceptions of Dr. Clement A. Finch, a guest lecturer, and Dr. Robert Hillman, the authors of the various chapters were all members of the faculty of The University of Rochester School of Medicine and Dentistry at the time that the course was presented.

Three important assumptions underlie the format and content of the book. The assumptions are that the reader (1) has a basic background and continuing interest in hematology, (2) is significantly interested in important recent advances that have been made in our understanding of the pathologic biochemistry and pathophysiology of major hematologic disorders, and, most importantly, (3) wishes to be informed about current therapy for the various disorders, particularly in the light of newer insights into pathophysiology.

Hematology for Internists is divided into parts dealing with anemia, problems of hemostasis, and myeloproliferative and lymphoproliferative disorders. Each part contains at least one chapter reviewing basic science and research contributions, to provide the clinician the understanding essential for rational diagnosis and treatment. The length of the chapters and the balance of emphasis within each chapter on diagnostic procedures versus therapeutic recommendations relate more to the extent of our current knowledge than to the statistical frequency of the disorders themselves.

This book emphasizes recent advances in the important areas of hematology rather than attempting to cover *all* topics or *all* advances. For this reason and because much of the material has been organized to emphasize pathophysiology, certain very important subjects such as iron deficiency and thalassemia do not appear as separate chapters. However, clues to the recognition of iron deficiency and the interaction of iron with erythropoietin are discussed in the chapter on clinical approaches to anemia, while thalassemia is discussed under the more general heading of Heinz body disorders. When diagnosis or therapy, or both, warrant, major disorders are grouped together; for example, chronic lymphocytic leukemia is discussed along with the management of lymphomas.

In addition to being selective about inclusion of topics in the interest of reasonable brevity, authors have been encouraged to express and amplify their own opinions regarding specifics of clinical management. By such selection and by avoiding presentation of all views on controversial subjects, the book admittedly has something of a Rochester flavor except for Chapter 1. Certainly we have passed over many who have made major contributions. However, it is hoped that the resultant relatively short text may thus be more readable and of more practical value to its intended audience—particularly if it is recognized that whenever opinion supplements facts in the text, the opinion is that of the particular author.

In order to save space and to avoid interrupting the text, most reference citations have been eliminated. The selected references found at the end of each chapter represent either pertinent general review articles or new contributions to the understanding and management of the disease under discussion. Certain key references are indicated in the text by author's name and date of publication, however. The appendix, a current bibliography of methodology in various areas of hematology, is included for readers who wish up-to-date references on various techniques important in the hematology laboratory.

The assistance of Carol B. Weed, my wife and secretary, is hereby gratefully acknowledged. Her hard work, sense of organization, and assistance in providing firm encouragement to the authors to complete their manuscripts have been invaluable.

R. I. W.

CONTENTS

II.   PROBLEMS OF HEMOSTASIS

III.   MYELOPROLIFERATIVE DISORDERS

IV. DISORDERS OF THE LYMPHATIC SYSTEM

CONTRIBUTING AUTHORS

Except as otherwise noted, all authors are at The University of Rochester School of Medicine and Dentistry, Rochester

RICHARD F. BAKEMEIER, M.D.
ASSOCIATE PROFESSOR OF MEDICINE

ARTHUR W. BAUMAN, M.D.
ASSOCIATE PROFESSOR OF MEDICINE

JOHN M. BENNETT, M.D.
ASSOCIATE PROFESSOR OF MEDICINE

ROBERT T. BRECKENRIDGE, M.D.
ASSOCIATE PROFESSOR OF MEDICINE

LAWRENCE N. CHESSIN, M.D.
CLINICAL ASSISTANT PROFESSOR OF MEDICINE

CLEMENT A. FINCH, M.D.
PROFESSOR OF MEDICINE, THE UNIVERSITY OF WASHINGTON SCHOOL OF MEDICINE, SEATTLE

KONG-OO GOH, M.D.
ASSOCIATE PROFESSOR OF MEDICINE AND OF ANATOMY

WILLIAM A. GREENE, M.D.
PROFESSOR OF MEDICINE AND OF PSYCHIATRY

PAUL F. GRINER, M.D.
ASSOCIATE PROFESSOR OF MEDICINE

THOMAS C. HALL, M.D.
PROFESSOR OF MEDICINE AND OF PHARMACOLOGY AND TOXICOLOGY

ROBERT S. HEUSINKVELD, M.D.
SENIOR INSTRUCTOR IN MEDICINE

ROGER S. HILL, M.D.
RESEARCH FELLOW, DEPARTMENT OF HAEMATOLOGY, ROYAL
POSTGRADUATE MEDICAL SCHOOL, LONDON

ROBERT S. HILLMAN, M.D.
ASSOCIATE PROFESSOR OF MEDICINE, THE UNIVERSITY OF WASHINGTON
SCHOOL OF MEDICINE, SEATTLE

LEON W. HOYER, M.D.
ASSOCIATE PROFESSOR OF MEDICINE, UNIVERSITY OF CONNECTICUT SCHOOL
OF MEDICINE, HARTFORD

FREDERICK A. KLIPSTEIN, M.D.
ASSOCIATE PROFESSOR OF MEDICINE, THE UNIVERSITY OF ROCHESTER
SCHOOL OF MEDICINE AND DENTISTRY, ROCHESTER, AND THE UNIVERSITY
OF PUERTO RICO, SAN JUAN

PAUL L. LACELLE, M.D.
ASSOCIATE PROFESSOR OF MEDICINE AND OF RADIATION BIOLOGY AND
BIOPHYSICS

JOHN P. LEDDY, M.D.
ASSOCIATE PROFESSOR OF MEDICINE

MARSHALL A. LICHTMAN, M.D.
ASSOCIATE PROFESSOR OF MEDICINE AND OF RADIATION BIOLOGY AND
BIOPHYSICS

ARNOLD I. MEISLER, M.D.
ASSISTANT PROFESSOR OF MEDICINE

DENIS R. MILLER, M.D.
ASSOCIATE PROFESSOR OF PEDIATRICS, CORNELL UNIVERSITY MEDICAL
COLLEGE, NEW YORK

GEORGE E. MILLER

CHIEF LABORATORY TECHNICIAN, HEMOPHILIA CENTER OF ROCHESTER AND MONROE COUNTY, ROCHESTER GENERAL HOSPITAL, ROCHESTER

SEYMOUR I. SCHWARTZ, M.D.

PROFESSOR OF SURGERY

DAVID A. SEARS, M.D.

ASSOCIATE PROFESSOR OF MEDICINE AND OF PHYSIOLOGY, THE UNIVERSITY OF TEXAS MEDICAL SCHOOL AT SAN ANTONIO, SAN ANTONIO

STANLEY B. TROUP, M.D.

PROFESSOR OF MEDICINE

ROBERT I. WEED, M.D.

PROFESSOR OF MEDICINE AND OF RADIATION BIOLOGY AND BIOPHYSICS

LAWRENCE E. YOUNG, M.D.

DEWEY PROFESSOR OF MEDICINE AND CHAIRMAN, DEPARTMENT OF MEDICINE

I
ANEMIAS

1. A CLINICAL APPROACH TO ANEMIA

Clement A. Finch
Robert S. Hillman

THIS PRESENTATION is a brief summary of a problem-solving approach to anemia adapted from the University of Washington Red Cell and Hematology laboratory manuals. Its purpose is to provide the physician with a pathophysiologic classification of anemia in which the functional disturbance of the erythron is emphasized. In this approach it is necessary to begin with a few general statements about the behavior of the erythron.

The normal *erythron* is composed of a generating tissue in the medullary cavities of the axial skeleton and a mass of circulating red cells. The relationship between the erythroid marrow and circulating red cells is shown in Table 1-1. Approximately 4 days are required for the immature red cell to undergo some four mitotic divisions and extrude its nucleus; additional time is spent as a maturing *reticulocyte* within the marrow. Finally, after entering the circulating blood, the reticulocyte requires 1 day or more to lose its reticulum. The mature red cell lives 120 days in the circulation, after which time it is destroyed by the reticuloendothelial cell.

Marrow activity is regulated by *erythropoietin*. This hormone determines the degree of proliferation of the marrow and also affects the rate of maturation. Under increased erythropoietin stimulus, immature erythroid cells increase in number within 2 or 3 days and the reticulocyte output from the marrow increases over the following 3 or 4 days. Total production will be 3 to 5 times base level within a week, provided adequate iron is available. In addition to the increased proliferation, *shift cells* (basophilic macroreticulocytes) appear in the circulation.

Iron supply for erythropoiesis normally is derived almost completely from broken-down erythrocytes. When increased amounts of iron are required for erythropoiesis beyond that available from red cell breakdown, iron must be mobilized from stores. Rates of erythropoiesis in man follow-

Table 1-1. *Relationship Between Erythroid Marrow and Circulating Red Cells*

Cell Type	Time Span (Days)	Relative Number
Nucleated RBC	5	1.5
Marrow reticulocytes	1.5	1.5
Blood reticulocytes	1	1
Adult RBC	120	100

Cell Type	Circulating Mass	Daily Turnover
Red cells	2000 ml	17 ml
Hemoglobin	660 gm	5.7 gm
Porphyrin pigment	23 gm	190 mg
Iron	2.2 gm	18 mg

Conversion constants: body hematocrit = 0.90 × venous hematocrit; iron per gram hemoglobin = 3.38 mg; daily red cell breakdown = 1/120 (or 0.83%); hemoglobin molecular weight = 66,000; protoporphyrin molecular weight = 566; urobilinogen molecular weight = 580; iron atomic weight = 56.

ing blood loss do not usually increase above 2 times normal because of the limitations of iron mobilization from stores. Higher rates of erythropoiesis are found in hemolytic states because of the ease with which the reticulo-endothelial cell can catabolize iron from nonviable red cells.

The normality of the erythron is usually judged by the concentration of red cells in the circulation. Usual values for normal subjects are shown in Table 1-2. *Anemia* is defined as a significant decrease in circulating hemoglobin, usually more than 10% of the accepted mean. Thus anemia is a

Table 1-2. *Concentration of Red Cells in Circulation in Normal Subjects*

Age	Hemoglobin (gm/100 ml)	Hematocrit (%)
Birth	17.0	50
1 to 3 months	14.0	42
3 months to 5 years	12.0	36
6 to 10 years	12.0	37
11 to 15 years	13.0	39
Adult male	15.5	47
Menstruating female	13.5	41
Pregnancy (last trimester)	12.0	37

laboratory diagnosis related to a population norm rather than to the physiology of the individual.

LABORATORY TESTS

The nature of anemia is determined both from qualitative abnormalities in individual cells as revealed by examination of the aspirated marrow, the blood film, and red cell indices and from those parameters that characterize the rate of blood production and destruction, the reticulocyte index, marrow E:G ratio (ratio of erythroid to granulocytic cells in the aspirated marrow), and bilirubin.

BLOOD SMEAR

An estimation should be made of the red cell size, and shape abnormalities should be identified. The following cell forms have particular significance: *shift cells,* which indicate increased erythropoietin stimulus; *true macrocytes,* which indicate a nuclear maturation defect (and, when accompanied by a hypersegmentation of granulocytes, indicate megaloblastic anemia); *hypochromic microcytes,* which indicate a block in hemoglobin synthesis; *spherocytes,* which indicate a hemolytic process. Other cell forms that suggest hemolysis are fragmentation, sickle cell, ovalocytes, and acanthrocyte and stomatocyte deformities. *Poikilocytosis* is significant as an indication of defective maturation process. A *myelophthisic blood picture,* including immature cells of all series, indicates disease within the marrow.

RED CELL INDICES

Measurements of hemoglobin, hematocrit, and red cell number permit calculations of cell size, hemoglobin concentration, and content. Basal values are shown in Table 1-3. These "normal" values are modified by erythropoietin and iron supply. Increased erythropoietin produces an increase in the MCV and decreases in the MCHC. For the increase in volume to occur, however, the plasma iron must be above 100 μg per 100 ml.

Table 1-3.   Basal Adult Values (Coulter Counter)

MCV	(mean cell volume in μ^3)	$\dfrac{Hct}{RBC}$	90 ± 8	$82 - 98$
MCH	(mean cell hemoglobin in $\mu\mu$g)	$\dfrac{Hgb}{RBC}$	30 ± 3	$27 - 33$
MCHC	(mean cell hemoglobin concentration in gm/100 ml)	$\dfrac{Hgb}{Hct}$	33 ± 2	$31 - 35$

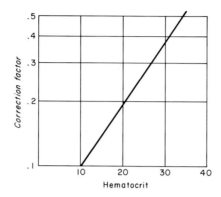

Figure 1-1. Chart for calculation of reticulocyte index. The reticulocyte index may be obtained by multiplying the patient's reticulocyte count by a correction factor derived from the patient's hematocrit.

RETICULOCYTE INDEX

The number of circulating cells containing reticulum provides a measure of red cell production. In order for this to be meaningful from a quantitative standpoint, the reticulocyte count must be corrected for the number of cells in circulation and for the maturation time of the reticulocyte in the peripheral blood. Increased erythropoietin produces a shift of reticulocytes from marrow to blood and prolongs the maturation time. Combined correction factors for various degrees of anemia are shown in Figure 1-1. In making the correction for shift, a predictable relationship between erythropoietin level and the degree of anemia is assumed. It is well to check the blood film to determine whether or not the expected degree of shift is present. Normal reticulocyte count is 1% or about 60,000 reticulocytes per cubic millimeter. The corrected reticulocyte count or reticulocyte index should be compared to the normal value of 1. This index indicates the number of reticulocytes entering the blood stream per day (effective erythropoiesis).

PLASMA IRON AND IRON-BINDING CAPACITY $PLL = \frac{PI-}{I-BC} = \frac{50-150}{280-380}$

Plasma iron level and the ratio of plasma iron to iron-binding capacity of the plasma indicate the adequacy of the iron supplied to marrow. Normal plasma iron fluctuates from 50 to 150 μg per 100 ml, and usually shows a diurnal fluctuation from 110 in the morning to 70 μg per 100 ml in the evening. Iron-binding capacity is usually stable at about 330 ± 50 μg per 100 ml. A plasma iron of less than 30 μg per 100 ml and a percent saturation of 15 or less indicate a deficient iron supply if erythropoiesis is at a basal level.

ICTERUS INDEX OR BILIRUBIN

The amount of pyrrole pigment in the plasma is normally between 4 and 8 units of icterus index or 0.4 to 0.8 mg of bilirubin. Values below this are useful in indicating decreased red cell breakdown.

BONE MARROW EXAMINATION

An approximation of the number of nucleated red cells may be obtained from the E:G ratio. Such a ratio is meaningful only if granulocyte production is normal as reflected by a normal circulating granulocyte count. The normal E:G ratio in marrow smears is 1 to 3. This indicates the degree of proliferation of erythroid cells within the marrow (total erythropoiesis). Qualitative changes in the red cell series which are important to recognize are megaloblastic alterations and sideroblastic changes (iron accumulations within the cytoplasm as determined by a Prussian blue iron stain). Reticuloendothelial iron stores should also be examined in marrow aspirate.

RED CELL LIFE-SPAN AND SPLENIC LOCALIZATION

^{51}Cr tagging of erythrocytes is useful for measuring both shortening of red cell life-span and, by in vivo counting, excessive accumulation of radioactivity in the splenic area. Normal ^{51}Cr life-span is 29 ± 3 days.

CLINICAL MANIFESTATIONS

With mild degrees of anemia (hemoglobin 10 to 14 gm per 100 ml) symptoms are usually not detected. If present, they are more often attributable to underlying disease than to anemia per se. At most, symptoms appear only on heavy exercise and reflect the compensatory overactivity of heart and lungs. They consist of palpitation, dyspnea, and sometimes excessive sweating. With moderate anemia there is increase of these symptoms and fatigue. In severe anemia tachycardia, wide pulse pressure and hyperpnea, sensitivity to cold, loss of appetite, weakness, and occasional syncope may be seen. In elderly people local vascular disease may sensitize certain tissues to the effect of anemic hypoxia and result in such manifestations as intermittent claudication and angina.

DIAGNOSIS

Anemia is due either to increased destruction of circulating red cells or to an abnormality in production (Fig. 1-2). The first of these, *hemolytic anemia,* is characterized by a reticulocyte index of 3 or more times normal. A reticulocyte index of less than 2 times normal indicates a disturbance in erythropoiesis related either to impaired proliferation or to an abnormality in the maturation process which is associated with excessive cell death prior to the reticulocyte stage. Either one of these abnormalities may result in a reticulocyte index of less than 2 times normal in the anemic patient. Distinction between them is made on the basis of smear, indices, and bilirubin. With *hypoproliferative anemia,* red cells are usually of normal size and shape with shift cells present if erythropoietin is increased, and bilirubin is often below normal. With *maturation abnormality* true macrocytosis or microcytosis may be found along with poikilocytosis, and bilirubin is normal or slightly increased.

Hypoproliferative Anemias

Hypoproliferative anemias are by far the most frequent type of anemia and are due to three main causes: an inadequate iron supply, decreased stimulation by erythropoietin, or marrow disease. Iron supply can be evaluated directly from the plasma iron and iron-binding capacity. Anemias due to decreased erythropoietin stimulation do not show the expected shift cells on smear. Marrow damage is usually associated with abnormalities in all the formed elements of the blood. Marrow examination often is required to establish the nature of the marrow dysfunction, e.g., aplasia, neoplastic infiltration, myelofibrosis.

Maturation Abnormalities

Most maturation abnormalities fall into the two main categories of macrocytic normochromic and microcytic hypochromic anemias. The former are considered to be due to abnormalities in nuclear development and are often caused by deficiencies of vitamin B_{12} or folic acid. They may be suspected by the presence of true macrocytes on smear (as differentiated from shift macrocytes) and by hypersegmentation of granulocytes. They are confirmed by the presence of megaloblastic changes in the marrow. Direct evidence of the two deficiency states may be obtained by their plasma levels. Microcytic hypochromic anemia may be caused by iron deficiency or by disorders of globin metabolism (thalassemias) or of porphyrin synthesis (pyridoxine and sideroblastic anemias). The globin and porphyrin abnormalities differ from iron deficiency in that there is a high plasma iron and accumulation of iron in the developing red cells (sideroblasts).

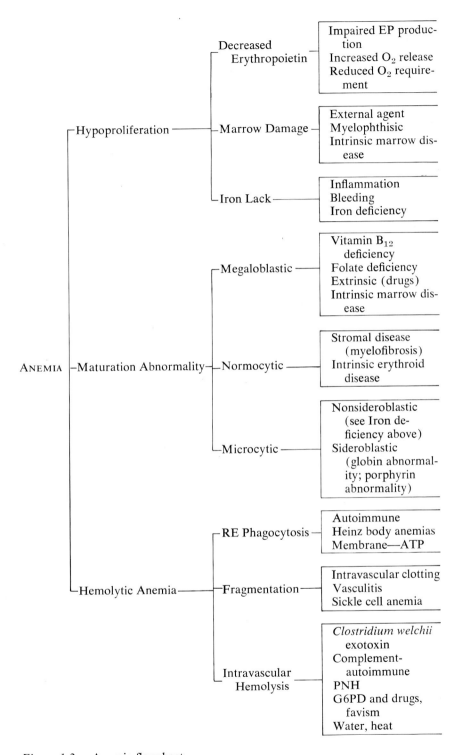

Figure 1-2. Anemia flowsheet.

Hemolytic Anemias

Hemolytic anemias may be approached through the pigment abnormalities produced by the excessive red cell breakdown. One group of anemias characterized by intravascular hemolysis may be recognized by the presence of hemoglobinemia and hemoglobinuria, hemosiderinuria, and methemalbuminuria (positive Schumm's test). A second group is characterized by red cell fragmentation and may have irregularly shaped red cells on smear, the hallmark of these disorders. By far the largest group is associated with reticuloendothelial destruction of red cells and may be due to a variety of causes. The Coombs' test is most useful in indicating that group of disorders that is associated with globulin coating of the red cell membrane, including the autoimmune hemolytic anemias. Defects in aerobic glycolysis and also certain unstable hemoglobins are characterized by excessive Heinz body formation, i.e., masses of denatured globin within red cells. This may be detected by supravital staining when masses are present in the circulation, or by incubation with or without oxidizing agents to bring out the tendency of hemoglobin to denature. Defects in anaerobic glycolysis may be suggested by excessive hemolysis of blood incubated at 37°C (incubation hemolysis test). Certain red cell membrane abnormalities such as hereditary spherocytosis may also show an abnormal incubation hemolysis test. Hypersplenism is an additional cause of excessive reticuloendothelial destruction of red cells.

The laboratory characterization of anemia along these lines in some instances provides a definitive diagnosis; for example, iron deficiency anemia. In other instances the identification of marrow damage or a type of hemolytic disease may be indication for a careful search for a specific etiologic agent. The ultimate objective of the physician is to understand the anemia in both physiologic and etiologic terms.

THERAPY

In this discussion remarks concerning therapy can be of only the most general sort. A decrease in oxygen supply of mild anemia is easily corrected by a slight increase in cardiac output and decreased affinity of hemoglobin for oxygen. The latter is effected by an increase in red cell 2,3 diphosphoglycerate. If cardiac function is normal, a hemoglobin level of 7 gm does not produce symptoms. However, severe degrees of anemia (level less than 4 gm) may seriously limit oxygen transport and place an increased burden on the heart. Although a red cell transfusion may correct this, the severely anemic patient is susceptible to circulatory overload and pulmonary edema. When transfusion seems advisable, plasma volume should be reduced before transfusion by the administration of rapid-acting diuretics or by the removal of an equal volume of blood. An exception to this is acute hemorrhage in which blood volume is depleted and reconstitution may be rapid and aggressive. In the severely anemic patient it is important to monitor pulmonary status during transfusion, including central venous pressure and auscultation of the lung fields for basilar rales. If specific therapy is available to which the patient's bone marrow may respond, it may be advisable to avoid the hazards of transfusion, which include not only overload but also hepatitis. If there is evidence of increased red cell breakdown, it is important to determine the nature of hemolysis, since transfused cells may live a very short time if an extrinsic hemolytic mechanism is present. Indeed, immunologic destruction may often be more severe against transfused cells than against the patient's own cells. Oxygen therapy may be helpful in the extremely anemic patient since plasma transport of oxygen in this situation may amount to 25% of the total oxygen transport.

Three deficiency states of particular importance because of their response to specific therapy are iron, folate, and vitamin B_{12} deficiencies. The presence of iron deficiency anemia usually means blood loss, and it may be more important to identify the cause of bleeding than to treat the anemia. It is always important to search for a drug which may have had an adverse effect on blood production or destruction. Immunologic mechanisms responsible for red cell destruction are often amenable to steroids or other suppressive drug therapy. Finally, discovering that the spleen is playing an important role in hemolysis can lead to improvement in the patient's status by splenectomy.

REFERENCES

Adamson, J. W., Eschbach, J., and Finch, C. A. The kidney and erythropoiesis. *Amer. J. Med.* 44:725, 1968.

Bainton, D. F., and Finch, C. A. The diagnosis of iron deficiency anemia. *Amer. J. Med.* 37:62, 1964.

Brain, M. C. The hemolytic-uremic syndrome. *Seminars Hemat.* 6:162, 1969.

Dacie, J. V., and Worlledge, S. M. Auto-Immune Hemolytic Anemias. In E. B. Brown and C. V. Moore (Eds.), *Progress in Hematology.* New York: Grune & Stratton, 1969. Vol. 6, pp. 82–120.

Finch, C. A. *Red Cell Manual.* Seattle: University of Washington, Division of Hematology, 1969.

Herbert, V. Megaloblastic anemias. Mechanisms and management. *D.M.,* Aug. 1965. P. 1.

Hillman, R. S. *Hematology Laboratory Manual.* Seattle: University of Washington, Division of Hematology, 1969.

Hillman, R. S., and Finch, C. A. Erythropoiesis: Normal and abnormal. *Seminars Hemat.* 37:62, 1967.

Horrigan, D. L., and Harris, J. W. Pyridoxine-Responsive Anemias in Man. In R. S. Harris, I. G. Wool, and J. A. Loraine (Eds.), *Vitamins and Hormones: Advances in Research and Applications.* New York: Academic, 1968. Vol. 26, p. 549.

Valentine, W. N. Hereditary hemolytic anemias associated with specific erythrocyte enzymopathies. *Calif. Med.* 108:280, 1968.

2. THE MEGALOBLASTIC ANEMIAS

Frederick A. Klipstein

PRINCIPAL ADVANCES during the past decade in the field of megaloblastic anemia have resulted from the development of techniques which permit precise delineation of the vitamin(s) responsible for the anemia and the pathophysiologic factors responsible for the development of these deficiencies. This chapter discusses the application of these techniques to the investigation of persons with this form of anemia, summarizes the normal physiology of folate and vitamin B_{12}, and describes those conditions which can be responsible for the development of a megaloblastic anemia.

CLINICAL ASPECTS

The clinical picture of megaloblastic anemia includes symptoms referable to the anemia itself, including weakness and easy fatigability, as well as symptoms of cardiovascular decompensation in advanced cases. Anorexia and weight loss are common. The megaloblastic changes also occur in epithelial cells throughout the intestinal tract and elsewhere (cervical cytology is usually abnormal). The tongue may be either sore and beefy red or smooth and atrophic. A few persons develop diarrhea. Some patients have a fever; although fever is usually low grade, temperatures may rise to as high as 104°F solely because of the presence of a megaloblastic anemia. The skin may become hyperpigmented.

Vitamin B_{12} deficiency, but *not* folate deficiency, can result in inadequate synthesis of myelin. The neurologic manifestations of vitamin B_{12} deficiency are variable. Paresthesia with numbness and tingling of the hands and feet is commonly the earliest neurologic symptom, and diminution of vibration and position sense the first sign of deficiency. In more advanced deficiency, mental changes ("megaloblastic madness") are common and the more severe neurologic manifestations of subacute combined degeneration become evident. It is essential for the clinician to be aware that (1) neurologic manifestations of vitamin B_{12} deficiency can be present in the absence of anemia and (2) treatment with folic acid can correct the anemia due to B_{12} deficiency yet permit the neurologic disorder to progress. For these reasons it is imperative for the physician to exclude the presence of vitamin B_{12} deficiency in nonanemic persons with neurologic abnormalities and to determine the exact cause of the megaloblastic anemia in each patient.

Several articles in the literature have suggested that folate deficiency may be responsible for mental symptoms, particularly in elderly individuals. The evidence for this is meager, principally subjective, and circumstantial; no relationship has been evident between the presence of folate deficiency and objective neurologic changes in epileptics taking diphenylhydantoin (Dilantin).

HEMATOLOGIC ASPECTS

The hematologic manifestations of deficiency of folate or vitamin B_{12} are indistinguishable. The initial change in the peripheral blood smear consists of the presence of macrocytes and hypersegmented polymorphonuclear leukocytes. As the deficiency becomes more prolonged and severe, anemia develops which is often associated with leukopenia and thrombocytopenia. Thus persons with a severe megaloblastic anemia usually present with a *pancytopenia*. In the bone marrow, megaloblastic changes may be confined to erythroid cells of intermediate maturity in mild deficiency states but in severe deficiency are present in cells varying from the most primitive to the very mature nucleated forms. The characteristic finding in these cells is a maturation arrest, also referred to as nuclear cytoplasmic dissociation, in which the nuclear appearance remains disproportionately immature in relationship to the cytoplasm. The biochemical abnormality responsible for this appears to be an accumulation of nuclear RNA due to reduced capacity to double the nuclear DNA complement, a step necessary for cell division. The presence of giant metamyelocytes is the other characteristic abnormality in the bone marrow.

Concomitant iron deficiency may mask morphologic changes of folate or vitamin B_{12} deficiency. Individuals with a combined deficiency of iron and vitamin B_{12} (as often occurs following gastrectomy) or of iron and folate (as may occur in malabsorption syndromes) usually have a dimorphic pattern of erythrocytes in the peripheral blood consisting of hypochromic erythrocytes and macrocytes, but—of diagnostic importance—hypersegmented polymorphonuclear leukocytes are also present. Megaloblastic changes in the bone marrow may be slight. Iron therapy results in only a partial hematologic response, and repeat bone marrow aspiration shows conversion to florid megaloblastic changes.

In addition to changes in the blood elements, persons with a megaloblastic anemia have a hemolytic component which usually results in elevation of the indirect-acting serum bilirubin concentration. Serum concentrations of the enzymes lactic dehydrogenase (LDH), 2-hydroxybutyrate dehydrogenase (HBDH), and muramidase are also elevated. Since the major portion of measurable muramidase activity is derived from degraded granulocytes, the elevated concentration of this enzyme suggests that neutropenia in megaloblastic anemia results primarily from increased turnover of granulocytes.

LABORATORY INVESTIGATIONS

Laboratory techniques available for the investigation of megaloblastic anemias are summarized in Table 2-1. For the sake of convenience, determinations pertaining to folate and vitamin B_{12} are discussed separately.

Table 2-1.   Laboratory Investigation of Megaloblastic Anemias

---

FOLATE

Deficiency
    Serum folate concentration
    Red blood cell folate concentration
    Plasma clearance of folic acid
    Urinary excretion of formiminoglutamic acid (FIGLU)

Absorption
    Microbiologic assay of serum after oral test dose
    Absorption of ^{3}H-labeled folic acid (^{3}H FA)

VITAMIN B_{12}

Deficiency
    Serum vitamin B_{12} concentration
    Urinary excretion of methylmalonic acid (MMA)

Absorption
    Absorption of ^{57}Co B_{12} tested in stool, urine, or by hepatic uptake

Related determinations
    Assay for intrinsic factor in gastric juice
    Determination of gastric acidity
    Serum assay for intrinsic factor or parietal cell antibodies
    Changes in serum-binding proteins of vitamin B_{12}
    Radiologic examination of the intestine

FOLATE

The somewhat abbreviated version of the folate metabolic pathway illustrated in Figure 2-1 is presented to call attention to two points of importance to the clinician. (1) Several microbiologic organisms are available for use in assays. Growth of these bacteria is dependent on different monoglutamate forms of folate; they do not respond to polyglutamate forms unless these forms are deconjugated by the addition of the enzyme folate deconjugase to the monoglutamate. Growth of the organism *Streptococcus faecalis* reflects the presence of folic acid (pteroylglutamic acid), that of *Lactobacillus casei* is supported by most folate monoglutamates including folic acid, tetrahydrofolic acid, and N^5-methyltetrahydrofolic acid, and that of *Leuconostoc citrovorum* requires the presence of formyl and formimino forms of folate. (2) Folate and vitamin B_{12} metabolism are interrelated in certain processes. In the conversion of homocysteine to methionine, the methyl group of N^5-methyltetrahydrofolic acid is transferred to cobalamin to form methyl B_{12} and then subsequently to homocysteine to form methionine. Thus deficiency of vitamin B_{12} may be responsible for changes in folate metabolism; this is reflected in the fact that some one-third of persons with B_{12} deficiency have an elevated serum folate concentration and formiminoglutamic acid (FIGLU) present in the urine.

Determinations to Detect Deficiency

The proper interpretation of these tests requires a knowledge of the sequence of events during folate deficiency. The maintenance of a normal serum concentration depends upon both body stores and a mechanism

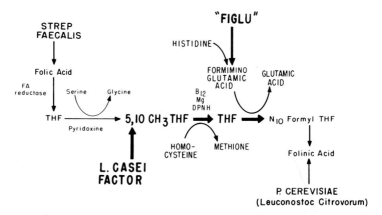

Figure 2-1. Simplified version of folate metabolism. *Streptococcus faecalis, Lactobacillus casei,* and *Leuconostoc citrovorum* refer to microorganisms whose growth reflects various different folate forms.

whereby incoming folate displaces hepatic folate into the blood. Sequential observations in persons placed on a diet devoid of folate have shown that the serum folate concentration falls within 2 weeks, hypersegmented neutrophils appear in the peripheral blood at 8 to 12 weeks, FIGLU appears in the urine after 14 weeks, the red blood cell folate level becomes reduced at 17 weeks, and megaloblastic changes appear in the bone marrow at 19 weeks.

SERUM FOLATE CONCENTRATIONS.   Serum folate concentration is measured by a microbiologic assay using *L. casei*. The principal folate form present in the serum and detected in this manner is N^5-methyltetrahydrofolic acid (Fig. 2-1). The introduction of commercially available assay mediums has simplified the performance of this assay to the point that it can be readily adopted for use in most general hematology laboratories. Food intake affects the serum concentration, and only fasting persons should be tested. The serum can be either assayed immediately or stored at $-20°C$ for up to 6 months without appreciable loss of folate activity. A radioisotopic assay for serum concentration using tritium-labeled folic acid has been developed, but its complexity precludes use in routine laboratories.

The normal range of serum folate activity differs according to the laboratory conducting the determination, but in most instances values in normal subjects are found to range from 7 to 20 mμg per milliliter, and values are less than 5 mμg per milliliter in deficiency states. Serum levels fall promptly in conditions associated with folate deficiency, and subnormal values may antedate folate depletion of tissues or hematologic manifestations of folate deficiency. Serum folate concentrations are also reduced by the administration of folate antagonists and may be spuriously subnormal in persons taking antibiotics (with the exception of tetracycline and nonabsorbable sulfa preparations). Serum folate concentrations are elevated above normal in persons receiving folic acid and in about one-third of those deficient in vitamin B_{12}.

RED BLOOD CELL FOLATE CONCENTRATION.   Red blood cell folate concentration is determined by assay, with *L. casei,* of a hemolysate of the whole blood. The RBC concentration in normal individuals ranges from 160 to 640 mμg per milliliter. The intact red blood cell appears to be relatively impermeable to folate compounds; thus the RBC folate concentration is a reflection of marrow folate stores at the time of erythrocyte production, and values correlate closely with hematologic manifestations of deficiency. The RBC folate concentration is reduced in all persons who have a megaloblastic anemia due to folate deficiency and in approximately one-third of nonanemic folate-deficient subjects. The RBC determination thus permits, in conjunction with the serum value, a more precise guide to the severity of folate deficiency; this determination cannot, however, be used alone to differentiate between deficiency of folate or vitamin B_{12}, since RBC folate levels are also subnormal in two-thirds of persons deficient in vitamin B_{12}.

URINARY EXCRETION OF FORMIMINOGLUTAMIC ACID. FIGLU is an intermediate product of histidine metabolism which requires the presence of tetrahydrofolic acid for its conversion to glutamic acid (Fig. 2-1). Hence its excretion in the urine provides indirect evidence for the presence of folate deficiency. The test is performed by electrophoresis on a 5-hour urine sample obtained following the oral administration of 15 gm histidine.

Most normal subjects have no detectable FIGLU in the urine, whereas persons with hematologic evidence of folate deficiency have been found to excrete more than 3.5 mg per hour and those with severe deficiency can excrete up to 80 mg per hour. The difficulty with this determination is that spuriously positive results can be obtained in two circumstances: (1) the absence of the enzyme formiminotransferase, which can occur in persons with liver disease or in mentally retarded children who have a congenital deficiency of this enzyme; (2) in approximately a third of persons who are deficient in vitamin B_{12}. Thus the test cannot be used alone to differentiate between folate and vitamin B_{12} deficiency.

Determination of Folate Absorption

The clinically applicable tests of folate absorption all employ an oral test dose of crystalline folic acid, varying from physiologic doses of 25 to 200 μg to a pharmacologic dose of 40 μg per kilogram of body weight. The various tests differ in whether serum, urine, or feces are analyzed and whether microbiologic or radioisotopic techniques are employed for this. With the exception of tests which employ fecal collections, all require preliminary saturation with folic acid, 15 mg parenterally, for 3 days prior to the study.

MICROBIOLOGIC TECHNIQUES. The easiest and most reliable technique is to determine serum folate concentrations using *S. faecalis* at hourly intervals for 3 hours after an oral test dose of 40 μg per kilogram of body weight. Normal subjects have a peak serum concentration of greater than 40 mμg per milliliter, and persons with impaired jejunal absorptive function are usually found to have lower values.

RADIOISOTOPIC TECHNIQUES. Tests to measure folic acid absorption by radioisotopic means, using either tritium or ^{14}C-labeled folic acid, were introduced in 1961. The most direct of these is the determination of radioactivity excreted in the feces following an oral test dose; however, the technical difficulties attendant on measuring radioactivity in fecal samples have restricted its use to research projects.

More amenable to use in the clinical laboratory is the assay of urinary radioactivity after an oral test dose. This test is performed by administering (following previous parenteral saturation with folic acid) an oral test dose of 40 μg ^{3}H-labeled folic acid (^{3}H FA) per kilogram of body weight concomitantly with a parenteral "flushing" dose of 15 mg of folic acid and ascertaining the amount of radioactivity excreted in the succeeding 24-hour urine collection. Normal subjects excrete from 26 to 58% of the oral test dose; values are usually reduced in persons with impaired jejunal absorptive capacity.

VITAMIN B_{12}

Determinations to Detect Deficiency

SERUM VITAMIN B_{12} CONCENTRATION.   Serum levels of this vitamin can be ascertained by microbiologic or radioisotopic techniques. The radioisotopic techniques are rapid but require expertise. Assay with either *Lactobacillus leishmannii* or *Euglena gracilis* are both reliable, and the availability of commercially prepared assay media makes these tests sufficiently simple for adoption for use in routine hematology laboratories. Assay with *L. leishmannii* has the advantage of requiring less elaborate equipment and the results are available after an overnight growth. Assay with *E. gracilis,* which is perhaps more precise, requires growth for 7 days before interpretation.

Serum values in normal subjects in most laboratories are found to range between 150 and 900 $\mu\mu$g per milliliter. In contrast to the serum folate concentration, the serum concentration of vitamin B_{12} is a more precise reflection of tissue stores since serum levels usually become depressed only after depletion of hepatic stores. Serum vitamin B_{12} concentrations of less than 100 $\mu\mu$g per milliliter are usually associated with hematologic manifestations of deficiency, and concentrations are usually less than 50 $\mu\mu$g per milliliter in persons who have neurologic complications of B_{12} deficiency.

Spuriously low concentrations have been reported in persons taking chlorpromazine. Excessively high serum concentrations are found in persons having renal failure, acute or chronic liver disease, polycythemia vera, chronic myelogenous leukemia, and other myeloproliferative disorders. The increased concentration in chronic myelogenous leukemia is a reflection of an increase in the plasma concentration of the vitamin B_{12}–binding alpha globulin. Alpha globulin is thought to be relatively inert in transferring vitamin B_{12} to erythroid precursors, and persons have been described with chronic myelogenous leukemia who had a megaloblastic anemia due to pernicious anemia in the presence of a normal serum concentration of vitamin B_{12}. A plasma carrier of B_{12} present exclusively in persons with polycythemia vera has also been identified recently.

Determination of Vitamin B_{12} Absorption

The availability of gamma-emitting radioisotopic forms of vitamin B_{12}—^{57}Co B_{12}, which has a half-life of 60 days, and ^{60}Co B_{12}, which has a half-life of 5 years—makes determinations of the absorption of this vitamin a relatively simple matter. Studies have shown that the absorption of radioactive cyanocobalamin in normal individuals is equivalent to the absorption of vitamin B_{12} incorporated into dietary meat. The tests employed all consist of administering an oral test dose of 0.5 to 1.0 μg ^{57}Co- or ^{60}Co-labeled vitamin B_{12} and determining the percentage of radioactivity present in various specimens thereafter.

WHOLE BODY. The whole body counter gives what is probably the most accurate measurement of the percentage absorbed by labeled cyanocobalamin, provided that unabsorbed radioactivity has been eliminated in the stool. With this technique, normal subjects are found to absorb more than 30% of a test dose, although considerable variation has been detected in repeat determinations in the same subject as well as in groups of normal individuals.

FECAL EXCRETION (HEINLE TEST). The fecal elimination test is another direct approach for determining quantitative absorption of vitamin B_{12}. Fecal collections must be extended for at least 5 days after the administration of the oral test dose. The average fecal *recovery* in normal subjects is 34%, and values exceed 60% in persons with malabsorption of vitamin B_{12}. Results in individual subjects are usually reproducible to within less than 10% variation.

HEPATIC UPTAKE (GLASS TEST). Since absorbed vitamin B_{12} is concentrated in the liver, determination of hepatic radioactivity 10 days after the oral test dose can be used as an index of vitamin B_{12} absorption.

URINARY EXCRETION (SCHILLING TEST). Normal subjects excrete more than 8% of an oral test dose of 1 μg radioactive vitamin B_{12} in the urine within 24 hours if a "flushing" dose of 1000 μg of vitamin B_{12} is administered parenterally 1 hour after the oral test dose, and persons with malabsorption of vitamin B_{12} excrete less than this amount. The technical simplicity and rapidity (24 hours versus 5 to 10 days for the three previous tests) of the Schilling test make it the determination of choice, although it must be recognized that this test includes the administration of a therapeutic (1000 μg) dose of vitamin B_{12}. The manner in which the Schilling test may be modified to give additional information is presented in Table 2-2. Antibiotic therapy usually consists of tetracycline, 1 gm per day, or another appropriate broad-spectrum antibiotic, for 10 days.

SERUM COUNTING. Normal subjects have been reported to have more than 15 cpm in 4 ml of serum, and persons with malabsorption fewer counts, at 8 hours after the oral administration of the radioactive test dose. This technique overcomes the difficulties imposed on the Schilling test by incomplete urine collection or renal insufficiency. At the present time its reliability needs further confirmation prior to acceptance for general usage.

Other Useful Determinations

ASSAY OF INTRINSIC FACTOR. Absence of intrinsic factor is usually documented by the demonstration that ^{57}Co B_{12} absorption is normal only when the radioactive vitamin B_{12} is given with a source of exogenous intrinsic factor. The presence of intrinsic factor can also be tested by determining whether a sample of gastric juice abets ^{57}Co B_{12} absorption when given to an individual with known pernicious anemia. Since 1963 more direct techniques of assaying intrinsic factor have been available. In a radioimmune technique the amount of intrinsic factor present in a standard volume of gastric juice is assessed by its ability to bind in vitro isotopically labeled vitamin B_{12}.

SERUM VITAMIN B_{12}–BINDING PROTEINS. Most of the vitamin B_{12} in normal serum is bound to an alpha globulin (transcobalamin I). When vitamin B_{12} is added to normal serum in vitro, however, it is bound predominantly to a beta globulin (transcobalamin II), presumably because the alpha globulin is saturated with endogenous B_{12}. It has been suggested that the beta globulin is the active transport protein whereas the alpha globulin functions mainly to conserve the vitamin. In B_{12} deficiency states, the alpha globulin is relatively unsaturated and added B_{12} attaches itself principally to this carrier.

Table 2-2. Modifications of the Schilling Test

Administer		Urinary Excretion of ^{57}Co B_{12}			
Orally	Intramuscularly	Normal	PA	Blind Loop	Sprue
1 μg ^{57}Co B_{12}	B_{12} 1000 μg	Normal	Low	Low	Low
1 μg ^{57}Co B_{12} + intrinsic factor	B_{12} 1000 μg	Normal	Normal	Low	Low
1 μg ^{57}Co B_{12} after antibiotic	B_{12} 1000 μg	Normal	Low	Normal	Low

Techniques are available for measuring the total plasma vitamin B_{12}–binding capacity (TBBC), the unsaturated vitamin B_{12}–binding capacity (UBBC), and percentage of TBBC and UBBC due to physiologically normal (or abnormal) alpha or beta vitamin B_{12}–binding globulins. Although the performance of these determinations is beyond the scope of the usual laboratory evaluation of persons with a megaloblastic anemia, their measurement is proving to be of interest in delineating pathophysiologic changes not only in B_{12} deficiency states but also in pregnancy, liver disease, and the myeloproliferative disorders.

ANTIBODIES.   Antibodies to either intrinsic factor or parietal cells are commonly found in the sera of patients with adult-type pernicious anemia. Although their presence cannot be construed as an indication of deficiency of vitamin B_{12}, they are of use in elucidating the pathogenesis of the deficiency.

Antibody to intrinsic factor.   Two types of antibody to intrinsic factor have been identified by the use of electrophoretic or charcoal absorption techniques. One type or both types together have been detected in the serum of 70% of patients with pernicious anemia. *Type I* (blocking antibody) blocks the binding of vitamin B_{12} to intrinsic factor when added to intrinsic factor before the B_{12}; this antibody blocks intrinsic factor–mediated B_{12} absorption in vivo when mixed in the sequence intrinsic factor plus antibody plus cyanocobalamin. *Type II* (binding antibody, precipitating antibody) reacts with intrinsic factor when B_{12} is attached and prevents the absorption of this complex.

Parietal cell antibody.   Antibody to parietal cells, detected by immunofluorescent techniques, has been found to be present in some 80% of patients with pernicious anemia. The presence of parietal cell antibody is independent of the presence or absence of intrinsic factor antibodies.

PRACTICAL HEMATOLOGIC EVALUATION

Clearly it is neither practical nor proper to apply all the tests cited to the investigation of the patient who presents with a megaloblastic anemia. The following are suggested guidelines.

1. The presence in the peripheral blood of macrocytes and hypersegmented polymorphonuclear leukocytes suggests that an anemia (or pancytopenia) is due to folate or B_{12} deficiency. This must be confirmed by a *bone marrow aspiration* which demonstrates megaloblastic changes.

2. The presence of concomitant iron deficiency, which may mask some of the morphologic characteristics of a megaloblastic anemia, must be considered. If the peripheral blood smear shows a dimorphic pattern (hypo-

chromia and macrocytes), serum iron determinations and iron stain of the bone marrow should be obtained.

3. The exact vitamin deficiency responsible for the megaloblastic anemia should be determined by *serum assay* for folate and B_{12}. If these determinations are not available locally, serum can be conveniently shipped in the frozen state to a commercial laboratory.

4. Subsequent work-up depends on whether folate or B_{12} deficiency is responsible for the anemia. The *history* and *physical examination* usually offer strong clues to the etiology of the megaloblastic anemia and to the appropriate diagnostic steps to be followed. Thus folate deficiency is most likely in pregnant or alcoholic subjects, or in those with a hemolytic anemia or taking anticonvulsant medications; vitamin B_{12} deficiency, on the other hand, is likely following a gastrectomy, in persons with regional enteritis, or in those who have had intestinal surgery. The work-up can continue while serum determinations are being performed.

5. If *vitamin B_{12} deficiency* is suspected, it should be pursued.

a. Tests for *gastric acidity* are usually initiated by means of the Diagnex Blue reaction. If the test is positive (i.e., no dye is excreted in the urine), then this should be confirmed by direct gastric aspiration following histamine stimulation.

b. The presence of *antibodies* to intrinsic factor or parietal cells should be ascertained if means are available.

c. *Radiologic studies* of the stomach and small intestine should be undertaken to check for the presence of gastric carcinoma, regional enteritis, strictures, fistulas, or blind loops.

d. *Vitamin B_{12} absorption* is usually assessed by the Schilling test and its modifications (Table 2-2). The disadvantage of the Schilling test is that a pharmacologic dose of 1000 μg of B_{12} is administered, so that in some instances it may be preferable to defer it until after therapeutic trials (see 7 below).

e. If bacterial overgrowth in the small intestine is suspected, *culture of jejunal aspirate* should be performed and the antibiotic sensitivity of the isolated organism determined.

6. If *folate deficiency* is suspected, it should be pursued.

a. Test of folic acid absorption is made if intestinal disease is present. This can most easily be accomplished by administering—following daily parenteral "saturation" with 15 mg folic acid for 3 days—an oral test dose and determining subsequent peak serum concentrations microbiologically (serum can also be shipped for these determinations). This test may be deferred if therapeutic trials are to be conducted. Other tests, such as jejunal biopsy and determinations of xylose and fat absorption, may be indicated.

7. Therapeutic trials have a practical value and deserve more wide-

spread usage than is usually the case, particularly in persons suspected of having primary folate deficiency. Pharmacologic doses of either folate or vitamin B_{12} produce a hematologic response irrespective of the vitamin deficiency causing the megaloblastic anemia, whereas physiologic doses of 1 μg B_{12} or 50 μg crystalline folic acid produce a response only when the vitamin responsible for the anemia is administered. Thus a hematologic response to 50 μg folic acid given orally daily for 10 days (larger doses up to 400 μg are required in instances of excessive demand) confirms the fact that folate was the primary cause of the megaloblastic anemia, whereas a response to 1 μg daily of vitamin B_{12} given parenterally for 10 days implicates that vitamin.

CAUTIONS

Two points of caution should be emphasized. (1) The demonstration of free hydrochloric acid in the stomach rules out the presence of pernicious anemia but does *not* exclude the diagnosis of vitamin B_{12} deficiency due to abnormalities of the distal intestine. (2) Evaluation of anemia restricted to determinations of serum folate and vitamin B_{12} concentrations does *not* give meaningful information. Folate deficiency particularly occurs in varying gradations of severity (see Fig. 2-2). Serum folate concentrations commonly become reduced in many disorders of chronic debility, but a reduced value can be interpreted as indicating that folate deficiency is responsible for the anemia *only when megaloblastic erythropoiesis is demonstrated.*

VITAMIN B_{12} DEFICIENCY STATES

Vitamin B_{12} is synthesized in nature exclusively by microorganisms and is present only in meat and dairy products, principally in various coenzyme forms, most or all of which are probably bound to peptides. These forms are metabolically inactive until this bond is split by proteolysis. Daily intake of vitamin B_{12} varies from 1 to 5 μg. In the stomach the vitamin (molecular weight, 1 million) combines with intrinsic factor, a glycoprotein secreted by the parietal cells that has a molecular weight in the range of 50,000 and is structurally related to blood group substance. The B_{12}–intrinsic factor complex passes down the length of the small intestine to the ileum where, in the presence of ionic calcium and a pH of 6 or greater, absorption takes place. The exact mechanism by which intrinsic factor facilitates B_{12} absorption remains incompletely resolved. The principal role of intrinsic factor appears to be to permit attachment of the B_{12}–intrinsic factor complex to the brush border of the mucosa. Intrinsic factor is released from B_{12} during absorption and does not pass through the mucosal cell. In addition to this active process, vitamin B_{12} in quantities greater than those normally present in the food may be absorbed by passive diffusion.

Absorbed vitamin B_{12} enters the blood at a slow rate; it first appears in the plasma 3 to 4 hours after a meal and reaches a peak level at 8 to 12 hours. Following absorption, vitamin B_{12} is attached to carrier proteins, principally beta globulin (transcobalamin II) traveling via the portal circulation to the liver, its principal storage site. Hepatic stores of B_{12} in normal subjects range from 1 to 5 mg.

Approximately 3 to 7 μg of vitamin B_{12} is excreted daily into the intestinal tract, principally in the bile, of which all but about 1 μg is reabsorbed in the ileum. Disruption of this enterohepatic cycle by reduced intrinsic factor secretion or ileal disease results in a loss of endogenous vitamin B_{12} which can contribute to the development of the deficiency.

Clinically important facts to remember about vitamin B_{12} include:

1. Aside from inadequate dietary intake (which rarely occurs in this country), deficiency is always secondary to disease of the intestinal tract.
2. Intestinal defects resulting in malabsorption of B_{12} occur in the stomach (absent intrinsic factor) or ileum.
3. Body stores of B_{12} are in the range of 1 to 5 mg—well over a thousandfold the daily intake (1 μg) and requirement (1 μg) of the vitamin. They are thus sufficient to supply needs for 3 years or more in the absence of any intake of this vitamin.

CONDITIONS RESPONSIBLE FOR DEFICIENCY

Inadequate Dietary Intake

Prolonged restriction of vitamin B_{12} from the diet, as is practiced by persons with certain religious preferences, results in the eventual development of deficiency of this vitamin, although when such individuals take a diet high in folate content (principally vegetables), they may have only slight or no hematologic abnormalities.

Malabsorption of Vitamin B_{12}

ABSENT SECRETION OF INTRINSIC FACTOR

Addisonian pernicious anemia. The factors leading to the development of gastric atrophy, achlorhydria, and absent secretion of intrinsic factor in this condition remain poorly defined. It is well recognized that there are predisposing racial and genetic factors. Pernicious anemia occurs more commonly among persons with blood group A than among those of any other group. Latent features, and sometimes the overt form, of pernicious anemia are common among relatives of affected persons.

Recent attention has been directed to immunologic abnormalities in pernicious anemia. Antibodies to intrinsic factor (of either the blocking or the binding type, or both) are present in the serum of some 70%, and antibody to parietal cells in over 80%, of persons with pernicious anemia. Antibody to parietal cells (but not to intrinsic factor) can also be detected in a quarter of relatives (many of whom have abnormalities of gastric morphology or function) of persons with pernicious anemia and in over 50% of persons who have chronic atrophic gastritis. The key question concerns the relationship of these serum antibodies to the pathogenesis of the gastric lesion. The answer is uncertain. In some individuals (as many as 50% in one series) either or both of these antibodies have been detected in gastric juice; it has been suggested that in this circumstance they may act to combine with residual intrinsic factor, thus preventing its facilitation of vitamin B_{12} absorption. This suggestion receives support from reports of cases of transplacentally transferred serum antibody to intrinsic factor in which the antibody was found transiently present in the newborn's gastric juice, where it appeared to be responsible for malabsorption of B_{12}. On the other hand, some individuals develop pernicious anemia in the absence of any antibody to gastric elements detectable in the serum, and pernicious anemia has been described in patients with immunoglobulin deficiency. Treatment with prednisone results in regeneration of the gastric mucosa and return of acid and intrinsic factor secretion to normal in some cases of pernicious anemia, but this occurs irrespective of the presence or absence of serum antibody to intrinsic factor.

The higher prevalence of pernicious anemia in persons with *primary hypothyroidism* has long been recognized, the incidence of coexisting disease running from 8 to 12% in two series. In addition, nearly one-half of persons with myxedema are achlorhydric. Both the stomach and the thyroid are endodermal in origin, and an immunologic relationship is apparent since a quarter of patients with myxedema are found to have antibodies to parietal cells and a quarter of persons with pernicious anemia have antibodies to thyroid tissue. There is also a higher prevalence of thyrotoxicosis among persons who have pernicious anemia than in the general population. (Folate deficiency should also be considered in evaluating persons with thyroid disease. Serum levels are commonly depressed and the plasma clearance abnormally rapid in persons with thyrotoxicosis, although to date megaloblastic anemia due to folate deficiency has not been reported. Megaloblastic anemia in several persons with hypothyroidism has been attributed to folate deficiency, although the pathogenesis of deficiency in this condition is obscure.)

Pernicious anemia has also been found in association with hypoparathyroidism or Addison's disease in several individuals.

Juvenile pernicious anemia.   Juvenile pernicious anemia is the term applied to infants who are unable to absorb vitamin B_{12} due to absent secretion of intrinsic factor. Gastric mucosa histology and hydrochloric acid secretion are normal in these infants, and they do not have antibodies to intrinsic factor or parietal cells in the serum. Similar milder defects of intrinsic factor secretion have been noted in the parents and siblings of some affected children, and it has been suggested that juvenile pernicious anemia may represent the homozygous inheritance of a gene responsible for deficient secretion of intrinsic factor.

The condition in infants with juvenile pernicious anemia must be differentiated from that seen in older children, usually aged 10 to 18 years, who also present with malabsorption of vitamin B_{12} due to absent intrinsic factor secretion, but who in addition have an atrophic gastric mucosa, achlorhydria, and often serum antibodies. Many of these children have an associated endocrinopathy (hypoparathyroidism, hypothyroidism, or Addison's disease), a situation which may be comparable to the increased incidence of myxedema in the adult population with pernicious anemia.

Gastric damage due to other causes.   Damage to parietal cells may reduce their capacity to secrete intrinsic factor leading to absorption of vitamin B_{12}. Radiotherapy, ingestion of certain chemicals such as lye, malignant neoplasia of the stomach, and the presence of certain intestinal disorders such as celiac disease and tropical sprue may all result in reduced gastric secretion.

Gastric resection.   Complete removal of the stomach (*total gastrectomy*) results in malabsorption of vitamin B_{12}, and evidence of deficiency becomes apparent some 3 or more years later when the hepatic supply of this vitamin becomes exhausted. Less well recognized are the consequences for vitamin B_{12} absorption of *subtotal gastrectomy* (especially the Billroth II procedure). Following this operation, some one-third of persons develop, usually after 5 years or more, atrophy of the gastric remnant with reduced or absent secretion of intrinsic factor, and as many as 20% may become deficient in vitamin B_{12}. In other individuals deficiency of vitamin B_{12} may result from bacterial overgrowth in the afferent loop.

CONSUMPTION OF VITAMIN B_{12} WITHIN THE GUT LUMEN

By bacteria. Conditions such as blind loops, strictures, or fistulas in which there is stasis of fecal flow can be associated with the proliferation of aerobic coliform organisms within the small intestine. Viable *Escherichia coli* are capable of assimilating vitamin B_{12}, thus rendering it unavailable for absorption in the ileum. Intrinsic factor serves to protect the vitamin partially, but incompletely, from bacterial uptake. The clinical significance of bacterial uptake of vitamin B_{12} as a cause of malabsorption can be documented by demonstrating that absorption of radioactive B_{12} returns to normal following a 10-day course of treatment with tetracycline.

By Diphyllobothrium latum.   The fish tapeworm, when present in the proximal jejunum, is capable of splitting the bound vitamin B_{12}–intrinsic factor complex and utilizing the vitamin, thus rendering it unavailable for absorption and utilization by the host. In Scandinavia over a quarter of the population is infested with tapeworm. More than 50% of carriers of this worm have a reduced serum concentration of vitamin B_{12}, and 3% are found to have a megaloblastic anemia. Gastritis of varying severity and hypochlorhydria are also common in infested persons. The histologic abnormalities show reversion toward normal following expulsion of the worm.

MALABSORPTION AT THE ILEUM.   Complete *ileal resection* aborts all absorption of vitamin B_{12} with consequent development of deficiency following depletion of body stores.

Regional enteritis.   Malabsorption of vitamin B_{12} occurs commonly in regional enteritis. It may be a result of ileal resection, impaired absorption through a diseased ileal mucosa, or the presence proximally of bacterial overgrowth due to blind loops, strictures, or enterocolic anastomosis. Not infrequently deficiency may be the result of a combination of these factors.

Gluten-induced enteropathy (celiac disease).   The intestinal lesion induced by gluten in sensitive individuals appears to be dosage-related; thus ileal abnormalities, with consequent malabsorption of vitamin B_{12}, are present in only about a third of cases. Folate deficiency is a more common cause of megaloblastic anemia in this condition, but some one-third of patients have a combined deficiency of both vitamins. Vitamin B_{12} absorption often improves following prolonged dietary restriction of gluten.

Tropical sprue.   During the early phase of tropical sprue, as seen mostly in visitors to the tropics, intestinal malabsorption may be confined to the jejunum, resulting in folate deficiency only. In the more commonly encountered chronic condition, the intestinal lesion involves the entire small intestine, and malabsorption of vitamin B_{12} is present in over 90% of such cases. Megaloblastic anemia in this circumstance is usually due to a combined deficiency of folate and vitamin B_{12}. Treatment with folic acid improves B_{12} absorption in a few but prolonged treatment with antimicrobials is required to return B_{12} absorption to normal in most cases.

Physiologic changes.   The attachment of the intrinsic factor–B_{12} complex to receptor sites on the ileal mucosa requires a pH of greater than 6 and the presence of ionic calcium. Excessive gastric acid secretion, as occurs in the Zollinger-Ellison syndrome, may sufficiently reduce the ileal pH so as to inhibit B_{12} absorption. In chronic pancreatitis not only is the intestinal pH lowered due to impaired pancreatic secretion of bicarbonate, but the intraluminal ionic calcium concentration is reduced as well. These changes can be associated with B_{12} malabsorption, which is correctable by feeding sodium bicarbonate or pancreatic extract.

Drugs.   Para-aminosalicylic acid (PASA) is capable of causing a decrease in vitamin B_{12} absorption with a resulting decline, during long-term PASA therapy, of the serum vitamin B_{12} concentration. This reaction appears to be selective since other tests of intestinal function usually remain normal in persons receiving the drug. The mechanism of inhibition is unknown, but concomitant treatment with folic acid has been shown to improve B_{12} absorption. Treatment with folic acid has likewise been reported to improve B_{12} absorption in several patients taking diphenylhydantoin who were found to have malabsorption of this vitamin.

The administration of either colchicine or neomycin may result in a generalized malabsorption, including that of vitamin B_{12}.

Other conditions.   Transient ileal malabsorption of vitamin B_{12}, correctable by treatment with cyanocobalamin, has been described in patients with deficiency of this vitamin due to pernicious anemia or vegetarianism, which fact suggests that B_{12} deficiency per se may produce ileal damage of sufficient severity to reduce absorption of the vitamin. Malabsorption of vitamin B_{12} occurs following radiation of the distal small intestine. It has also been described in persons with protein-calorie malnutrition; in such persons the malabsorption of B_{12} has been attributed to the protein-calorie deficiency.

FOLATE

DIETARY INTAKE

Folates are present in nearly all foodstuffs; yeast, liver, and green vegetables have a particularly high content. Folate is labile, however, unless protected by the presence of ascorbic acid. Prolonged cooking (especially boiling) can appreciably reduce the content in foodstuffs. The average daily diet (prior to cooking) usually contains from 500 to 1000 μg of folate. Most of this folate is in polyglutamate form; that is, the folate molecule is conjugated with up to 7 glutamate molecules, forming a heptaglutamate; there is very little (less than 50 μg) "free," monoglutamate folate in the diet. Thus the bulk of dietary folate is not immediately available for utilization.

ABSORPTION

Folate is absorbed in the jejunum. Crystalline folic acid is readily absorbed by active transport; this process is relatively efficient since from 60 to 85% of a physiologic test dose (25 to 200 μg) is absorbed in normal persons. Polyglutamate forms, on the other hand, are considerably less well absorbed. The precise mechanism involved in their absorption is uncertain, but it is thought that they require preliminary deconjugation to the triglutamate or monoglutamate form prior to absorption. An enzyme (folate de-conjugase) capable of doing this is present in the intestinal mucosa.

STORAGE

Following absorption, folate is rapidly cleared by the portal circulation to the liver, where it is stored principally in the form of N^5-methyltetrahy-drofolic acid. Hepatic stores range from 5 to 10 mg, approximately a hundredfold the amount absorbed (50 to 100 μg) and utilized (50 to 100 μg) per day.

DIFFERENCES BETWEEN FOLATE AND VITAMIN B_{12}

The key differences between folate and B_{12} are that folate

1. Can be destroyed in the diet by cooking
2. Requires deconjugation prior to absorption
3. Is absorbed in the jejunum
4. Is hepatically stored in quantities equal to only a 3-months' requirement

CONDITIONS RESPONSIBLE FOR DEFICIENCY

Inadequate Dietary Intake

Mild degrees of folate deficiency due to inadequate dietary intake are more common than is usually suspected. Such certainly appears to be the case among elderly and debilitated persons in Great Britain. This may be related to the fact that the average British diet is lower in folate content than the American, partly because of the tendency in that country to cook by prolonged boiling. This dietary factor is probably responsible for the fact that overt folate deficiency—that is, with concomitant megaloblastic changes—is more common among British subjects with conditions such as rheumatoid arthritis, malignancy, and epilepsy requiring anticonvulsant medications than in persons with these conditions living in the United States.

Severe forms of folate deficiency associated with a megaloblastic anemia can occur in several groups:

DIETARY FADDISTS.   Persons who markedly restrict their dietary intake, usually just to carbohydrate; this commonly includes elderly people who are "tea and toast-ers."

ALCOHOLICS.   Folate deficiency is common in alcoholics, with or without liver disease. The factors responsible for this are complex, but deficiency is due principally to inadequate dietary intake often coupled, in persons with liver disease, with an excessive requirement for folate by the bone marrow, secondary to hemolysis or blood loss. Impaired hepatic ability to metabolize folate does not appear to be of importance in the pathogenesis of folate deficiency, but in some instances alcohol itself appears to play an inhibitory role in the hematologic response to folate.

SCURVY. Inadequate intake of folate appears to be one factor responsible for megaloblastic anemia in scurvy, since treatment with a physiologic dose of 50 μg crystalline folic acid has resulted in a hematologic response in persons in whom treatment with vitamin C was ineffective hematologically.

POSTGASTRECTOMY. Megaloblastic anemia due to folate deficiency following gastrectomy usually occurs within several weeks after operation and most often in persons who had a difficult postoperative course. Inadequate dietary intake appears to be the principal factor responsible for deficiency in this circumstance. The absorption of crystalline folic acid is usually normal in such persons, although polyglutamate folate absorption has yet to be tested.

INFANCY. Folate deficiency among infants in temperate zones usually occurs before 2 years of age and is seen principally in *premature infants* and in those whose diet consists largely of goat's milk, a rather poor source of folate. Megaloblastic anemia due to folate deficiency is common in the tropics in children who have *kwashiorkor*.

Malabsorption of Folate

The absorption of folate has usually been assessed by studies of crystalline folic acid absorption; the absorption of polyglutamate forms of folate, which may well be of more physiologic importance, has been tested in relatively few instances. Malabsorption of folate can occur in the following conditions:

GLUTEN-INDUCED ENTEROPATHY (CELIAC DISEASE). Malabsorption of crystalline folic acid and deficiency of folate occur in the majority of persons with celiac disease. Gluten restriction usually results in reversal of the folic acid absorption to normal.

TROPICAL SPRUE. Abnormalities of villous structure and intestinal function are usually less severe in tropical sprue than in celiac disease. Absorption of pharmacologic doses of crystalline folic acid is impaired in one-half of cases with this disorder, and these subjects are usually folate-deficient. The absorption of polyglutamate folate has been subnormal in the several patients tested. This observation, plus the findings that some subjects with tropical sprue who are folate-deficient have normal absorption of physiologic doses of crystalline folic acid, and that some patients may respond to an oral dose of 50 μg of crystalline folic acid per day, suggest that polyglutamate malabsorption is responsible for folate deficiency in these individuals.

REGIONAL ENTERITIS.   Folate deficiency occurs in a small proportion of patients with active Crohn's disease. This appears to be due to a combination of factors—inadequate dietary intake, malabsorption, and perhaps excessive utilization of the vitamin.

INTESTINAL RESECTION.   Folic acid absorption remains normal following intestinal resection unless all but a few feet of jejunum are removed; deficiency due to malabsorption can occur following more extensive intestinal resection.

OTHER DISORDERS.   Malabsorption of crystalline folic acid has been described in scattered cases of persons with involvement of the small intestine by *lymphoma, scleroderma, amyloid,* or *Whipple's disease* as well as in subjects with malabsorption associated with *hypoparathyroidism* and *diabetes mellitus.* Folate malabsorption in these disorders rarely produces folate deficiency of sufficient severity to result in a megaloblastic anemia.

BACTERIAL OVERGROWTH.   Whereas in conditions of stasis such as blind loops or strictures the coliform organisms found in the proximal small intestine can utilize vitamin B_{12}, they synthesize folate. Therefore the condition of bacterial overgrowth does *not* result in folate deficiency, and persons with the condition often have elevated serum concentrations of folate.

Excessive Requirement for Folate

Folate stores go into negative balance whenever the requirement exceeds the normal intake of 50 to 100 μg per day. The increased demand may be secondary to hyperactivity of erythropoiesis of the tissues, increased metabolic demand, or excessive loss.

INCREASED ERYTHROPOIESIS.   Persons with a mild hemolytic anemia often have a subnormal serum folate concentration; those with a severe hemolytic anemia (where the demand may result in as much as a sevenfold increase in bone marrow production) may become sufficiently depleted to result in a megaloblastic anemia. This has been described in cases of sickle cell anemia and its variants (sickle-C, sickle-thalassemia), thalassemia, hereditary spherocytosis, paroxysmal nocturnal hemoglobinuria, and acquired hemolytic anemia due to various causes. It is important to recognize that persons with such a condition may have a megaloblastic bone marrow in the presence of an elevated reticulocyte count. The anemia in this circumstance responds to doses of 300 μg per day or more of folic acid.

Folate determinations (serum folate concentration and the plasma clearance of folic acid) are often abnormal in persons who have polycythemia, acute erythremic myelosis (Di Guglielmo syndrome), and myeloid metaplasia, although megaloblastic anemia due to deficiency of folate is uncommon in these disorders.

INCREASED TISSUE DEMANDS

Pregnancy. Parasitism by the fetus increases folate requirement during pregnancy such that by the third trimester it approximates 300 μg per day and is even higher in women carrying twins. Approximately one-third of pregnant women in this country develop a reduced serum folate concentration during the third trimester, and a certain proportion develop an overt megaloblastic anemia. The exact incidence of megaloblastic anemia of pregnancy in this country is uncertain; what is certain is that its prevalence has risen since folic acid was withdrawn from routine antenatal vitamin supplements. The prevalence in Great Britain appears to be in the range of nearly 1%, and that in certain undeveloped countries may be as high as 7%. Evidence has been presented which suggests that both abruptio placentae and antepartum bleeding may occur more commonly in women who are deficient in folate.

Neoplastic disease. Serum folate concentrations are frequently subnormal in persons with neoplastic disease of either the hematopoietic or other tissues, and on occasion such persons may be found to have a megaloblastic anemia. The severity of the folate deficiency appears to relate in general to the extent of the neoplastic disease.

Skin disease. The rapid turnover of skin associated with certain dermatologic disorders may be of sufficient magnitude to result in abnormal folate determinations although, to date, megaloblastic anemia has not been described in this condition. Malabsorption of crystalline folic acid has been noted in a few individuals with dermatitis herpetiformis.

INCREASED METABOLIC DEMANDS.

Homocystinuria is an inborn error of methionine metabolism in which deficiency of the enzyme cystathionine synthetase results in failure of conversion of homocysteine to methionine. The methyl group required for this conversion is usually derived from N^5-methyltetrahydrofolic acid (Fig. 2-1). Increased homocysteine-methionine transmethylation in homocystinuria results in a reduced serum concentration of folate, and such subjects are also found to have an abnormally rapid plasma clearance. The urinary excretion of FIGLU, however, is consistently negative; this may be due to inhibition of FIGLU formation by the high blood levels of homocysteine and methionine.

EXCESSIVE EXOGENOUS LOSS.　Folate deficiency with megaloblastic erythropoiesis has been documented in some patients with terminal uremia who were being treated by maintenance hemodialysis. Poor dietary intake and loss of considerable quantities of folic acid through the dialysis appear to be responsible for this.

Drugs

The administration of certain drugs may result in a megaloblastic anemia due to folate deficiency. In some instances the locus of interference in folate metabolism is well established; in others, it is unknown.

FOLATE ANTAGONISTS.　Drugs such as aminopterin and amethopterin combine with the enzyme dihydrofolate reductase, thereby blocking the reduction of folic acid to tetrahydrofolic acid and further steps in folate metabolism. The prolonged administration of such drugs regularly results in the development of a megaloblastic anemia.

ANTIMETABOLITE DRUGS.　Agents used in the chemotherapy of neoplastic disease which interfere with DNA synthesis regularly produce a megaloblastic anemia. Drugs in this category include the purine antagonist 5-fluorouracil, the cytosine antagonist 1-β-D-arabinofuranosylcytosine, and hydroxyurea. Megaloblastic anemia has been attributed to vinblastine sulfate in one instance.

PYRIMETHAMINE (DARAPRIM).　Pyrimethamine, which acts as a weak folate antagonist, produces a megaloblastic anemia in a high proportion of persons given a dosage of 25 mg per day for 2 months (as in the therapy for toxoplasmosis) but not in the usual prophylactic dose for malaria of 25 mg weekly.

ANTICONVULSANTS.　Some 50% of epileptics taking either diphenylhydantoin (Dilantin) or primidone (Mysoline) have a subnormal serum folate concentration, and subjects taking either these or the structurally related drugs nitrofurantoin (Furadantin), glutethimide (Doriden), or various barbiturates have developed a megaloblastic anemia due to folate deficiency. The anemia in these persons responds either to withdrawal of the drug or to a physiologic dose (25 to 50 μg) of crystalline folic acid per day.

The mechanism by which the anticonvulsant and related drugs induce folate deficiency is unknown. The similarity of their structure to the folate molecule (Fig. 2-2) has suggested a metabolic block, but in vitro studies

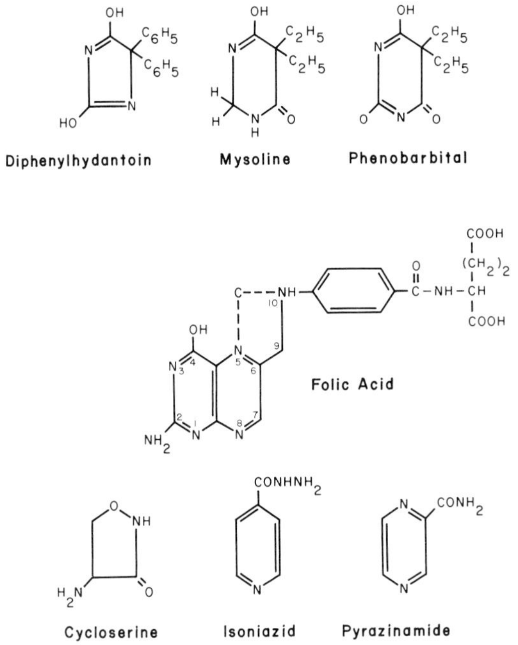

Figure 2-2. Formulas for folic acid and those anticonvulsant and antituber-culosis drugs whose administration may be associated with the development of folate deficiency. Basic acceptor site in the folic acid molecule for one-carbon moieties (such as methyl, methylene, formyl, and formimino groups) is at the N5,10 position indicated by the broken lines. (From F. A. Klipstein et al., *Blood* 29:697, 1967.)

have failed to demonstrate inhibition. Scattered patients have been reported to have mild malabsorption of crystalline folic acid, but this could not account for the deficiency. Two recent reports have incriminated reduced folate deconjugase (assayed microbiologically) within the intestinal mucosa, with resultant malabsorption of polyglutamate folate, as the cause of folate deficiency, but these results have not been confirmed by studies that used isotopically labeled folate polyglutamate.

ANTITUBERCULOSIS DRUGS. Mild folate deficiency has been reported to be common in persons with tuberculosis in England. This may be secondary to poor nutrition; but additional studies in the United States have shown that serum folate concentrations are often depressed, and megaloblastic anemia due to folate deficiency may occasionally occur, in well-nourished persons with tuberculosis who are taking the combination of isoniazid and cycloserine. Cycloserine and, to a lesser extent, isoniazid and pyrazinamide thus appear to act as mild folate antagonists, in addition to their better-recognized effect on pyridoxine metabolism. These drugs also bear a structural relationship to the folate molecule (Fig. 2-2), and cycloserine has been shown in vitro to have an inhibitory effect on folate metabolism which can be nullified partially by the addition of pyridoxine.

ORAL CONTRACEPTIVES. Megaloblastic anemia due to folate deficiency has been reported in a group of women taking oral contraceptive medications of various kinds although no regular relationship between serum folate concentrations and oral contraceptives has been demonstrated in groups of nonanemic women. The absorption of crystalline folic acid in these subjects is normal, but that of folate polyglutamate has been found to be reduced.

OTHER DRUGS. Megaloblastic anemia due to folate deficiency has been described in, and attributed to, ingestion of triamterene in two cases and chronic arsenic poisoning in one.

Unknown

RHEUMATOID ARTHRITIS. Some two-thirds of persons with rheumatoid arthritis studied in England have a subnormal serum folate concentration, one-third have a depressed red blood cell folate concentration, and one out of five has been reported to have megaloblastic changes in the bone marrow. In the United States persons with this disorder commonly have a subnormal serum concentration of folate, but hematologic abnormalities are rare. The changes in folate determinations are not restricted to persons with rheumatoid arthritis but are present in individuals with gout and other forms of arthritis. The responsible factors are unknown. Crystalline folic acid absorption is normal in this condition. It is possible that increased tissue replacement may play a role.

SIDEROBLASTIC ANEMIA. Persons with sideroblastic anemia commonly have abnormal folate determinations and mild megaloblastic changes in the bone marrow, as discussed in Chapter 3.

TREATMENT

The minimum amount of crystalline folic acid available commercially in a capsule is 5 mg. In view of the fact that this exceeds the physiologic requirement by a hundredfold, daily oral administration of this dosage is adequate in all cases of megaloblastic anemia due to folate deficiency, and there is no cause or justification for giving larger amounts of folic acid orally or for giving this vitamin parenterally.

Vitamin B_{12} should be given parenterally. A dosage of 30 μg per month is sufficient to supply the body's needs, but it seems preferable under ordinary circumstances to administer initially 1000 μg daily (up to 90% of this dose will be lost in the urine) for 5 days to partially replete hepatic stores in persons with a megaloblastic anemia due to deficiency of this vitamin. Maintenance therapy of 100 μg monthly is then adequate.

REFERENCES

Baker, S. J.   Human vitamin B_{12} deficiency. *World Rev. Nutr. Diet.* 8:62, 1967.

Butterworth, C. E.   The availability of food folate. *Brit. J. Haemat.* 14:339, 1968.

Butterworth, C. E., Baugh, C. M., and Krumdieck, C.   A study of folate absorption and metabolism in man utilizing carbon-14-labeled polyglutamates synthesized by the solid phase method. *J. Clin. Invest.* 48:1131, 1969.

Chanarin, I.   *The Megaloblastic Anaemias.* Oxford, Eng.: Blackwell, 1969.

Chanarin, I., Anderson, B. B., and Mollin, D. L.   The absorption of folic acid. *Brit. J Haemat.* 4:156, 1958.

Folate deficiency in the elderly (editorial). *Brit. Med. J.* 1:649, 1967.

Hall, C. A.   Transport of vitamin B_{12} in man. *Brit. J. Haemat.* 16:429, 1969.

Hampers, C. L., Streiff, R., Nathan, D. G., Snyder, D., and Merrill, J. P.   Megaloblastic hematopoiesis in uremia and in patients on long-term hemodialysis. *New Eng. J. Med.* 276:551, 1967.

Herbert, V.   Current concepts in therapy: Megaloblastic anemia. *New Eng. J. Med.* 268:201, 1963.

Herbert, V.   Drugs Effective in Megaloblastic Anemias. In L. S. Goodman and A. Gilman (Eds.), *The Pharmacological Basis of Therapeutics* (4th ed.). New York: Macmillan, 1970.

Herbert, V.   Megaloblastic anemias: Mechanisms and management. *D. M.,* Aug. 1965.

Herbert, V.   Diagnostic and prognostic values of measurement of serum vitamin B_{12}–binding proteins. *Blood* 32:305, 1968.

Hines, J. D., Hoffbrand, A. V., and Mollin, D. L.   The hematologic complications following partial gastrectomy: A study of 292 patients. *Amer. J. Med.* 43:555, 1967.

Hoffbrand, A. V., Stewart, J. S., Booth, C. C., and Mollin, D. L.   Folate deficiency in Crohn's disease: Incidence, pathogenesis and treatment. *Brit. Med. J.* 2:71, 1968.

Johns, D. G., and Bertino, J. R.   Folates and megaloblastic anemia: A review. *Clin. Pharmacol. Ther.* 6:372, 1965.

Kitay, D. Z.   Folic acid deficiency in pregnancy. *Amer. J. Obstet. Gynec.* 104:1067, 1969.

Klipstein, F. A.   Subnormal serum folate and macrocytosis associated with anticonvulsant drug therapy. *Blood* 23:68, 1964.

Klipstein, F. A.   Folate deficiency secondary to disease of the intestinal tract. *Bull. N.Y. Acad. Med.* 42:638, 1966.

Klipstein, F. A.   Progress in gastroenterology: Tropical sprue. *Gastroenterology* 54:275, 1968.

Klipstein, F. A., Berlinger, F. G., and Reed, L. J.   Folate deficiency associated with drug therapy for tuberculosis. *Blood* 29:697, 1967.

Klipstein, F. A., and Lindenbaum, J.   Folate deficiency in chronic liver disease. *Blood* 25:443, 1965.

Lindenbaum, J., and Klipstein, F. A.   Folic acid deficiency in sickle cell anemia. *New Eng. J. Med.* 269:1, 1963.

MacGibbon, B. H., and Mollin, D. L.   Sideroblastic anemia in man: Observations on seventy cases. *Brit. J. Haemat.* 11:59, 1965.

McIntyre, O. R., Sullivan, L. W., Jeffries, G. H., and Silver, R. H.   Pernicious anemia in childhood. *New Eng. J. Med.* 272:981, 1965.

McLean, F. W., Heine, M. W., Held, B., and Streiff, R. R.   Relationship between the oral contraceptive and folic acid metabolism. *Amer. J. Obstet. Gynec.* 104:745, 1969.

Omer, A., and Mowat, A. G.   Nature of anaemia in rheumatoid arthritis: IX. Folate metabolism in patients with rheumatoid arthritis. *Ann. Rheum. Dis.* 27:414, 1968.

Rosenberg, I. H., Streiff, R. R., Godwin, H. A., and Castle, W. B.   Absorption of polyglutamic folate: Participation of deconjugating enzymes of the intestinal mucosa. *New Eng. J. Med.* 280:985, 1969.

Samloff, I. M., Kleinman, M. S., Turner, M. D., Sobel, M. V., and Jeffries, G. H.   Blocking and binding antibodies to intrinsic factor and parietal cell antibody in pernicious anemia. *Gastroenterology* 55:575, 1968.

Schilling, R. F.   A new test for intrinsic factor activity. *J. Lab. Clin. Med.* 42:946, 1953.

Spurling, C. L., Sacks, M. S., and Jiji, R. M.   Juvenile pernicious anemia. *New Eng. J. Med.* 271:995, 1964.

Sullivan, L. W., and Herbert, V.   Studies on the minimum daily requirement for vitamin B_{12}: Hematopoietic responses to 0.1 microgm. of cyanocobalamin or coenzyme B_{12}, and comparison of their relative potency. *New Eng. J. Med.* 272:340, 1965.

Wangel, A. G., Callender, S. T., Spray, G. H., and Wright, R.   A family study of pernicious anaemia: I. Autoantibodies, achlorhydria, serum pepsinogen and vitamin B_{12}. *Brit. J. Haemat.* 14:161, 1968.

3. SIDEROBLASTIC ANEMIAS

David A. Sears

THE SIDEROBLASTIC or iron-loading anemias are a heterogeneous group of disorders characterized by a poorly understood disturbance of iron metabolism that frequently results in hypochromic anemia and increased total body iron. The morphologic feature that defines this group of diseases is the presence in the bone marrow of nucleated red cells containing large granules of stainable iron arranged about the cell nucleus, so-called ringed sideroblasts. Names that have been applied to members of this group of anemias include sideroachrestic anemia (Heilmeyer), refractory normoblastic anemia (Dacie), chronic refractory anemia with sideroblastic bone marrow (Bjorkman), refractory anemia with hyperplastic bone marrow—Type 1 (Vilter), hereditary sex-linked hypochromic anemia (Rundles and Falls), primary refractory anemia (Bomford and Rhodes), and Di Guglielmo syndrome or chronic Di Guglielmo disease (Dameshek). As is suggested by the existence of this profuse nomenclature, underlying pathogenetic mechanisms have not been elucidated.

In the normal individual the developing bone marrow normoblast takes up iron in excess of its immediate requirements for hemoglobin synthesis. This iron is temporarily stored in the cytoplasm as ferritin or other aggregates which stain with the usual Prussian blue iron stain. Estimates of the proportion of nucleated red cells in normal marrow that contain these granules range up to 90%. However, these siderotic inclusions are few (often only 1 or 2 per cell), small, and may be difficult to see. The normoblasts containing stainable iron are called *sideroblasts* and are, of course, a normal constituent of marrow. Sideroblasts are not seen in the marrows of patients with iron deficiency. As normoblasts mature, the iron is consumed for hemoglobin synthesis. At the reticulocyte stage the proportion of cells containing stainable siderotic granules is 1% or less. Ferritin can be identified by electron microscopy in a majority of reticulocytes but is apparently not aggregated sufficiently to produce Prussian blue positivity.

39

The mature red cell contains neither stainable iron nor ferritin. The spleen seems to be important in removal of iron from nonnucleated red cells, either through the "pitting" mechanism described by Crosby or by temporary sequestration of reticulocytes, during which time the last traces of iron are consumed in hemoglobin synthesis. Nonnucleated red cells containing stainable iron granules are called *siderocytes* and are seen most commonly in splenectomized patients. They are not a common finding in the sideroblastic anemias but may be present in very small numbers.

The *abnormal sideroblast* that characterizes the sideroblastic anemias contains larger, more readily visible, Prussian blue–positive granules which are arranged in a perinuclear distribution, hence the term *ringed sideroblast*. This iron, consisting of ferritin and unstructured aggregates, is contained in mitochondria, in contrast to the iron in normal sideroblasts which is scattered throughout the cytoplasm. The possible significance of the mitochondrial location will be discussed. The ringed sideroblast often manifests other cytoplasmic abnormalities such as poor hemoglobinization and vacuolization.

Large siderotic granules in red cells may be visible on an ordinary Wright's stained blood smear as basophilic inclusions, so-called Pappenheimer bodies. This is a rare finding, and without iron stains these inclusions are difficult to distinguish from other sorts of punctate basophilia.

CLASSIFICATION

The sideroblastic anemias have been classified in various ways. Since little is understood about the etiology or pathogenesis of these disorders, any classification, such as the one in Table 3-1, must be considered tentative.

The primary hereditary cases usually appear in young adult males; many of these are pyridoxine-responsive. Female "carriers" have occasionally

Table 3-1. Classification of Sideroblastic Anemias

Primary or idiopathic
  Hereditary (sex-linked hypochromic anemia)
  Acquired (refractory sideroblastic anemia)

Secondary
  Drugs or toxins (e.g., isoniazid, cycloserine, pyrazinamide, chloramphenicol, alcohol, lead)
  Other diseases (e.g., myeloproliferative diseases, leukemia, lymphoma, cancer, rheumatoid arthritis, porphyria, pernicious anemia, malabsorption syndromes, hemolytic anemias, myxedema)

---

shown some features of the disorder. The primary acquired group consists of the nonfamilial cases in which an offending drug or underlying disease cannot be identified and would include, for example, the preleukemia and preaplasia patients. In the secondary cases associated with certain drugs, toxins, or other diseases, the sideroblastic anemia is a complication that usually does not dominate the clinical picture. The relative incidence of the various types of sideroblastic anemia is not known. In 70 cases described by MacGibbon and Mollin, half were primary and half secondary. Fewer than 10% were clearly hereditary. The recent studies of Hines and Grasso have emphasized the frequency of sideroblastic changes in alcoholic patients.

[handwritten annotation: N n HM normocytic / RTC ↓ / SI ↑ % saturation of transferrin ↑]

HEMATOLOGIC FEATURES

The hematologic features of the sideroblastic anemias are variable, but the characteristic findings most common to the primary sideroblastic anemias are as follows:

1. Hypochromic and microcytic in primary types; more often normochromic or "dimorphic" (i.e., two red cell populations, one hypochromic, one normochromic) in secondary types
2. Reticulocyte percentage usually low
3. Serum iron and percent saturation of transferrin usually increased
4. Marrow erythroid hyperplasia, ringed sideroblasts, defective hemoglobinization, often megaloblastic
5. Increased clearance rate and turnover of plasma iron with decreased red cell incorporation
6. Red cell life-span normal or slightly decreased
7. Tissue siderosis (not invariable)

The morphologic characteristics of the blood smear and marrow may be indistinguishable from those of iron deficiency. Obviously the serum iron determination and evaluation of marrow iron differentiate the two processes. The tissue siderosis commonly present may be of the massive proportions seen in idiopathic hemochromatosis and identical to it histologically. Many sideroblastic anemia patients have been transfused, and a history of previous iron therapy is not uncommon. These will, of course, augment the siderosis, but it is clear that iron-loading occurs also in patients unexposed to these sources of excess iron. Hepatic fibrosis has been observed in a few patients, and iron has been found at autopsy in other organs, including the pancreas and myocardium.

Ferrokinetic studies demonstrate the classic characteristics of ineffective erythropoiesis, i.e., increased turnover of plasma transferrin-bound iron but diminished incorporation of the iron into circulating red cells. That plasma iron is actually delivered to marrow sites has been shown by radioisotopic studies with body surface counting. Interestingly, elevations of serum lactic acid dehydrogenase have not been observed in primary sideroblastic anemia. The normal or only slightly shortened red cell life-span and the absence of increased levels of hemoglobin F or A_2 help distinguish the sideroblastic anemias from thalassemia, which shares many of the other features. Splenomegaly is a variable feature of the sideroblastic anemias.

PYRIDOXINE, HEME SYNTHESIS, AND MITOCHONDRIA

Considerable interest has centered on the pyridoxine responsiveness of some patients with sideroblastic anemia in the belief that this characteristic must hold some clue to the mechanisms of the anemia. From one-third to half of all patients with either primary or secondary types exhibit pyridoxine responsiveness. The response to pyridoxine is itself variable. A few patients have responded to what may be physiologic doses of the vitamin (2 mg per day or less), but the majority require doses of at least 10 times this amount and some as much as 200 mg per day. These and many other observations make it clear that, with few exceptions, the patients who respond to pyridoxine do not have simple pyridoxine deficiency. Neither dietary deficiency of the vitamin, defective absorption, nor increased excretion has been demonstrated. The patients lack other manifestations of deficiency of the vitamin such as neuropathy, dermatitis, and glossitis.

The response to pyridoxine, especially in the hereditary group of patients, is incomplete. While the hemoglobin level improves with therapy, often returning to normal levels, the abnormal red cell morphology is, at best, only partially repaired, and hypochromia and poikilocytosis persist. Some patients have maintained their hematologic improvement for long periods after pyridoxine was stopped; a few others have become unresponsive to the vitamin. With pyridoxine therapy the serum iron usually falls initially but may rise again while therapy is continued. Ringed sideroblasts continue to be evident in the marrow, and tissue siderosis persists. Splenomegaly, if present, usually does not disappear with pyridoxine therapy. In a few cases of secondary sideroblastic anemia, both the anemia and the ringed sideroblast abnormality have disappeared completely after therapy with pyridoxine and folic acid. In other instances the abnormalities have disappeared with remission of the associated disease.

Though patients lack other clinical manifestations of pyridoxine deficiency, metabolic abnormalities related to the vitamin can sometimes be demonstrated. Pyridoxal phosphate is involved in the tryptophan–nicotinic acid metabolic pathway as cofactor for two enzymes, kynureninase and kynurenine transaminase. This pathway can be "stressed" by administration of an oral tryptophan load and abnormalities discovered by quantifying urinary excretion of intermediate metabolites. Xanthurenic acid and certain kynurenine derivatives may be excreted in increased amounts in pyridoxine deficiency. Some abnormality in tryptophan metabolism has been found in about half the pyridoxine-responsive patients tested.

Since the morphologic features of sideroblastic anemia suggest a defect in hemoglobin synthesis, the role of pyridoxine in heme synthesis has been of particular interest. The pathway of heme synthesis is shown in Figure 3-1. Pyridoxal phosphate is cofactor for δ-aminolevulinic acid synthetase, the enzyme catalyzing the first step in the synthetic pathway. There is little direct evidence that the pathway of heme synthesis is disturbed in pyridoxine-responsive anemia. However, one report has described decreased incorporation of glycine into heme in vitro by marrow cells from a patient. Studies by Vavra and Poff in a group of patients with sideroblastic anemia

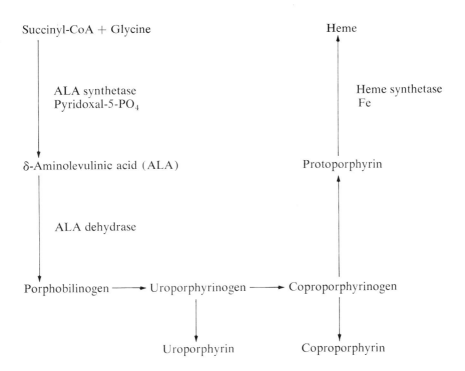

Figure 3-1. Pathway of heme synthesis.

showed no impairment of incorporation of δ-aminolevulinic acid into heme. Measurements of red cell coproporphyrin and protoporphyrin levels have demonstrated abnormalities but no consistent pattern. Lead, which can produce sideroblastic anemia, is known to interfere with heme synthesis at several levels, including that of δ-aminolevulinic acid synthetase.

Because iron can be chelated by pyridoxal phosphate and because excessive iron inhibits the condensation of glycine and succinate in vitro, it has been proposed that iron excess might interfere with pyridoxine function in sideroblastic anemia. The possibility that iron-loading is the primary defect seems now to have been excluded by observations on patients whose excessive body iron was removed by repeated phlebotomy. Even after depletion of tissue iron, the red cell defects and pyridoxine requirement persisted.

Since the active coenzyme form of pyridoxine is pyridoxal-5-phosphate, the possibility of a defect in the conversion of the dietary to the coenzyme form has been considered. German workers have reported a single patient who responded better to treatment with pyridoxal phosphate than pyridoxine, and unpublished observations on 3 patients by Hines and Love also suggest the possibility of a defect in conversion of pyridoxine to pyridoxal phosphate. Methods recently developed by Hines and Love for accurate measurement of pyridoxal phosphate in body fluids should be useful in evaluating this possibility further. Such a mechanism may be important in patients with sideroblastic anemia secondary to treatment with the antituberculosis drugs. Isoniazid (INH), for example, is an inhibitor of the enzyme pyridoxal kinase, which catalyzes the phosphorylation of pyridoxal. INH is known to complex directly with pyridoxal and may inhibit action of the vitamin in this way also.

Attention has been directed to mitochondrial function in the sideroblast because mitochondria are the site of the massive iron deposition and have been observed by electron microscopy to have distinct morphologic abnormalities including swelling, vacuolization, and loss of internal structure. Likewise certain of the enzymes of the heme synthesis pathway are localized to mitochondria, including δ-aminolevulinic acid synthetase (for which pyridoxal-5-phosphate is cofactor) and the iron-incorporating enzyme, heme synthetase. Harris and his colleagues have reported the interesting observations that reticulocyte mitochondria prepared from pyridoxine-deficient rabbits and from 2 human subjects with pyridoxine-responsive sideroblastic anemia incubated with appropriate substrates in vitro did not take up and release iron unless pyridoxal phosphate was added to the medium. After the subjects (rabbits and humans) were treated with pyridoxine, the uptake and release of iron by the reticulocyte mitochondrial preparations were normal.

Many of the observations on the sideroblastic anemia patients with pyridoxine responsiveness hint at some metabolic disturbance in utilization of the vitamin. It has been suggested that an increased pyridoxine requirement might come about through "hyperutilization," much as patients with marked marrow erythroid hyperplasia seem to have an increased folic acid requirement. In support of this hypothesis a single report can be cited of an infant with sickle cell disease who had a hypochromic anemia and developed reticulocytosis on treatment with pyridoxine. On the other hand, Horrigan and Harris suggest the possibility that in pyridoxine-responsive sideroblastic anemia some other erythropoietic factor is lacking and that this deficiency can be partially compensated for by pyridoxine. They cite a well-studied patient whose response to pyridoxine was potentiated by an indole compound isolated from crude liver extract. In isolated instances a variety of other substances have been reported to induce reticulocytosis or enhance the response to pyridoxine, including ascorbic acid, tryptophan, and histidine.

FOLIC ACID

A number of authors, particularly those in England, have described a striking incidence of disturbances of folate metabolism in both the primary and secondary types of sideroblastic anemia. In one series half of the primary cases and three-fourths of the secondary cases had megaloblastic marrow changes, and serum folate levels were low in 80% of both groups. However, a much smaller percentage had a hematologic response to folic acid therapy, and the response was rarely complete. The mechanism of folate deficiency in the sideroblastic anemias is not clear. There is seldom dietary deficiency, except perhaps in the alcoholic patients, or evidence of malabsorption. It has been suggested that folic acid requirements may be increased in sideroblastic anemia due to the marrow erythroid hyperplasia.

Responses to folic acid and pyridoxine have been additive in some patients. A metabolic site at which folic acid and pyridoxine are related is in the conversion of serine to glycine, a reaction for which pyridoxal-5-phosphate is cofactor and in which a one-carbon fragment is generated. Tetrahydrofolic acid functions in various one-carbon transfer reactions and may be the intermediate recipient of this one-carbon unit.

TREATMENT

The foregoing discussion of the possible roles of pyridoxine and folic acid in the sideroblastic anemias has indicated the advisability of a therapeutic trial of these two vitamins in these disorders. In a very few patients empirical trial of crude liver extract or the other nutrients mentioned may be justified. In the secondary cases associated with drugs or toxins, discontinuation of the offending agent results in disappearance of the sideroblastic changes. Reversal of the sideroblastic process due to antituberculosis drugs has been achieved with pyridoxine therapy without stopping the drugs. In the cases of sideroblastic anemia secondary to other diseases, the major clinical problems are generally those of the underlying disease.

In the primary forms of sideroblastic anemia one must consider phlebotomy therapy to remove the excessive iron stores. The rationale for such therapy is the extreme siderosis that has been observed in liver, myocardium, pancreas, and other organs, and the conviction that such siderosis is at least potentially harmful. Interestingly, the incidence of diabetes in these patients is higher than that in the general population. There is evidence that tissue siderosis may have played a role in the death of some patients with sideroblastic anemia.

In the few patients who have been bled to remove excess iron, the amount removed has ranged from 6 to 16 gm (as compared with normal body stores of about 1.5 gm). In 2 well-studied cases Weintraub and his colleagues found it possible to remove 2 to 3 units of blood per week initially. The hemoglobin concentration decreased by about 2 gm per 100 ml but then leveled off, despite continued phlebotomy, until iron stores were depleted. Thus the erythroid marrow retained its reserve capacity to respond to bloodletting but still did not raise the patients' hemoglobin levels completely to normal on pyridoxine therapy.

Since sideroblastic anemia may be a hereditary disorder, and since the familial patients seem particularly predisposed to accumulation of large excesses of body iron, it is important to investigate family members, much as would be done in idiopathic hemochromatosis.

The sideroblastic or iron-loading anemias are a heterogeneous group of hereditary and acquired disorders, the pathogenesis of which is obscure but in which iron metabolism, heme synthesis, mitochondrial function, or a combination of these is disturbed in erythropoietic tissue, producing the morphologic hallmark of the disorder, the ringed sideroblast. The secondary varieties may be seen in association with a variety of drugs, toxins, and underlying diseases. Red cells often appear hypochromic and microcytic, but there may be a "dimorphic" or even normal blood picture. Ineffective erythropoiesis is characteristic. Defects in pyridoxine or folic acid metabolism or both may exist, and a therapeutic trial of these vitamins is always warranted, at least in the primary cases. Tissue siderosis may be marked, particularly in the primary forms, and removal of excess iron by phlebotomy is advisable. The hereditary, apparently sex-linked character of many of the primary cases indicates the need for family studies.

REFERENCES

Dacie, J. V., and Mollin, D. L.   Siderocytes, sideroblasts, and sideroblastic anemia. *Acta Med. Scand.* (Suppl. 445):237, 1966.

Hines, J. D.   Reversible megaloblastic and sideroblastic marrow abnormalities in alcoholic patients. *Brit. J. Haemat.* 16:87, 1969.

Hines, J. D., and Grasso, J. A.   The sideroblastic anemias. *Seminars Hemat.* 7:86, 1970.

Horrigan, D. L., and Harris, J. W.   Pyridoxine-responsive anemia: Analysis of 62 cases. *Advances Intern. Med.* 12:103, 1964.

Horrigan, D. L., and Harris, J. W.   Pyridoxine-responsive anemias in man. *Vitamins Hormones* 26:549, 1968.

Proceedings of the Symposium on Sideroblastic Anemia held during the Annual Meeting of the British Society for Haematology, London, Mar. 20, 1964. *Brit. J. Haemat.* 11:41, 1965.

Vavra, J. D., and Poff, S. A.   Heme and porphyrin synthesis in sideroblastic anemia. *J. Lab. Clin. Med.* 69:904, 1967.

Weintraub, L. R., Conrad, M. E., and Crosby, W. H.   Iron-loading anemia: Treatment with repeated phlebotomies and pyridoxine. *New Eng. J. Med.* 275:169, 1966.

4. DETERMINANTS OF ERYTHROCYTE SURVIVAL IN HEMOLYTIC STATES: INDICATIONS FOR SPLENECTOMY

Robert I. Weed

SHORTENING OF erythrocyte life-span below the normal time of 120 days is potentially of serious consequence. Acute hemolysis with anemia may result in tissue hypoxia or may be associated with disseminated intravascular coagulation as is occasionally seen in paroxysmal nocturnal hemoglobinuria, presumably related to release of phospholipid thromboplastic material from the lysed cells. On the other hand, chronic low-grade hemolysis may not even result in anemia, since the bone marrow has a six- to eightfold capacity to compensate. However, chronic hemolysis often results in cholelithiasis and cholecystitis, as in some middle-aged patients who may have a diagnosis of hereditary spherocytosis made as an incidental finding during evaluation for their gallbladder disease. Of the various types of anemia found in the United States, fewer than one-eighth can be classified as primarily hemolytic disorders, i.e., those associated with normal cell production but shortened survival attributable to acquired or environmental defects. If, however, one broadens the consideration of hemolysis to include anemic disorders in which a hemolytic component can be demonstrated, then two-thirds of anemic disorders must be considered to have hemolytic components.

In certain cases, such as iron deficiency, the hemolytic component becomes overt only when the iron deficiency is severe, and the same appears

This work was supported by U.S. Public Health Service Research Grant HE-06241 and the U.S. Atomic Energy Project at the University of Rochester. It has been assigned publication no. UR-49-1298.

49

to be the case in megaloblastic anemias such as pernicious anemia. In inflammation, for example, the anemia is most commonly a combination of decreased production and some increase beyond the normal rate of destruction. In disorders such as thalassemia, ineffective erythropoiesis is found. This is measured by the erythrocyte iron turnover (EIT) utilizing isotopic ^{59}Fe (EIT = plasma iron turnover $\times$ erythrocyte utilization). However, even in the disorders of hemoglobin synthesis a significant share of ineffective erythropoiesis may, in fact, represent intramarrow hemolysis before the cells ever appear in the peripheral blood. The same may be true of iron deficiency in which it is now clear that some element of ineffective erythropoiesis occurs even in milder cases. Thus it is of critical importance to understand what determines red cell life-span under normal circumstances and to consider how this may be altered in any anemic state and, in particular, to consider the special role of the spleen in overt hemolytic anemias in which consideration of splenectomy may be of considerable clinical importance.

PATHOPHYSIOLOGY OF HEMOLYSIS

Within the past 15 years much attention has been focused on the pathologic biochemistry of the red cell apparent in the various hemoglobinopathies, in enzyme deficiencies of the Embden-Meyerhof pathway leading to faulty maintenance of red cell adenosine triphosphate (ATP), and in defects of the pentose phosphate shunt which interfere with the ability of the red cell to maintain reduced glutathione and resist exposure to the stress of oxidant drugs. However, it has recently become increasingly clear that the pathologic physiology of shortened life-span related to these underlying biochemical defects can be best understood in terms of altered physical properties of the red cell. Cellular deformability is a critical property essential to permit an erythrocyte, whose normal greater diameter exceeds 8μ, to pass for 120 days through capillaries which range from 3 to 12 μ in diameter as well as through the splenic cords which have apertures in the basement membrane separating cords from sinuses as small as 0.5μ in diameter.

Another critical cellular parameter is membrane "stickiness," i.e., the predisposition to adhere to another erythrocyte, to a phagocyte, or to a vessel wall. Rouleaux formation or red cell aggregation enhanced by fibrinogen and gamma globulin, inhibited by albumin and alpha globulin, is a weak type of cell–cell interaction which occurs normally under conditions of stagnation but is easily disrupted by shearing stresses of normal circulatory flow. Pathologic macroglobulins may produce a nonspecific aggregation that leads to small vessel occlusion. The negatively charged sialic acid groups on the cell membrane normally act to inhibit cell–cell aggregation, but these repulsive forces may be overcome by certain antibodies which produce agglutination by reacting with specific antigen sites on the red cell, particularly in a plasma environment, with resultant rapid removal by spleen and liver. In microangiopathic disorders such as the hemolytic–uremic syndrome or metastatic carcinoma, small vessel injury with fibrin deposition may lead to formation of strands connecting red cells to vessel walls, with subsequent fragmentation of such a red cell when buffeted by circulatory flow.

MECHANISMS OF HEMOLYSIS

Although hemolysis in the test tube implies breakdown of the cell membrane with release of hemoglobin, hemolysis in vivo indicates a shortened red cell life-span, without implication as to the mechanism of cell removal or destruction, or both. Three major hemolytic mechanisms operate in vivo.

MAINTENANCE OF VOLUME.   Maintenance of normal red cell volume requires an appropriate balance between normal membrane permeability and the ATP-dependent Na-K active transport mechanism which balances the tendency of the red cell to accumulate cations because of the colloid osmotic effect of intracellular hemoglobin. Theoretically, injury of the membrane, by producing a membrane defect less than the dimensions of hemoglobin (32.5 A in effective diffusion radius), results in colloid osmotic swelling and lysis of the cell. Alternatively, if antibody and complement (C) produce a membrane defect larger than the hemoglobin molecule itself, hemoglobin is released directly. Practically, however, the hemolysis seen in incompatible transfusions—i.e., produced by isoantibody, the acid hemolysis of paroxysmal nocturnal hemoglobinuria, and the hemolysis of paroxysmal cold hemoglobinuria—are all associated with membrane defects which are larger than the hemoglobin molecule itself and which result in direct escape of hemoglobin. Enzymatic damage such as occurs with the phospholipase produced by clostridial organisms also produces direct release of hemoglobin. However, it must be recognized that the disorders mentioned are relatively rare clinically and other hemolytic mechanisms are much more common.

ERYTHROPHAGOCYTOSIS.   Erythrophagocytosis is a second mechanism for red cell destruction by macrophages within the spleen and elsewhere in the reticuloendothelial system. Erythrophagocytosis can be demonstrated to a variable extent upon examination of the spleen in most hemolytic disorders, and in severe hemolysis, particularly immune hemolytic disease, erythrophagocytosis may be seen in the marrow and in a peripheral blood preparation (particularly buffy coat). Phagocytosis is a complex phenomenon which depends on (1) chemotaxis or attraction between damaged red cells and the phagocyte, (2) adhesion between the cells concerned, (3) ingestion of the red cell or portions of the latter and, finally, (4) digestion. Apart from the C-dependent release of hemoglobin, shortened survival of antibody-injured red cells presumably depends upon alterations in cell surface properties which predispose them to agglutination or to phagocytosis or partial phagocytosis. Phagocytosis of just a portion of the cell must be considered a form of cellular fragmentation insofar as the consequences of fragmentation may be a progressively sphered and increasingly rigid cell which has a further shortening of its life-span.

3   FRAGMENTATION.   The most important of the various hemolytic mechanisms is that of red cell fragmentation, which may be defined as loss from the cell of a piece of membrane which may or may not contain hemoglobin. Such a loss does not necessarily imply immediate in vivo or in vitro hemolysis, but it does have important implications for the subsequent survival of the cell. Fragmentation loss of a piece of membrane or even a piece of membrane enclosing a portion of cellular content does not necessarily imply immediate phagocytosis of the cell but rather may lead to progressive sphering which will ultimately limit the ability of the cell to survive within the circulation.

ERYTHROCYTE DEFORMABILITY

The first determinant of red cell deformability is that of shape. The biconcave disc shape of the normal erythrocyte is absolutely essential for maintenance of normal deformability. The normal excess of surface area to volume makes it possible for erythrocytes to pass normally through channels up to 14 μ in length with as small a diameter as 2.8 μ, as illustrated diagrammatically in Figure 4-1A, or shorter channels with diameters down to 0.5 μ as are found in the spleen. Any increase in cell volume or decrease in surface area or "effective" surface area results in the production of a more spherical cell that is less able to bend or deform in order to negotiate narrow channels in the microcirculation. Thus spherocytes, whether found in hereditary spherocytosis or in immune hemolytic anemia, are limited in their survival by the critical ratio of surface area to volume, as shown in Figure 4-1B. A third major pathophysiologic mechanism determining loss of red cell deformability is an increasing stiffness of the membrane itself related to a decrease in intracellular ATP.

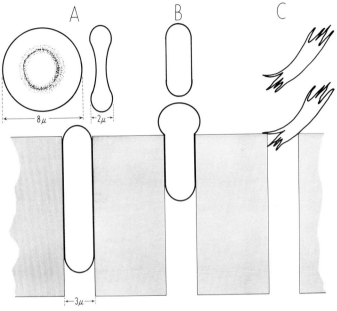

Figure 4-1. Erythrocyte passage through 2.8 μ channels. (A) Normal bicon-cave cell deforms into a 14 μ cylinder and passes easily. (B) A partially sphered cell cannot negotiate the passage because of a decreased surface area to volume ratio. (C) A sickle cell cannot deform to pass because of its rigid contents.

Figure 4-2 illustrates the various pathophysiologic pathways giving rise to cellular rigidity and the fragmentation which may be part of that patho-physiology or the consequence of it. Pathway A illustrates the fact that abnormal hemoglobins such as SS or CC, under conditions of low oxygen tension or hyperosmolarity, respectively, may give rise to increased intracel-lular viscosity or rigidity with resultant secondary loss of cellular deforma-bility. The projecting tips of sickle cells are sufficiently rigid to be frag-mented from such cells during passage through the microcirculation, and such fragmentation may even result in cation leak with colloid osmotic lysis of the parent cell. Pathway B illustrates the possible consequences of intra-cellular formation of Heinz bodies. The disorders leading to Heinz body production are discussed in Chapter 6. If present in sufficient quantities, such rigid intracellular inclusions limit cell passage through restricted re-gions such as the splenic pulp circulation. If only occasional intracellular precipitates occur, they may be pitted from the cells as they pass through the spleen. The resultant morphologic consequences of this may be produc-tion of teardrop cells or cells which appear to have a bite-shaped defect and which are in turn made more rigid by the damage; therefore their own sub-

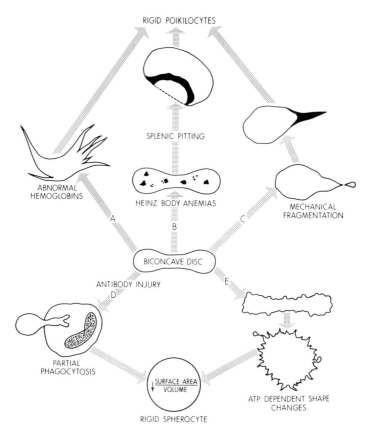

RIGID POIKILOCYTES

SPLENIC PITTING

ABNORMAL
HEMOGLOBINS

HEINZ BODY ANEMIAS

MECHANICAL
FRAGMENTATION

A

B

C

BICONCAVE DISC

ANTIBODY INJURY

E

D

PARTIAL
PHAGOCYTOSIS

SURFACE AREA
VOLUME

ATP DEPENDENT SHAPE
CHANGES

RIGID SPHEROCYTE

Figure 4-2. Pathogenesis of erythrocyte rigidity and fragmentation (see text). (From R. I. Weed, The Cell Membrane in Hemolytic Disorders. In E. R. Jaffé [Ed.], *Proceedings of the XIIth Congress of the International Society of Hematology*, New York, 1968.)

sequent survival may be compromised. Extrinsic trauma such as that seen in prosthetic heart valve hemolysis or the syndromes of microangiopathic hemolysis results in fragmentation of cells which undoubtedly leads to subsequent shortening of life-span of the damaged cells. Extensive fragmentation and schistocytosis are often evident on the blood smear. Pathway D illustrates the form of fragmentation seen in association with antibody injury, i.e., partial phagocytosis with resultant increased sphering of the residual nonphagocytosed portion of the cell. Finally, in Pathway E can be seen the disc–sphere transformation which is known to occur with ATP depletion and occurs in hereditary spherocytes even at normal ATP levels.

Erythrocyte ATP is known to be a critical determinant of survival and it is now clear that this is so not only because ATP, if present in sufficient concentration, prevents the disc-to-sphere shape change but also because it maintains internal fluidity of the cell and intrinsic membrane deformability. Thus any enzyme defect that impairs maintenance of critical levels of ATP leads to shortening of red cell life-span.

LABORATORY EVALUATION OF LOSS OF RED CELL DEFORMABILITY

The first and simplest clue to alteration in red cell deformability can often be obtained by careful examination of the peripheral blood smear. Any significant departure in red cell morphology from the normal smooth contoured biconcave cell, identifiable on the Wright's stained smear by virtue of its area of central pallor, should suggest the possibility of fundamental alterations in cellular physical properties that will predispose to shortened life-span. As mentioned, morphologic identification of significant spherocytosis allows a prediction of shortened red cell life-span and should stimulate a search for all the causes of spherocytosis. The presence of crenated disc or spherocytic forms which are variously referred to as burr cells, spur cells, pyknocytes, or spicule cells, while resulting from a variety of fundamental abnormalities, in all may imply loss of normal cell deformability. Likewise, fragmentation with small hemoglobin-containing fragments or larger cells that appear to have pieces missing not only should suggest that a significant hemolytic process is operating, but the fact that such damaged cells retain their abnormal or bizarre shape rather than reassuming a smooth contour suggests that their contents or their membranes, or both, have themselves been altered.

The osmotic fragility test, although based on many assumptions, provides a measure of the relationship of surface area to volume of red cells being tested and therefore of their ability to deform and pass through the spleen. Thus if red cell volume in plasma is normal or near normal, an increase in osmotic fragility indicates that there is either a decrease in surface area or a decrease in effective surface area (resistance to swelling). Conversely, decreased osmotic fragility implies an increase in the surface area to volume ratio either as the cells exist in plasma or as they are swollen in the procedure itself.

Tests of red cell filterability either with Millipore,* Nucleopore,† or certain select types of ordinary filter paper provide an overall measure of red cell deformability. If red cell filterability is decreased, indicating loss of cellular deformability, then the osmotic fragility test should be utilized to further categorize the abnormality. If deformability is abnormal and osmotic fragility is increased, then the defect must be attributed to spherocyte formation, which should be suggested on the blood smear. Abnormalities in

---

* Millipore Filter Corp., Bedford, Mass.
† General Electric, Vallecitos, Cal.

the physical state of intracellular hemoglobin, however, cause a decrease in filterability without change or with a decrease in osmotic fragility. This phenomenon is illustrated in Figure 4-1C.

ROLE OF THE SPLEEN

The spleen poses several important and critical challenges to pathologic red cells. Normal arterial blood flow supplying red cells to the splenic pulp may pass directly from terminal arterioles to the splenic venous sinuses via a shunting mechanism. Alternatively, the terminal arteriolar flow may pass into the splenic pulp, through the cords, and then pass through the basement membrane separating cords from sinuses back into the splenic venous sinuses and return to the general circulation, as illustrated in Figure 4-3. Figure 4-3 also illustrates that the threats of circulation through the splenic cord include (a) the anatomic requirement for deformability imposed by the high endothelial cells at the terminal arteriole, (b) the necessity for squeezing through the potential space which lies between the phagocytes of the splenic cord, and (c) the specifically restrictive requirement for defor-

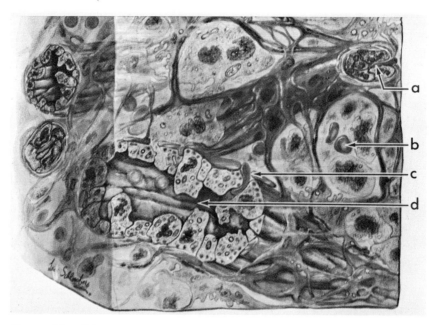

Figure 4-3. Diagrammatic representation of the ultrastructure of splenic red pulp (see text). Terminal arteriole (*a*), red cells in the splenic cord (*b*), red cell traversing lumen in basement membrane (*c*), splenic sinus (*d*). (From L. Weiss, *Amer. J. Anat.* 113:51, 1963.)

mation through the 0.5 to 5.0 μ openings in the basement membrane separating cords from sinuses. Obviously any predisposition to aggregation as in the case of agglutinated cells, increase in intrinsic cellular rigidity for any of the reasons discussed, or enhancement of red cell adhesiveness to cordal macrophages predisposes to phagocytosis within the cords.

In addition to these splenic threats, it is now clear that the architecture of the bone marrow is similar to that of the spleen in certain important respects. Hematopoiesis and maturation occur within hematopoietic cords, but erythrocyte and granulocyte precursors at the reticulocyte and metamyelocyte stage, respectively, must migrate from the hematopoietic cords through an adventitial layer and a basement membrane separating cords from marrow sinuses, much as mature cells must be able to migrate from splenic cords into the sinuses. Thus in order to begin life in the circulation, immature erythrocytes must achieve a degree of deformability and dimensions comparable to those of mature red cells which will permit passage into the general circulation. Thus both hypothetical and practical consideration of the indications for splenectomy requires insight into the stage in cellular maturation at which intrinsic or extrinsic defects begin to affect the physical properties of the cells. Particularly in congested spleens, lowered pH and oxygen tension in the pulp represent important threats. Both decreased pH and low Po_2 (less than 25 mm Hg) make even normal red cells rigid. The lowered pH and Po_2 of the splenic pulp do not induce critical changes in normal cells but, when superimposed on cellular rigidity already present in abnormal erythrocytes, may make it impossible for the pathologic cells to escape once they enter the pulp.

INDICATIONS FOR SPLENECTOMY

Table 4-1 lists hemolytic states in which splenectomy may be of benefit whether or not it is the treatment of choice. The table also includes an indication of the mechanism of splenic damage and the results to be expected. It can be seen that the best results can be anticipated when the red cell changes that predispose to splenic destruction occur after the erythrocytes leave the bone marrow and enter the general circulation. As one might anticipate, splenectomy in the face of intramedullary damage or destruction can provide only amelioration, at best.

Thus splenectomy is clearly indicated as a preferred form of therapy in hereditary spherocytosis and elliptocytosis with significant hemolysis, to avoid the complications of long-term hemolysis. In autoimmune hemolytic disease the results are generally good—particularly if the cells are coated with gamma globulin, if the patient's disease is steroid responsive, and if the spleen is enlarged. However, since lymphoma, chronic lymphocytic leuke-

Table 4-1. Splenectomy in Hemolytic Anemia

Disorder	Pathophysiology of Splenic Injury	Cellular Abnormality Present in Marrow Precursor	Expected Result
Hereditary spherocytosis	Splenic "conditioning" aggravates tendency for RBC to become sphered and rigid	No	Clinical cure
Hereditary elliptocytosis with significant hemolysis	Same as in hereditary spherocytosis	?	Clinical cure
Acquired "autoimmune" hemolytic anemia	Antibody injury predisposes to partial phagocytosis → sphering	No	Variable results
"Idiopathic hypersplenism"	?	No	Good result
Sickle cell disease	Rigid sickle cells fragment and are trapped in hypoxic splenic pulp	Yes	Amelioration in children if spleen is enlarged; no benefit in adults with small, infarcted spleen
S-T, S-C diseases	Same as in sickle cell disease	Yes	Amelioration of hemolysis
Thalassemia major	Fragmentation pitting of Heinz bodies from cells or trapping if entire cell is sufficiently rigid	Yes, with intramedullary hemolysis (ineffective erythropoiesis)	Amelioration of hemolysis (and transfusion requirement)
Unstable hemoglobin syndromes	Same as in thalassemia major	Yes, with intramedullary hemolysis (ineffective erythropoiesis)	Amelioration of hemolysis (and transfusion requirement)
Pyruvate kinase deficiency	Reticulocytes and shrunken, rigid pyknocytes are trapped in the spleen	Yes, but aging in the circulation aggravates the cellular abnormality	Usually significant amelioration
"Hypersplenism" associated with myeloproliferative disorders	Trapping and fragmentation of abnormal cells in an anatomically abnormal spleen	Yes, in myeloproliferative disorders	Amelioration
Lymphomas	Same as in "hypersplenism"	Depends on whether there is bone marrow involvement	Amelioration

mia, or lupus erythematosus may underlie autoimmune hemolysis, these diseases should be sought and primary treatment directed toward them, if indicated. In addition some patients may remit while under treatment with corticosteroids, either related to therapy or because of spontaneous subsidence of the process. Obviously these patients do not need early splenectomy. In general, therefore, splenectomy in autoimmune disease should be reserved for patients who relapse upon cessation of steroid therapy or who require more than a very small dose (greater than 5 to 10 mg daily) to prevent recurrence of anemia after an initial 6-week trial.

For the other diseases indicated in Table 4-1, splenectomy is never curative but may have sufficient value in minimizing transfusion requirements to warrant serious consideration.

Evaluation of splenic function in the face of a hemolytic state may be helpful in predicting the possible benefit to be expected from splenectomy. Splenic contribution to hemolysis can be appraised by labeling of red cells with ^{51}Cr sodium chromate, reinjection, and following cell survival in conjunction with surface counting over liver, spleen, heart, and occasionally sacrum. Consideration should be given to whose blood shall be used for the splenic uptake studies. In patients with hereditary or acquired anemias in whom a major element of splenic destruction seems likely, the patient's own cells should be used. In patients who become a problem because they seem to be destroying transfused cells at an increasing rate, fresh cells from a normal donor should be used.

The number of publications which disagree over details of precise technique for splenic surface counting attest to some of the technical problems inherent in the technique. It is beyond the scope of this chapter to discuss such details; nevertheless certain generalizations are justified. First of all, the key problem relates to geometry, i.e., location and size of the spleen and liver and placement of the counter probe. The technique recommended by Hughes-Jones and Szur attempts to take into account initial differences between liver and spleen and compare subsequent counts with the precordium as a control, thereby arriving at an estimate of excess spleen counts. This technique emphasizes the importance of an increasing splenic count reaching a critical value in relation to the liver at the half-time (T$\frac{1}{2}$) for red cell survival. Likewise, a rising spleen to liver ratio at the T$\frac{1}{2}$ is evidence of significant splenic sequestration. If splenic accumulation is demonstrated, the studies provide support for a decision to undertake splenectomy.

Even though no evidence of splenic sequestration is found, however, splenectomy may still be beneficial at times. An example is the situation in which plasma volume is expanded and splenic red cell pools occur, as in certain cases of cirrhosis with portal hypertension or Gaucher's disease. Patients with "idiopathic hypersplenism" may benefit from splenectomy without evidence of organ sequestration, and in pyruvate kinase deficiency splenectomy may be beneficial even though excess hepatic uptake is suggested. Excess hepatic uptake appears to be explained either by splenic damage to the cells which are then destroyed in the liver, or by the red cells actually lysing within the splenic circulation although the labeled hemoglobin passes on to the liver. Thus splenic sequestration studies must be considered as one part of the evaluation of the patient but not the absolute criterion for splenectomy.

COMPLICATIONS OF SPLENECTOMY

Apart from moderate postoperative complications, most patients with normal bone marrows develop thrombocytosis which may reach levels of 500,000 to 1 million platelets per cubic millimeter 3 weeks postoperatively and leukocyte counts up to 30,000 per cubic millimeter. Neither of these necessarily poses any threat, although if steroid therapy is being administered, the platelets occasionally reach levels that may present cause for concern. Red cell changes include the appearance of Howell-Jolly bodies (nuclear remnants), occasional nucleated red cells, siderocytes, and target cells. These morphologic changes may be useful in evaluating patients who have a relapse in the severity of their hemolysis within a year after splenectomy. Disappearance of Howell-Jolly bodies and other postsplenectomy changes from the blood of such patients suggests the presence of an accessory spleen which should be removed. Postsplenectomy infectious complications are no more of a problem in adults with hemolytic anemia than the incidence of infection in nonsplenectomized adults with the same disorder.

REFERENCES

Bowdler, A. J., and Prankerd, T. A. J.   Splenic mechanisms in the pathogenesis of anaemia. *Postgrad. Med. J.* 41:748, 1965.

Burton, A. C.   Role of geometry, or size and shape, in the microcirculation. *Fed. Proc.* 25:1753, 1966.

Dacie, J. V.   The haemolytic anaemias: A brief review of recent advances. *Seminars Hemat.* 6:109, 1969.

Hughes-Jones, N. C., and Szur, L.   Determination of the sites of red cell destruction using Cr[51]-labelled cells. *Brit. J. Haemat.* 3:320, 1957.

Jaffé, E. R.   Clinical profile: Hereditary hemolytic disorders and enzymatic deficiencies of human erythrocytes. *Blood* 35:116, 1970.

Jandl, H. J., Simmons, R. L., and Castle, W. B.   Red cell filtration in the pathogenesis of certain hemolytic anemias. *Blood* 28:133, 1961.

LaCelle, P. L.   Alteration of erythrocyte membrane deformability in stored blood. *Transfusion* 9:238, 1969.

LaCelle, P. L.   Alteration of membrane deformability in hemolytic anemias. *Seminars Hemat.* 7:355, 1970.

Ponder, E. *Hemolysis and Related Phenomena.* New York: Grune & Stratton, 1948.

Weed, R. I. Disorders of red cell membrane: History and perspectives. *Seminars Hemat.* 7:249, 1970.

Weed, R. I. The importance of erythrocyte deformability. *Amer. J. Med.* 49:147, 1970.

Weed, R. I., and Bowdler, A. J. Metabolic dependence of the critical hemolytic volume of human erythrocytes: Relationship to osmotic fragility and autohemolysis in hereditary spherocytosis and normal red cells. *J. Clin. Invest.* 46:1137, 1966.

Weed, R. I., LaCelle, P. L., and Merrill, E. W. Metabolic dependence of red cell membrane deformability. *J. Clin. Invest.* 48:795, 1969.

Weed, R. I., and Reed, C. F. Membrane alterations leading to red cell destruction. *Amer. J. Med.* 41:681, 1966.

Weiss, L. The structure of fine splenic arterial vessels in relation to hemoconcentration and red cell destruction. *Amer. J. Anat.* 111:131, 1962.

Weiss, L. The structure of bone marrow: Functional interrelationships of vascular and hematopoietic compartments in experimental hemolytic anemia: An electron microscopic study. *J. Morph.* 117:367, 1965.

5. THE LABORATORY EVALUATION OF HEMOLYSIS

Denis R. Miller

DURING THE PAST DECADE we have witnessed, among other events, a vast proliferation of knowledge concerning the hemolytic anemias. Accordingly, the clinician must possess a firm understanding of the many possible etiologies of hemolysis. Despite the complexity of erythrocyte structure and function, the laboratory is able to provide many relatively simple aids to the diagnosis of hemolytic anemia. A systematic approach utilizing general tests that indicate hemolysis should be performed during the initial evaluation of the patient. These include standard measurements of erythrocyte indices, reticulocyte count, bilirubin, and haptoglobin; serologic tests for antibodies; and an examination of the bone marrow. Of invaluable importance is a critical examination of the peripheral blood for erythrocyte morphology, which can provide many of the clues for further studies.

A complete evaluation of the hereditary hemolytic anemias requires a systematic evaluation of the erythrocyte membrane, the hemoglobin molecule, and the intracellular enzymes and intermediates of cell metabolism. The determinations of osmotic fragility, autohemolysis, hemoglobin electrophoresis, and assays of enzymes and glycolytic intermediates provide most of these answers. Erythrocyte survival and organ sequestration studies are of great practical importance when splenectomy is being considered. Screening tests for enzymopathies and hemoglobinopathies should be utilized whenever possible because of their accuracy and simplicity in providing direction for further and more complicated studies.

A systematic approach to the clinical differentiation and laboratory eval-

This work was supported in part by U.S. Public Health Service Grants AM-13947 and CA-11174, and the Clinical Research Center, Division of Research Facilities and Resources (RR-44).

63

uation of hemolysis requires an appreciation of the varied etiologies of accelerated erythrocyte destruction. Hemolysis may be congenital or acquired and may be associated with intracorpuscular and extracorpuscular defects or may be caused by the interaction of intracorpuscular and extracorpuscular factors. An abbreviated classification of these defects is listed in Table 5-1. Any of the three main components of the erythrocyte—the membrane, the hemoglobin molecule, or the intracellular enzymes and substrates involved in the metabolic activities of the cell—may function abnormally with resultant premature cell death. Extracorpuscular abnormalities may have an immunohemolytic basis or may be associated with nonimmune mechanisms such as infectious agents, drugs, burns, splenomegaly, mechanical hemolysis with prosthetic heart valves, and microangiopathic states such as thrombotic thrombocytopenic purpura or the hemolytic uremic syndrome.

Intracorpuscular and extracorpuscular factors may conspire to produce hemolysis in paroxysmal nocturnal hemoglobinuria, favism, and lead poisoning. Other anemias, not primarily hemolytic in nature, are associated with ineffective erythropoiesis and shortened erythrocyte survival. These include vitamin B_{12} and folate deficiencies, aplastic anemia, leukemia, and iron deficiency anemia.

Table 5-1. A Simplified Classification of Hemolysis

Intracorpuscular defects
  Abnormalities of membrane (hereditary spherocytosis, hereditary elliptocytosis, stomatocytosis, phospholipid defects)
  Abnormalities of hemoglobin (hemoglobinopathies, thalassemia syndromes, unstable hemoglobin hemolytic anemias, erythropoietic porphyria)
  Abnormalities of enzymes (pentose phosphate shunt, Embden-Meyerhof pathway, and nonglycolytic enzyme and substrate defects)

Extracorpuscular defects
  Immunohemolytic anemias (transfusion reactions, autoimmune hemolytic anemia, paroxysmal cold hemoglobinuria, drug-induced immunohemolytic anemia, hemolytic disease of the newborn)
  Nonimmune mechanisms (infectious agents, burns, drugs, associated with splenomegaly, mechanical, microangiopathic)

Interaction of intracorpuscular and extracorpuscular factors
  Paroxysmal nocturnal hemoglobinuria and complement
  G6PD deficiency and favism
  Heme synthesis and lead poisoning
  Ineffective erythropoiesis and vitamin B_{12} deficiency
  Acanthocytosis and a-β-lipoproteinemia

GENERAL LABORATORY AIDS TO DIAGNOSIS OF HEMOLYSIS

A simplified, schematic approach to the patient with hemolytic anemia is presented in Figure 5-1. Relatively simple studies, available in most clinical laboratories, provide general evidence for hemolysis. Although anemia is usually present, some patients with well-compensated hemolytic disease may have normal values for packed cell volume, hemoglobin, and red blood cell counts. Reticulocytosis with or without normoblastemia is invariably found. A calculation of the absolute number of reticulocytes provides an accurate measurement of the severity of the hemolytic process and the degree of compensation.

Erythrocyte morphology is an invaluable aid to the diagnosis of hemolysis, and the need for careful scrutiny of a Romanowsky-stained peripheral

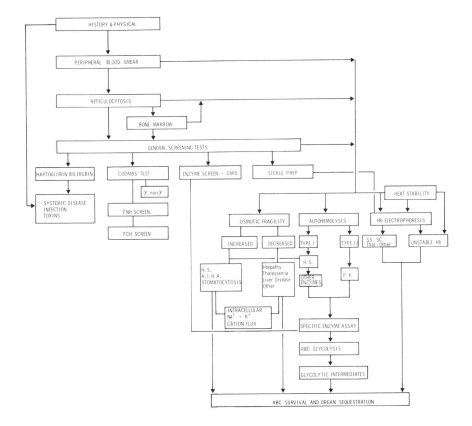

Figure 5-1. A simplified approach to the evaluation of hemolytic anemia.

blood slide cannot be stressed enough. Readily apparent abnormalities will be observed, such as spherocytes (hereditary spherocytosis, autoimmune hemolytic anemia, burns, or chemicals), elliptocytes, stomatocytes, acanthocytes (a-β-lipoproteinemia), schistocytes or fragmented erythrocytes (microangiopathic hemolytic anemia), spiculated spherocytes (erythrocyte enzyme deficiencies associated with defective energy metabolism), and poikilocytosis, basophilic stippling, hypochromia, and microcytosis (thalassemia). Some of these are illustrated in Figure 5-2.

In well-compensated hemolytic anemias the examination of the bone marrow reflects the peripheral reticulocytosis and polychromatophilia. The characteristic finding is usually one of marked normoblastic (and occasionally macronormoblastic) erythroid hyperplasia and a decrease or occasionally an inversion of the normal myeloid–erythroid ratio of 3 to 1. In the presence of folic acid deficiency complicating the hemolytic anemia, the erythroid precursors may be megaloblastic. Deficiencies of folate, iron, or vitamin B_{12} suppress erythropoiesis. An iron stain of marrow spicules is of immense help in evaluating iron stores.

Increased erythrocyte destruction is associated with increased metabolism and excretion of products of hemoglobin breakdown. These abnormal findings include hyperbilirubinemia (indirect fraction) and increased fecal urobilinogen levels. Determinations of fecal urobilinogen are rarely performed because of the difficulties associated with stool collections, the reported discrepancies between the degree of hemolysis and the measured fecal urobilinogen, and the availability of more accurate radioisotope procedures. Measurement of endogenous carbon monoxide production, which is increased in patients with hemolytic anemia, permits the detection of hemolysis but is reserved for the research laboratory.

With acute intravascular hemolysis, such as that occurring after the ingestion of certain oxidant drugs (phenylhydrazine) or with glucose-6-phosphate dehydrogenase (G6PD) deficiency, *methemalbumin* is found in the plasma. This hematin-albumin compound can be detected by the Schumm's test in which a hemochromogen is formed upon the addition of concentrated ammonium sulfide to plasma.

The measurement of *haptoglobin,* an alpha$_2$ globulin produced by the liver, is extremely useful. Each mole of this protein binds 1 or 2 moles of hemoglobin released into the circulation during hemolysis. The haptoglobin-hemoglobin complex is removed from the circulation by the reticuloendothelial system, and the levels of free haptoglobin may be markedly diminished or even absent. Haptoglobin can bind about 50 to 140 mg of hemoglobin per 100 ml of plasma. When the plasma hemoglobin levels saturate the haptoglobin-binding capacity of the plasma, or if haptoglobin production is compromised by liver disease, hemoglobinemia and hemoglobinuria

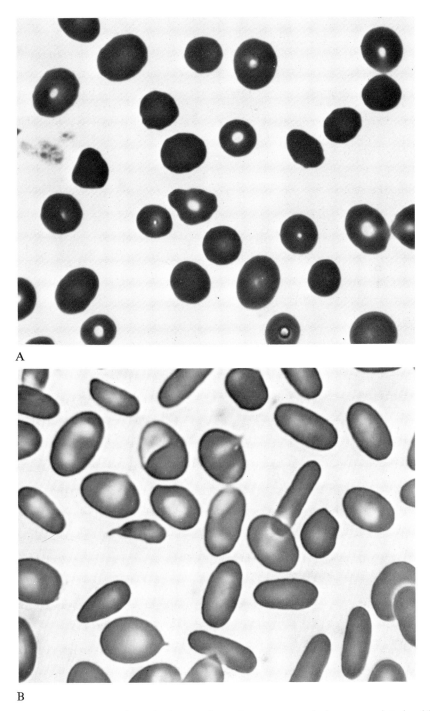

Figure 5-2. Examples of abnormal erythrocyte morphology associated with hemolytic anemia: (A) Hereditary spherocytosis; (B) Hereditary elliptocytosis.

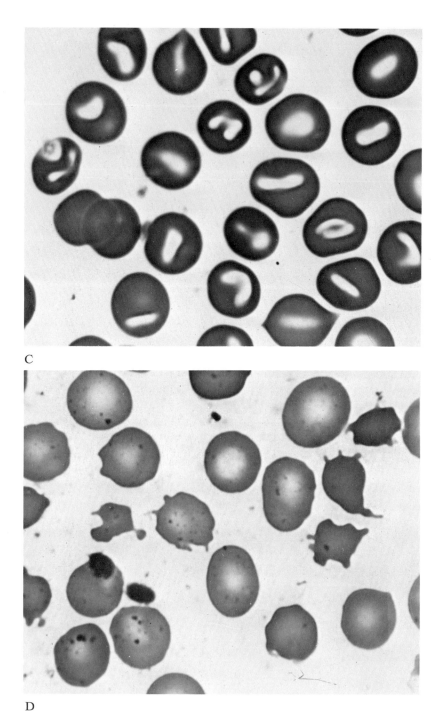

C

D

Figure 5-2 (Continued). (C) Hereditary stomatocytosis; (D) Acanthocytosis in a-β-lipoproteinemia.

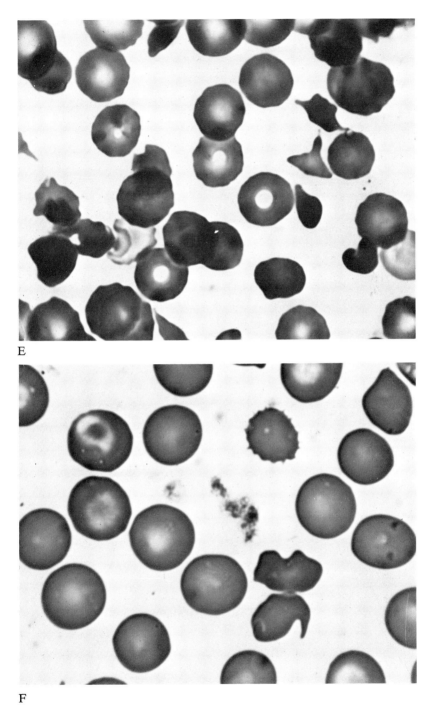

E

F

(E) Hemolytic uremic syndrome; (F) Pyruvate kinase deficiency.

may be detected. Since haptoglobin is an acute phase reactant, levels may increase in response to inflammatory diseases such as rheumatoid arthritis and systemic lupus erythematosus. In these states, associated with minor degrees of hemolysis, the haptoglobin concentration may be normal.

Hemopexin, the heme-binding beta globulin (glycoprotein) of human serum, is decreased or absent in patients with severe hemolytic disease. As with haptoglobin, it appears that the hemopexin-heme complex is eliminated by the reticuloendothelial system.

In patients with chronic hemolysis, such as in paroxysmal nocturnal hemoglobinuria (PNH) or in the thalassemia syndromes, *hemosiderin* may be detected by staining the urinary sediment with potassium ferrocyanide. The ferric iron derived from hemoglobin deposited within the renal tubule cells stains bluish-brown in this test and may be helpful in estimating the chronicity of hemolysis in patients with an apparent acute hemolytic process. This is particularly true in PNH or in patients with prosthetic heart valves associated with hemolysis. To summarize these events, hemolysis results in the liberation of hemoglobin from the erythrocyte into the plasma. Acute intravascular hemolysis is associated with the appearance of methemalbumin. If hemolysis persists, plasma hemoglobin (greater than 5 mg per 100 ml) complexes with haptoglobin and is removed from the circulation by the reticuloendothelial system. If the haptoglobin-binding capacity is saturated, hemoglobin appears in the urine, and if hemolysis is chronic, hemosiderin may be found in the urinary sediment.

Serologic tests for the presence or absence of abnormal antibodies on the erythrocyte surface or in the serum should be performed. A potent antiglobulin (Coombs') serum should be used. Both gamma-Coombs' and non-gamma-Coombs' sera should be tested since the presence of nongamma globulins such as complement or transferrin on the surface of the erythrocyte may result in a positive antiglobulin reaction not related directly to the immune hemolytic anemia. The subject of autoimmune hemolytic anemia is reviewed in detail in Chapter 9.

Since the clinical signs and symptoms of PNH may not resemble the classic description of this disease, screening tests for PNH should be performed in any patient presenting with atypical hemolytic anemia, pancytopenia, or aplastic anemia. These include the well-known acid hemolysis (Ham) test. Whereas PNH erythrocytes are hemolyzed in acidified serum (pH 6.5 to 7.0) at 37°C, normal cells are resistant to hemolysis in this pH range. The simple but accurate sugar water test of Jenkins and Hartmann is detailed in the text of Dacie and Lewis. The Donath-Landsteiner test for cold hemolysis and measurements of the cold agglutinin titer should be included in these serologic studies. It is often necessary to employ a wide range of temperatures and pH and to test erythrocytes in various suspending media (saline, albumin, or after enzyme treatment) in order to detect the presence of antibodies. The reader is referred to more detailed texts for a complete discussion of the acquired hemolytic anemias (Dacie, Part II).

Once the laboratory diagnosis of hemolysis is established with the general studies outlined here, more specific investigations should be performed.

SPECIAL INVESTIGATIONS FOR INTRACORPUSCULAR DEFECTS

OSMOTIC FRAGILITY

The osmotic fragility test has been useful for over 30 years in detecting hereditary spherocytosis. The patterns observed in other representative congenital and acquired hemolytic anemias are listed in Table 5-2.

Other states associated with increased osmotic fragility include hemolytic disease of the newborn and stomatocytosis after exposure to certain toxic chemicals or in burned patients. Decreased osmotic fragility may be seen in patients with liver disease, sickle cell anemia, and other hemoglobinopathies, and with thalassemia and iron deficiency anemia. Osmotic fragility should be measured with fresh blood and after sterile incubation at 37°C for 24 hours, since abnormalities may not be detected in fresh cells. With incubation and the resultant deprivation of glucose, the substrate required for the maintenance of metabolic activities, energy production, and membrane integrity, a defective population of cells may be noted. A small population of cells with increased fragility may be seen in pyruvate kinase deficiency hereditary hemolytic anemia, or in asymptomatic patients with hereditary spherocytosis. Markedly decreased fragility of the entire cell

Table 5-2. Osmotic Fragility Patterns in Hemolytic Anemia

Diagnosis	Osmotic Fragility	
	Fresh	Incubated
Hereditary spherocytosis	Increased	Markedly increased
Autoimmune hemolytic anemia	Increased	Markedly increased
Pyruvate kinase deficiency	Normal	Small "tail" increased
Thalassemia major	Slightly decreased	Decreased
Unstable hemoglobinopathy	Normal or slightly decreased	Markedly decreased

population is observed in hemoglobin Köln, an unstable hemoglobin hemolytic anemia.

AUTOHEMOLYSIS

The osmotic fragility test is usually performed with sterile defibrinated blood. Blood prepared this way may be used for measurements of autohemolysis, a useful but nonspecific screening test for intracorpuscular defects. The test should be performed on all patients in whom an intrinsic defect is suspected, since the results obtained will provide information for further specific studies. When defibrinated blood is incubated under aseptic conditions for 48 hours at 37°C, with or without nutrient additives (saline, glucose, adenosine, inosine, or ATP at pH 6.8), the degree and correction of hemolysis follow patterns which aid in differentiating some of the hemolytic anemias. With normal blood, autohemolysis in saline is less than 3.5%; with additives, hemolysis is usually less than 1.0%.

Dacie found that whereas the addition of glucose corrected the increased autohemolysis in some patients with nonspherocytic hemolytic anemia (Type I), glucose had no effect or even increased the autohemolysis in other patients, in whom neutralized ATP corrected the autohemolysis (Type II pattern). Subsequently these patients were found to have erythrocyte pyruvate kinase (PK) deficiency. If the test is performed meticulously and with normal controls, much useful information may be obtained, the most important of which is the identification of patients with erythrocyte PK deficiency, since the Type II pattern with ATP correction is characteristic of this entity. This is significant since after G6PD deficiency hemolytic anemia, PK deficiency is the next most common enzymopathy.

Autohemolysis patterns in various hemolytic disorders are presented in Table 5-3. Deficiencies of pentose phosphate shunt enzymes, unstable hemoglobin hemolytic anemias, and deficiencies of most Embden-Meyerhof pathway enzymes, excluding PK, are associated with Dacie Type I autohemolysis patterns. Except for certain severe autoimmune states associated with spherocytosis, ATP *and* glucose decrease the autohemolysis in all anemias except PK deficiency. The general screening tests, osmotic fragility curves, and autohemolysis patterns provide or exclude diagnoses of immune hemolysis and hereditary spherocytosis. If the etiology of the hemolytic anemia remains unresolved, erythrocyte metabolism may be examined next.

ERYTHROCYTE GLYCOLYSIS

The anaerobic (Embden-Meyerhof or EM) and aerobic (hexose monophosphate or HMP) pathways of erythrocyte metabolism are illustrated in

Table 5-3.   Autohemolysis in Various Hemolytic Disorders

Diagnosis	Degree of Hemolysis			Dacie Pattern
	Saline	Glucose	ATP[a]	
Normal RBC	3.5%	1.0%	1.0%	—
Autoimmune hemolytic anemia (with sphero-cytosis)	↑	Variable	Marked ↓	II
Hereditary spherocytosis	↑	Marked ↓	Marked ↓	I
G6PD deficiency	Normal or slight ↑	Slight to Moderate ↓	Slight to Moderate ↓	I
Pyruvate kinase deficiency	Moderate ↑	Moderate ↑	Marked ↓	II
Unstable hemoglobin	Slight ↑	Normal	Normal	I
Hexokinase deficiency[b]	Slight ↑	Normal	Normal	I

↑ = increase; ↓ = decrease.
[a] pH = 6.8.
[b] And deficiencies of phosphoglucose isomerase, triose phosphate isomerase, and phosphoglycerokinase.

Figure 5-3. Over 90% of glycolysis in the mature erythrocyte proceeds through the anaerobic pathway in which, ideally, 2 moles of lactate and a net of 2 moles of ATP are produced for each mole of glucose utilized. To date, deficiencies of hexokinase, glucosephosphate isomerase, phosphofructokinase, triose phosphate isomerase, glyceraldehyde phosphate dehydrogenase (GPD), phosphoglycerate kinase (PGK), and PK have been defined in the EM pathway.

Recently a branch of the EM pathway, the 2,3-diphosphoglycerate (2,3-DPG) or Rapoport-Luebering shunt has been identified. The main product of the shunt, 2,3-DPG serves as a regulator of hemoglobin-oxygen dissociation and a modulator of erythrocyte glycolysis. These are considered in detail in Chapter 10. The ATP generated at the PGK and PK steps is utilized to maintain membrane integrity and to serve as a substrate for cation pumping and as a cofactor for other glycolytic enzymes (hexokinase, phosphofructokinase) and nonglycolytic enzymes (glutathione synthetase). The NADH (DPNH)* generated at the GPD step serves as a cofactor for NADH-dependent methemoglobin reductase, the primary enzyme responsible for reducing methemoglobin.

Although the HMP shunt accounts for less than 10% of erythrocyte glycolysis under physiologic conditions, it protects the cell's proteins (hemoglobin, enzymes, and membrane) against oxidative denaturation by gen-

* Diphosphopyridine nucleotide, reduced form.

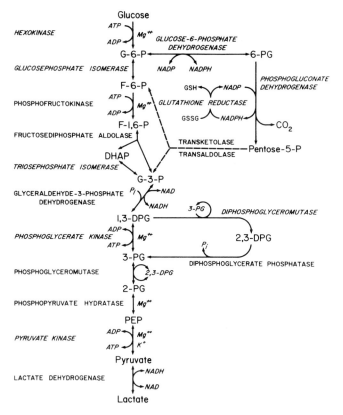

Figure 5-3. The anaerobic (Embden-Meyerhof) and aerobic (hexose monophosphate) pathways of erythrocyte glycolysis. Known enzyme deficiencies associated with hemolytic anemia are indicated by italics. (From W. N. Valentine, *Calif. Med.* 108:280, 1968.)

erating NADPH (TPNH)* and maintaining glutathione in the reduced form (GSH). Carbon dioxide is generated through HMP activity which can be stimulated with appropriate oxidative stresses such as the exposure to oxidant drugs. Deficiency of the first enzyme of the HMP pathway, G6PD, is the most common metabolic abnormality of man. Other deficiencies, including 6-phosphogluconic dehydrogenase, GSH reductase, GSH peroxidase, and GSH synthetase (congenital GSH deficiency) have been described but are extremely uncommon.

EVALUATION OF HEXOSE MONOPHOSPHATE SHUNT ACTIVITY

A number of simple, reliable, and inexpensive screening tests for G6PD

* Triphosphopyridine nucleotide, reduced form.

deficiency are available. The principle of most of the tests is dependent upon the failure of the G6PD-deficient erythrocyte to generate NADPH. Normally the NADPH generated would (1) reduce dyes such as brilliant cresyl blue (to a colorless state) or tetrazolium (to a purple formazan), (2) reduce methemoglobin, or (3) produce fluorescence. In our laboratory the methemoglobin reduction test is an accurate method for identifying deficient males and females. Although carrier heterozygotes could be identified also, there is no method that is entirely flawless for this group. One useful method is a histochemical test based on the inability of the G6PD-deficient cell to reduce nitrite-induced methemoglobin. Slides are prepared and methemoglobin-containing (G6PD-deficient) cells appear as empty "ghosts" when counterstained with erythrosin. The typical appearance of normal and G6PD-deficient cells is seen in Figure 5-4. An equal distribution of stained cells and ghosts would be seen in a G6PD heterozygote.

The spectrophotometric assay of G6PD and other glycolytic enzymes requires carefully prepared, leukocyte-free hemolysates and an accurate instrument. The principle of the assay is based on the linked reduction or oxidation of pyridine nucleotides and the resultant increase or decrease in absorbency, respectively. To avoid spurious results, carefully controlled assay conditions are required—pH, substrate and cofactor concentrations, and temperature.

The G6PD activity in the erythrocytes of a patient who has recently had an acute hemolytic episode and has a reticulocytosis may be in the low-normal or heterozygote range rather than in the deficient range (10 to 15% of normal activity). However, since G6PD activity reflects cell age and since the activity is markedly increased in reticulocytes, presumptive evidence for G6PD deficiency may be gained if the enzyme activity is not commensurate with the youth of the cell population. The simultaneous assay of G6PD activity in a control patient with a reticulocytosis often helps to circumvent this dilemma. G6PD activity decreases with cell age. Thus the quantitative assay of enzyme activity in young and old cells may also assist in detecting G6PD deficiency in the patient with a reticulocytosis. Since younger cells are lighter and older (deficient) cells are heavier, the centrifugation of cells at high speed permits separation of the cells. The G6PD activity of old (bottom layer) erythrocytes in the G6PD-deficient patient is significantly lower than that in a normal control.

If large numbers of patients are examined, a reliable screening test is as useful—as accurate and far less time-consuming and expensive—as the quantitative assay performed when the results of the screening test are equivocal. The screening test should be the method of choice to detect G6PD deficiency. In our experience false-positive results with the methemoglobin reduction test have been encountered in patients with unstable hemoglobin hemolytic anemia (hemoglobin Köln). Thus the test may be useful to screen for two entities. The ascorbate test of Jacob and Jandl,

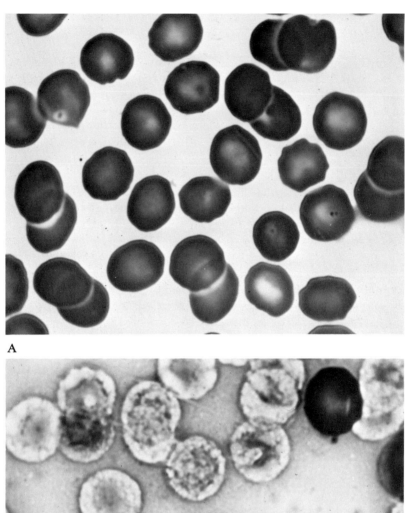

A

B

Figure 5-4. A histochemical method for the identification of G6PD deficiency. (A) Normal erythrocytes are stained with erythrosin. (B) G6PD-deficient cells appear as ghosts after elution of methemoglobin.

originally designed to detect G6PD deficiency, is not specific and may be abnormal in other types of hemolytic anemia due to metabolic deficiencies. These include GSH peroxidase deficiency, GSH reductase deficiency, pyruvate kinase deficiency, and certain unstable hemoglobinopathies (Köln).

As of 1970 approximately 50 genetic variants of G6PD deficiency associated with severe, moderate, mild, or no hemolytic anemia have been described. By standard assay techniques, G6PD activity ranged from less than 1% to 100% of normal. Special biochemical techniques are required for their characterization, including studies of electrophoretic mobility, thermostability, enzyme kinetics with determinations of Michaelis constants (Km), pH optima, serologic characteristics, and substrate utilization.

GSH deficiency and instability were the first metabolic abnormalities described in primaquine sensitivity before the exact biochemical defect was discovered by Carson et al. in 1956. Relatively simple methods are available for detecting GSH, and although decreased and unstable GSH is not specific for G6PD deficiency, the test is useful. Decreased GSH concentrations may be associated with congenital deficiency of GSH (glutathione synthetase deficiency), severe liver disease, unstable hemoglobinopathies, uremia, and the ingestion of oxidant drugs.

The presence of Heinz bodies (precipitated, denatured hemoglobin) may be detected in the peripheral blood during an acute hemolytic crisis in a patient with G6PD deficiency or in a normal individual after phenylhydrazine ingestion. Phase microscopy or supravital staining (with cresyl violet or methylene blue) must be used to identify the Heinz bodies, which usually appear as large single or small multiple coccoid bodies in the cell periphery. They are also seen in the erythrocytes of splenectomized patients with the unstable hemoglobin syndromes, many premature infants who have decreased GSH peroxidase activity, normal newborn infants, and patients with asplenia.

Congenital hemolytic anemias associated with GSH reductase and GSH peroxidase deficiencies have been described. Specific quantitative enzyme assays are required for their detection, although a fluorescent screening test for GSH reductase has been devised.

Overall HMP shunt activity can be evaluated by measuring $^{14}CO_2$ evolution from glucose-^{14}C. Although this must be considered a research laboratory procedure, it provides important information about the functional capabilities of the HMP shunt, especially when shunt activity is stimulated by methylene blue or ascorbate. The use of glucose-carbon labeled in several positions provides information about total HMP shunt activity ($^{14}C_1$), recycling activity ($^{14}C_2$), and Krebs cycle or mitochondrial activity ($^{14}C_6$). Normal erythrocytes show increased HMP shunt activity and $^{14}CO_2$ evolution with oxidative stress.

Normal erythrocytes and reticulocytes in autoimmune hemolytic anemia, hereditary spherocytosis, and PK deficiency have increased HMP shunt activity. However, in HMP shunt enzyme deficiencies, decreased $^{14}CO_2$ production is observed under physiologic conditions and with shunt stimulation. Representative values in these hemolytic anemias are presented in Table 5-4.

EVALUATION OF THE EMBDEN-MEYERHOF (ANAEROBIC) PATHWAY

Just as $^{14}CO_2$ evolution from glucose-^{14}C permits an evaluation of HMP shunt activity, measurements of glucose utilization and lactate production provide important information concerning overall erythrocyte glycolysis. Since a reticulocytosis of 10 to 20% may double the rate of glycolysis, defective glycolytic activity may be suspected when glycolysis is not commensurate with the degree of reticulocytosis associated with the hemolytic anemia. Glucose utilization and lactate production can be measured enzymatically, but the incubation conditions must be rigidly controlled with regard to temperature, pH, and inorganic phosphate concentration, since the glycolytic rate increases with elevations of all three.

Measurements of glycolytic intermediates and of adenine nucleotides are now possible with either enzymatic methods linked to the reduction of pyridine nucleotides or, less accurately, with column chromatography. Increased concentrations of glycolytic intermediates help to localize the defective glycolytic enzyme. Determinations of 2,3-DPG and ATP are the most important. Of the glycolytic intermediates within the erythrocyte, 2,3-DPG is present in the greatest concentration. Blockade below the Rapoport-Luebering cycle, as in PK deficiency, results in markedly increased levels of 2,3-DPG that cannot be explained by reticulocytosis alone. Conversely, the 2,3-DPG levels in hexokinase deficiency and 2,3-DPG mutase deficiency are lower than normal.

Since the main product of glycolysis is energy in the form of ATP, measurements of ATP concentration and stability permit an evaluation of erythrocyte energy metabolism. In PK deficiency, ATP concentration is low relative to the reticulocyte count and the concentration may diminish by 30 to 40% after short-term (4-hour) incubation periods. This reflects the blockade at the PK step, at which a diminished quantity of ADP is converted to ATP. These parameters of erythrocyte metabolism in several types of hemolytic anemia are recorded in Table 5-4.

Pyruvate kinase deficiency hemolytic anemia is the most common enzyme deficiency of the EM pathway. However, compared to the estimated 100,-000,000 human beings with G6PD deficiency, approximately 100 cases of PK deficiency have been reported. Only isolated single cases or families with the other EM enzyme deficiencies have been described. Most large

Table 5-4. *Erythrocyte Metabolism in Hemolytic Anemias*

Condition	Reticulocytes	Glucose Utilization (μM/ml RBC/hr)	Lactate Production (μM/ml RBC/hr)	ATP (μM/ml RBC)	2,3-DPG (μM/ml RBC)	CO_2 Evolution ($^{14}C_1$) [a] (μM/ml RBC/hr)	
						No M.B.[b]	M.B.
Normal	0.5–1.5	2.13 ± 0.09	4.19 ± 0.17	1.70 ± 0.06	4.2 ± 0.18	0.044–0.062	1.12–1.62
Acquired hemolytic anemia	33	4.50	7.35	1.95	6.0	Increased	
Hereditary spherocytosis	15.0	3.34	6.90	2.20	5.2	Increased	
G6PD deficiency	10	3.72	4.28	Normal (unstable)	Increased	Decreased	
PK deficiency	17.8	2.61	4.87	1.99 (unstable)	8.4	Increased	
Hb Köln	8.0	3.45	7.65	0.905	5.2	Increased	

[a] Data from Yunis and Yasmineh, 1969, pp. 34–35.
[b] M.B. = methylene blue.

university centers and community hospitals are capable of detecting G6PD deficiency. It is unlikely that the same hospitals have the ability to assay the 19 enzymes involved in glycolysis, the 15 glycolytic intermediates, and the various cofactors and nucleotides. It is doubtful that such a capability is practical or advisable. A more rational approach in evaluating the patient with a defect in glycolysis would be to exclude the common defects and transport a sample of the patient's blood and that of a suitable control to a specialized hematology research laboratory which is actively engaged in studies of erythrocyte metabolism. Several such centers are in existence across the country and are listed in the appendix to this chapter.

As with G6PD deficiency, a heterogeneity is developing within the PK deficiency hemolytic anemias. A number of mutants, each with different maximal activity, Michaelis constants, and pH optima have been described. A similar heterogeneity can be expected in the other enzyme deficiencies already described and in those not yet discovered.

EVALUATION OF HEMOGLOBINOPATHIES

A full presentation of the hemoglobinopathies is given in Chapter 7. The abnormal erythrocyte morphology, decreased osmotic fragility, and normal autohemolysis patterns are useful diagnostic clues to the hemoglobinopathies. The sickle cell preparation and hemoglobin electrophoresis should be performed. Although paper electrophoresis is useful for the detection of many common hemoglobinopathies (SS, SC, CC disease), other methods provide better separation of the minor hemoglobin components (A_2 and fetal hemoglobin) and are necessary to diagnose the thalassemia syndromes. These include starch-gel, starch block, cellulose acetate, and agarose-gel electrophoresis. The first two are more laborious procedures but provide excellent separation of A_2 and F.

Fetal hemoglobin may be determined quantitatively by the alkali denaturation method or qualitatively by a relatively simple histochemical test based on the insolubility of hemoglobin F at an acid pH. Raised levels of Hb F are seen in thalassemia (up to 90 to 95%), hereditary persistence of Hb F, and sickle cell disease and the other hemoglobinopathies. Slightly elevated levels (3 to 8%) have been recorded in other hemolytic anemias, including enzyme deficiency states, PNH, aplastic anemia, leukemia, and hereditary spherocytosis.

Another relatively simple but useful screening procedure for α-thalassemia syndromes is performed by incubating erythrocytes in a 0.2% solution of brilliant cresyl blue for 30 minutes at 37°C. Precipitated Hb H, a tetramer of β-chains, appears as small inclusions throughout the cell.

The unstable hemoglobin hemolytic anemias can be detected in the laboratory by demonstrating the presence of a heat-labile hemoglobin fraction which precipitates on incubation of a hemolysate at 50°C. These abnormal hemoglobins account for 10 to 20% of the total hemoglobin. The altered electrophoretic migration (best demonstrated on starch gel at pH 8.6) is not caused by a net change in the charge of the molecule but by spontaneous denaturation of the unstable hemoglobin. This instability is caused by an amino acid substitution altering and affecting the heme-binding site (Hb Köln: β^{98}Val → Met), the overall globin conformation (Hb Gun Hill: β^{91-97} deleted), or the site of subunit (α- and β-chain) interaction (Hb Philly: β^{35}Tyr → Phe). These substitutions produce an unstable, denaturable molecule. The heat lability results from heme-globin dissociation and eventual precipitation of the unstable globin moiety. Often slowly migrating free α-chains are seen in Hb Köln. The other laboratory features of Hb Köln, the most common of these rare but important diseases, include increased glycolytic and HMP shunt activities; slightly decreased GSH; slightly elevated methemoglobin, which increases with incubation; dipyrroluria, a urinary pigment produced by the breakdown of heme; decreased osmotic fragility, and the presence of Heinz bodies in the postsplenectomy state.

Chromatography and peptide fingerprinting are required for the complete characterization of the amino acid substitution responsible for the hemoglobinopathies, including the unstable hemoglobins. With radioisotope techniques, globin chain production rates can be measured in the thalassemia syndromes. Again, these are research laboratory techniques, but fetal hemoglobin staining, hemoglobin electrophoresis in a suitable medium, the heat-denaturation test, the Heinz body preparation, and brilliant cresyl blue tests should provide the diagnosis for all but a rare hemoglobinopathy.

ABNORMALITIES OF THE MEMBRANE

Abnormalities of the erythrocyte membrane associated with abnormal ion transport may occur in many hemolytic anemias. Determinations of intracellular cation content and measurements of cation flux using isotopes of Na^+ and K^+ may demonstrate these defects of membrane function. Increased permeability to sodium has been described in hereditary spherocytosis and abnormal increased "leakiness" (efflux) of potassium has been documented in PK-deficient erythrocytes and in Hb Köln. A number of other hemolytic anemias are associated with abnormalities of cation transport. A recent syndrome of stomatocytosis associated with increased intracellular Na^+, decreased intracellular K^+, and markedly increased sodium pumping has been described also. Often these changes in cation content reflect the abnormalities of osmotic fragility and the ability of the cell to maintain ATP levels. For example, hereditary stomatocytosis is associated with increased osmotic fragility and markedly increased intracellular sodium content.

The deformability and filterability of erythrocytes may be altered by increased membrane rigidity, as in spherocytosis, or by the intracellular formation of Heinz bodies, as in G6PD deficiency or Hb Köln.

Abnormalities of the erythrocyte lipids often reflect abnormalities of the plasma lipids. This is true in a-β-lipoproteinemia and in obstructive liver disease.

The total lipid content of young erythrocytes and reticulocytes is increased but the relative proportions of the phospholipids are not influenced by cell age. Thus changes in phospholipids in hemolytic anemia probably represent the increased physiologic lipid levels in the reticulocyte per se and not a primary defect. A nonspherocytic hemolytic anemia associated with increased total lipid and increased lecithin (phosphatidylcholine) has been described. Specific alterations of erythrocyte lipids related to hemolysis have not yet been described, although the increased peroxidation of membrane lipids by hydrogen peroxide in liver disease, in a-β-lipoproteinemia, and in premature infants with hemolytic anemia has been attributed to vitamin E (tocopherol) deficiency. Other factors (e.g., GSH peroxidase deficiency) may be involved, however.

Energy required for cation pumping is provided by the hydrolysis of ATP through a Mg^{++}-K^{+}-Na^{+}–dependent membrane ATPase. A single case of ATPase deficiency associated with congenital nonspherocytic hemolytic anemia has been described, but cation flux studies were not performed. More refined techniques, including electron microscopy, have been used to examine the erythrocyte membrane, but insufficient knowledge concerning the interaction of membrane structure and function limits our understanding of many of these defects.

SECONDARY HEMOLYTIC ANEMIAS

Increased rates of erythrocyte destruction, as determined by standard hematologic methods, have been found in patients with malignant diseases, renal and vascular diseases, aplastic anemia, iron deficiency anemia, lead poisoning, infections (bacteremia, viremia, and parasitemia), folate and vitamin B_{12} deficiency, various collagen diseases, and with prosthetic heart valves. Some entities are associated with altered metabolism and shape of the erythrocyte (e.g., increased glycolytic activity and ATP concentration with erythrocyte fragmentation in uremia), with altered activities of certain enzymes and intermediates (e.g., increased GSH in iron deficiency anemia), and with abnormalities in the synthesis of hemoglobin (e.g., the effects of chemotherapy in the treatment of acute leukemia). These alterations may not be the primary cause of shortened erythrocyte survival but are contributory factors.

Measurements of serum vitamin B_{12} and particularly folate in patients with hemolytic anemia are useful since deficiencies of either may decrease the erythropoietic response. Similarly, although serum iron levels are usually normal or increased in patients with hemolytic anemia, iron deficiency may also inhibit erythropoiesis.

ERYTHROCYTE SURVIVAL AND ORGAN SEQUESTRATION STUDIES

Erythrocyte survival (with ^{51}Cr-labeled cells) and in vivo organ sequestration studies can be combined in the patient as a single procedure if adequate surface counting equipment is available. The sequestration studies may indicate the main site(s) of hemolysis and supply information about the pathogenesis of hemolysis. Details and further consideration of these studies are presented in Chapter 4.

REFERENCES

Beutler, E. *Hereditary Disorders of Erythrocyte Metabolism.* New York: Grune & Stratton, 1968.

Carson, P. E., and Frischer, H.   Glucose-6-phosphate dehydrogenase deficiency and related disorders of the pentose phosphate pathway. *Amer. J. Med.* 41:744, 1966.

Dacie, J. V.   *The Haemolytic Anaemias* (2d ed.). Part I: *The Congenital Anaemias.* Chapter I. General Features of Increased Haemolysis: Blood Picture and Methods of Investigation for the Haemolytic Anaemias. New York: Grune & Stratton, 1960. Pp. 1–83.

Dacie, J. V.   *The Haemolytic Anaemias* (2d ed.). Part II: *The Autoimmune Haemolytic Anaemias.* New York: Grune & Stratton, 1963.

Dacie, J. V., and Lewis, S. M.   *Practical Haematology* (4th ed.). New York: Grune & Stratton, 1968.

Fairbanks, V. F., and Hernandez, M. N.   The identification of metabolic errors associated with hemolytic anemia. *J.A.M.A.* 208:316, 1969.

Hillman, R. S.   *Hematology Laboratory Manual.* Seattle: University of Washington Press, 1969.

Hoffman, J. F.   The red cell membrane and the transport of sodium and potassium. *Amer. J. Med.* 41:666, 1966.

Huehns, E. R., and Bellingham, A. J.   Diseases of function and stability of haemoglobin. *Brit. J. Haemat.* 17:1, 1969.

Jaffé, E.   Clinical profile: Hereditary hemolytic disorders and enzymatic deficiencies of human erythrocytes. *Blood* 35:116, 1970.

Jandl, J. H.   Leaky red cells. *Blood* 26:367, 1965.

Keitt, A. S.   Pyruvate kinase deficiency and related disorders of red cell glycolysis. *Amer. J. Med.* 41:762, 1966.

Yunis, J. J., and Yasmineh, W. G.   *Biochemical Methods in Red Cell Genetics.* New York: Academic, 1969.

APPENDIX

The list below includes names and addresses of workers in research laboratories in the United States who are engaged in the investigation of hereditary hemolytic anemias that result from deficiencies of erythrocyte enzymes.

Dr. E. Beutler	City of Hope Medical Center Duarte, Cal. 91010
Dr. G. J. Brewer	Simpson Memorial Institute University of Michigan Ann Arbor, Mich. 48104
Dr. E. R. Jaffé	Albert Einstein College of Medicine Bronx Municipal Hospital Center Bronx, N.Y. 10461
Dr. D. R. Miller	New York Hospital–Cornell Medical Center New York, N.Y. 10021
Dr. D. G. Nathan	Children's Hospital Medical Center Boston, Mass. 02115
Dr. F. A. Oski	Children's Hospital of Philadelphia Philadelphia, Pa. 19146
Dr. E. R. Simon	University of New Mexico College of Medicine Albuquerque, N.M. 87106
Dr. K. R. Tanaka	Harbor General Hospital Torrance, Cal. 90509
Dr. A. Yoshida	University of Washington College of Medicine Seattle, Wash. 98105
Dr. J. J. Yunis	University of Minnesota College of Medical Sciences Minneapolis, Minn. 55455

6. THE HEINZ
BODY DISORDERS

Paul L. LaCelle

APPROXIMATELY 100 years ago an acquired anemia characterized by cyanosis, brownish discoloration of fresh blood, and the presence of intracellular inclusion bodies was observed in industrial workers exposed to coal-tar derivatives. Heinz in 1890 described the experimental induction of an inclusion body anemia in frogs and rabbits by injection of aliphatic and aromatic amines, as well as by the phenylhydrazine derivatives implicated earlier by von Curtis as etiologic agents. Heinz observed the inclusions to be spherical, refractile bodies free-floating in the cell and noted, by spectroscopic means, the presence of methemoglobin.

During World War I an increased incidence of "cyanotic hemolytic poisoning" was recognized in individuals contacting nitro derivatives and, with the advent of sulfanilamide and congeners, hemolysis was noted in a minor fraction of patients receiving these drugs. Antimalarials were found to cause hemolysis, particularly in Negroes, and subsequently Emerson, Ham, and Castle, noting that these groups of toxic agents were compounds capable of electron transport, suggested that the hemolytic activity might be the result of their capacity as oxidants.

Although the earliest form of a Heinz body disorder thus was associated with oxidative erythrocyte damage, present knowledge suggests a broader functional definition to permit grouping of several hemolytic states according to a common mechanism of destruction rather than by specific etiology. Therefore Heinz body disorders include the anemias and compensated hemolytic states resulting from oxidative denaturation of hemoglobin, the unstable hemoglobin hemolytic anemias, and hemolytic disorders in which there is unbalanced synthesis of hemoglobin. Table 6-1 lists the abnormali-

This work was supported by U.S. Public Health Service Research Grant HE-06241-09 and the U.S. Atomic Energy Project at the University of Rochester. It has been assigned publication no. UR-49-1302.

ties of the pentose pathway, unstable hemoglobins, and unbalanced synthesis of hemoglobin which underlie the clinically apparent Heinz body disorders. Various names have been given to define specific abnormalities, e.g., congenital Heinz body hemolytic anemia (CHBHA) or unstable hemoglobin hemolytic anemia (UHHA); however, Heinz body disorder remains as a convenient name describing the group of abnormalities and indicates the common mechanism of accelerated erythrocyte destruction.

THE HEINZ BODY AND THE MECHANISM OF HEMOLYSIS

The Heinz body may be broadly defined as an intracellular globin precipitate which alters cellular properties sufficiently to shorten the erythrocyte life-span. As suggested in Table 6-1, the composition of the Heinz body depends on the particular defect; i.e., in pentose phosphate pathway defects and in the unstable hemoglobin the inclusion body is denatured hemoglobin, with mixed disulfides of glutathione and sulfhemoglobin as possible constituents, whereas in β-thalassemia the inclusions are insoluble α-chains. The size of the Heinz body is variable, ranging from the 1 to 2 μ size often observed following splenectomy in thalassemia or unstable hemoglobins, to the very fine, uniformly distributed submicroscopic particles typical of hemoglobin H disease. Figure 6-1, a phase photomicrograph, illustrates

Table 6-1. Heinz Body Disorders

Abnormalities of the pentose phosphate pathway		
G6PD deficiency		
GSH reductase deficiency		
GSH deficiency		
Unstable hemoglobin		
β-chain	Genova	Sabine
abnormalities	Tacoma	Köln
	Philly	Wien
	Hammersmith	Boras
	Zürich	Freiburg
	St. Mary's	Gun Hill
	Sydney	Leiden
	Santa Ana	Seattle
α-chain	Torino	
abnormalities	Sinai (Hasharon)	
	Bibba	
Unbalanced synthesis of hemoglobin		
Thalassemia		
Hb H		
Hb Lepore		

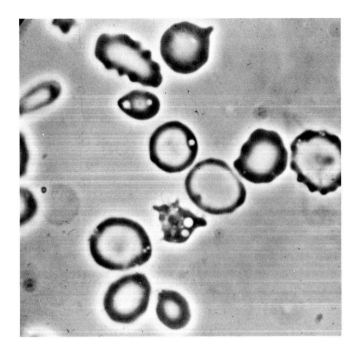

Figure 6-1. Heinz bodies in erythrocytes from a patient with β-thalassemia (phase, × 2000).

Heinz body–containing cells in β-thalassemia following splenectomy. Although Heinz originally described them as freely movable, unattached spheres, these inclusion bodies, particularly smaller peripheral ones, are also associated with the membrane—as studies of erythrocyte ghosts demonstrate—and, if present in sufficient quantities, render the membrane considerably less deformable than in the normal state.

The initiation of biochemical events leading to Heinz body formation, both in Heinz body disorders involving red cell–enzyme defects and presumably also in the unstable hemoglobin states, probably involves oxidation of the globin chains in the region of heme attachment. Subsequently formation of mixed disulfide linkage involving glutathione may occur, and finally, as protein conformational change exposes the molecule to further oxidation, precipitation of hemoglobin in Heinz bodies occurs. It is thought that Heinz bodies thus formed may become intimately associated with the cell membrane, possibly by disulfide linkages, and lead to alteration of the normal mechanical properties of the membrane.

It is of importance to recognize that occasional Heinz bodies may rarely be found in some normal persons, especially in infants, and may occur in significant numbers in normal individuals if sufficient oxidant stress is encountered. A classic example of the latter is seen in the case of excessive phenacetin ingestion; however, splenic destruction reduces the number of observable Heinz body–containing cells in this instance, and in most cases none may be evident in a conventionally stained peripheral blood smear. Dapsone in therapeutic doses is associated with Heinz body formation and mild hemolysis in normal individuals.

The normal erythrocyte has a biconcave disc shape, with an extremely flexible membrane whose surface area is almost twice that required to enclose the volume, a fact which permits the cell to adapt to the configuration of small channels (capillaries 3 to 12 μ in diameter) and to pass through the small apertures (0.5 to 5 μ) in the basement membrane separating the splenic cords from the sinuses. Figure 6-2 indicates the histology of the circulation in the splenic red pulp: in the upper portion are two endarterioles terminating in the splenic cords, and in the lower portion a sinus emptied of cells (for clarity's sake) is depicted. The highly deformable normal erythrocytes are able to squeeze between the cells lining cords and pass through apertures in the basement membrane into the sinuses and hence into the venous circulation. Less than 2% of the splenic circulation passes through the cord to a sinus; however, this portion of the microcirculation may be especially hazardous for abnormal cells, as is illustrated by many disorders in which patients benefit from splenectomy.

The mechanism of destruction in Heinz body disorders appears directly related to the presence of the relatively rigid Heinz bodies within the cell. When the cell contains relatively large inclusions, it has been observed that these are "pitted" from the cell; i.e., the rigid Heinz body and adjacent membrane are torn from the erythrocyte in the splenic circulation where the Heinz body–containing portion may be unable to pass from the splenic cord into the sinuses. The remainder of the cell may proceed into the general circulation as a teardrop or a scallop-shaped poikilocyte. Since the normal erythrocyte membrane is readily deformable, the maintenance of the poikilocytic shape after "pitting" indicates that alteration of plasticity of the membrane or adjacent hemoglobin, or both, has occurred during the spontaneous repair of the membrane at the injury site. Actually local rigidity of membrane in poikilocytes has been observed in vitro, utilizing a micropipette to measure local changes in deformability found particularly in the region adjacent to irregularities in contour of the cell surface. Pitting has been observed in experimental Heinz body anemia, β-thalassemia major, and hemoglobin H disease. It may be postulated that the relatively rigid poikilocytes resulting from the tearing off of a Heinz body fragment will have limited capacity to pass again through the capillary circulation or, particularly, to survive recirculation through the splenic cords, and thus are predisposed to premature destruction.

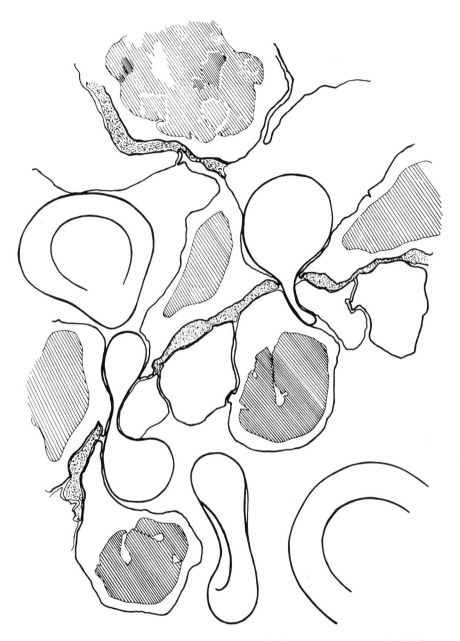

Figure 6-2. Histology of the splenic cords and sinuses. A cross-sectional view indicating a cord with termination of two end-arterioles and adjacent sinus. Erythrocytes shown in transit through the basement membrane (*stippled area*) separating the cord and sinus. For sake of clarity, only a few cells are depicted in the arteriole and sinuses.

The process of pitting or fragmentation has the second important consequence of decreasing the surface area of the membrane, resulting in a more
spherical volume configuration. A sphere is a geometrically rigid shape;
hence a cell of this shape is less able to deform to the requirements of
microcirculatory channels. The production of spherocytes is often observed
in Heinz body disorders.

If present in sufficient quantities the rigid, relatively homogeneously dis-
persed Heinz bodies may make the entire cell so inflexible that it is not
pitted but rather is trapped in the spleen, where it is destroyed.

Abnormal ion permeability is observed in hemolytic disorders, including
Heinz body disorders, and appears to be a general secondary membrane
phenomenon which is not responsible for significant change in cell shape or
for sequestration in the reticuloendothelial system. Thus, whether altered
ion permeability is a mechanism disposing to early cell destruction in Heinz
body–containing erythrocytes is not yet clear.

HEINZ BODY DISORDERS DUE TO PENTOSE PHOSPHATE PATHWAY DEFECTS

The mature erythrocyte has as its major role the transport of molecular
oxygen, without itself being oxidized. It is uniquely fitted for the task by
having as its energy source the anaerobic glycolytic pathway; i.e., it has a
minimal essential flow of electrons. As protection against oxidizing agents
whose introduction into the system would permit transport of electrons and
resultant oxidation, beginning with those intracellular constituents having
relatively low oxidation potentials, the erythrocyte maintains a defensive
antioxidant system, the pentose phosphate pathway (hexose monophosphate shunt). This shunt system, the phosphogluconate pathway represented in Figure 5-3, maintains a supply of NADPH by reduction of
NADP; NADPH can serve as a direct reducing agent and, further, serves to
maintain glutathione and hemoglobin in their reduced states.

The major abnormalities of this pathway are well known. The most common is, of course, G6PD deficiency; a second, a deficiency of glutathione
reductase (GSSG-R), is much less frequently encountered, as is also the
case of deficiency of GSH synthesis. Abnormalities of methemoglobin reductase (not pictured in Figure 5-3; this enzyme regenerates hemoglobin
from methemoglobin, utilizing a mole of NADPH) occur rarely and dis-
pose to high levels of methemoglobin, but not to Heinz body formation.
The GSH-linked enzyme glutathione peroxidase appears to have a direct
role in reducing potential oxidants which would otherwise oxidize the hemoglobin molecule directly, leading to sulfhydryl group oxidation, formation of glutathione-mixed disulfides, and eventual heme-protein precipitation as Heinz bodies. Catalase, also a detoxifying agent for peroxides, is

not an essential protective enzyme, for in individuals with hereditary absence of this enzyme, neither Heinz body formation nor hemolysis is noted.

It is evident that the protection afforded the cell by the pentose phosphate pathway is finite, and if sufficient stress is encountered even normal cells are susceptible to oxidation. This is seen clearly in cases of phenacetin overdose, in vitro incubation in phenylhydrazine, and with dapsone. Other oxidant drugs are potentially hazardous to normal individuals if the dose is sufficient, the difference between the effect in the normal person as compared to the G6PD-deficient patient being the difference in amount of protection afforded by the respective pentose phosphate pathways of their erythrocytes.

G6PD deficiency, the most extensively studied enzyme defect of the pentose phosphate pathway, has been associated with drug-induced Heinz body anemia, nonimmunologic hemolytic disease of the newborn, favism, and some cases of congenital nonspherocytic hemolytic anemia. In fully expressed variants of G6PD deficiency in males, enzyme levels are reduced to zero to 15% of normal in the Negro and zero to 8% in Caucasians and Chinese. Similar ranges have been noted in the fully expressed homozygous state in females. At least 25 G6PD variants exist with a broad range of enzyme activities: only slight reduction is seen, for example, in Joliet II, but enzyme activity is virtually absent in the case of Chinese II. The heterozygote female as well may have only partial expression with broad variations in enzyme levels.

Heinz bodies may be readily produced in vitro by incubation with oxidants; however, in G6PD deficiency as well as in the other defects of the pentose phosphate pathway, Heinz body–containing cells are only infrequently seen in blood from such individuals. This suggests that the alteration of the erythrocyte by the presence of the Heinz body is so significant that these rigid portions of the cell are virtually always removed in the spleen as rapidly as they are formed.

Abnormalities of glutathione reductase are relatively rare but lead to hemolysis when this essential protective enzyme cannot maintain normal levels of reduced glutathione. In affected individuals, who are often of Dutch, German, or French ancestry, as is the case with glutathione abnormalities, enzyme levels of approximately 50% of normal are noted.

Table 6-2 lists several drugs capable of causing hemolysis. At least 40 drugs have been reported to have this potential. It is important to recognize that hemolysis may also occur in infectious disorders in the absence of drugs, having been observed frequently in hepatitis and pneumonitis. Acidosis may cause hemolysis and significant hemolysis is commonly associated with diabetic acidosis in patients having enzyme defects.

The Heinz body disorders associated with defects in the erythrocyte glycolytic pathways have been restricted to the abnormalities of the pentose

Table 6-2.   Some Agents Reported to Produce Hemolysis in Patients with G6PD Deficiency

Antimalarials	*Antipyretics and analgesics*
Primaquine	acetylsalicylic acid
pamaquine	acetanilid
Pentaquine	acetophenetidin (phenacetin)
plasmoquine	antipyrine (*C*)
quinocide	Aminopyrine (*C*)
quinacrine (Atabrine)	p-aminosalicylic acid
quinine (*C*)	
	Sulfones
Sulfonamides	
Sulfanilamide	*Others*
N^1-acetylsulfanilamide	dimercaprol (BAL)
sulfacetamide (Sulamyd)	methylene blue
sulfamethoxypyridazine (Kynex, Midicel)	naphthalene
salicylazosulfapyridine (Azulfidine)	phenylhydrazine
sulfisoxazole (Gantrisin)	acetylphenylhydrazine
Sulfapyridine	probenecid
	vitamin K (large doses of
Nitrofurans	water-soluble analogs)
nitrofurantoin (Furadantin)	chloramphenicol (*C*)
furazolidone (Furoxone)	quinidine (*C*)
furaltadone (Altafur)	fava beans (*C*)
nitrofurazone (Furacin)	chloroquine
	nalidixic acid (NegGram)
	tolbutamide (Orinase)

(*C*): to date, only Caucasians.

phosphate pathway. The hemolysis associated with pyruvate kinase deficiency, for example, appears to relate to the cells' inability to maintain normal amounts of ATP, and the mechanism of destruction probably relates to the adverse effect on cell shape and deformability resulting from the decrease in ATP levels. Heinz bodies are not seen in such a disorder.

HEINZ BODY DISORDERS DUE TO UNSTABLE HEMOGLOBINS

The stability of the adult hemoglobin molecule ($\alpha_2\beta_2$) appears to depend on the integrity of the heme-binding site and the maintenance of normal globin conformation and of the sites of subunit interaction. The globin molecule, a highly ordered structure (approximately 75% in the helical form), has an excess of amino acids having hydrophobic side chains. A conformation is maintained in which hydrophilic side chains are exteriorly placed and interact with water, whereas the hydrophobic chains are arranged in close association interiorly with exclusion of water. The solubility thus depends on normal configuration of the hemoglobin tetramer. Short-range van der Waals forces stabilize the molecule by hydrophobic bonding interiorly; however, the fact that mild heating of normal hemoglobin causes precipitation indicates that water is not totally excluded. The presence of heme in the "pocket" formed by the E and F helices (cf. Fig. 6-3), and its important interaction with the globin molecule via the histidine residue (α-87 or β-92) in the F helix, contribute substantially to hemoglobin stability. The importance of the heme-binding site in the pocket is suggested by the constancy of the amino acids occupying this position in the various hemo-globins. It is also indicated by the significant alteration of hemoglobin sta-bility and decreased affinity for heme which result when amino acids of dif-ferent dimensions are substituted, with resultant modification of van der Waals bonding leading to differing dimensions of the heme pocket. Further stabilization is afforded hemoglobin by subunit interaction between α- and β-chains, especially in the $\alpha\beta$ dimer; and alteration of positions of subunit interaction by amino acid substitution leads to decreased stability.

The mechanism of Heinz body formation in the unstable hemoglobins appears to relate directly or indirectly to increased heme-globin dissoci-ation, a proposal supported by the finding of increased heme flux (rate of heme association and dissociation with globin) in hemoglobin Köln and a reduced heme to globin ratio observed in Hb Köln and Gun Hill. Increased heat lability of unstable hemoglobin is associated with the increased heme-globin flux with the resultant decrease of molecular stability, and it has been observed that the unstable hemoglobins, which precipitate at 50°C, may produce white, i.e., virtually heme-free, globin precipitates. Release of heme from globin permits access of water to the heme pocket and permits methe-moglobin formation and release of an oxidative product (possibly HO_2, the peroxide radical), which enhances oxidative changes leading to denatured hemoglobin. It has been postulated that the β-93 cysteine, at least in Hb Köln, forms a mixed disulfide with glutathione, with resultant heme release and subsequent oxidative change of the molecule. Globin lacking heme tends toward decreased solubility and an alteration in conformation which will expose further sulfhydryl groups to oxidation. The net result is a Heinz body, comprising denatured hemoglobin-methemoglobin and glutathione in mixed disulfide linkages.

Hb Köln is the most extensively studied of the unstable hemoglobins with abnormalities of amino acids at the site of heme binding; Hb Zürich, Ham-mersmith, Sydney, Sabine, and Kansas represent abnormalities affecting heme binding and have disease manifestations varying from the very severe hemolysis of Hammersmith to that of Zürich, in which oxidative stress is required to make the hemolysis clinically manifest. The majority of un-stable hemoglobins are β-chain defects, as noted in Figure 6-3 and in Table

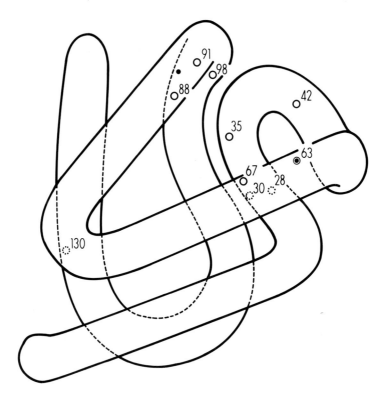

Figure 6-3. A representation of the β-chain of human hemoglobin, with approximate loci (o) of amino acid substitutions in some unstable hemoglobins associated with Heinz body hemolytic disorders, indicates histidines proximal and distal to heme. Not depicted are Hb E and the deletions, Freiburg, Gun Hill, and Leiden. 28, Genova; 30, Tacoma; 35, Philly; 42, Hammersmith; 63, Zürich; 67, Sydney; 88, Santa Ana; 91, Sabine; 98, Köln; 130, Wien.

7-1 (see also Table 10-1). Torino and Bibba are hemoglobins having α-chain substitutions affecting the heme-binding site. Hb Freeburg, Gun Hill, and Leiden represent disorders in which overall globin stability is affected due to crucial amino acid deletions. Overall conformational abnormality is seen in Santa Ana, Sabine, and Bibba. Hb Philly and Tacoma have reduced $\alpha_1\beta_1$ contacts due to amino acid replacements; in the latter only in vitro instability is seen.

Clinically the unstable hemoglobin Heinz body disorders are hemolytic ones, presenting in the heterozygote from infancy. They are characterized by the typical red cell inclusions, especially after splenectomy, and usually have splenomegaly and dipyrroluria.

In Hb Köln anemic crises may be superimposed upon the chronic hemolytic process; however, this is not a feature of other unstable hemoglobin disorders described thus far. Hemolysis with some degree of jaundice is usual in the unstable hemoglobin disorders, and even in Hb Zürich slight hemolysis is evident in the quiescent stage, i.e., in the absence of oxidant drugs. Of the more than 20 unstable hemoglobins described to date, approximately half present as very mild disorders.

The peripheral blood smear may contain microspherocytes, and polychromatophilia is prominent. The proportion of methemoglobin is variable, from virtual absence in Zürich to 12% in Bibba. The proportion of unstable hemoglobin in reported cases has varied from 10 to 43%; however, these low percentages may be due to splenic or intramarrow destruction of many cells containing abnormal hemoglobin.

Starch-gel electrophoresis is the most sensitive current method for detection of unstable hemoglobins, particularly if differing buffer pH values are selected and if oxyhemoglobin or methemoglobin derivatives are evaluated. Not all unstable hemoglobins have altered electrophoretic patterns; in fact, noncharged substitutes are noted in some of the most severe disorders. The presence of free α-chains is a constant finding in the unstable hemoglobins possessing β-chain abnormalities. Heating to observe differential precipitation of abnormal hemoglobins and evaluating oxygen dissociation of abnormal hemoglobins are also methods of screening hemoglobins suspected of instability. Determination of the molecular defect, of course, requires the assistance of a laboratory prepared to undertake amino acid sequence analysis.

HEINZ BODY DISORDERS DUE TO UNBALANCED SYNTHESIS OF HEMOGLOBIN

There are more than 100 known variants of human adult Hb A ($\alpha_2\beta_2$ tetramer); approximately one-third comprise alterations in α-globin chains, and the remainder are β-chain abnormalities. The underlying genetic abnormalities are of three general types: (1) point mutation, as exemplified by β-6 valine in Hb S, and substitutions observed in unstable hemoglobins; (2) unequal crossing over, e.g., Hb Lepore possessing α-globin chains plus chains consisting of N-terminal Δ and C-terminal β portions; (3) undefined genetic defects resulting in partial or complete block of synthesis of a specific chain. The last is descriptive of the thalassemia syndromes, including α, β, δ, $\beta\delta$. In such disorders no qualitative abnormality occurs; rather, decreased quantities of normal polypeptide chains are formed.

Four homologous pairs of genetic loci are concerned with production of globin tetramer subunit production in normal human erythroblasts. These loci—α, β, Δ, γ—may be jointly or severally affected in a thalassemia lesion, leading to reduced amounts of a globin subunit. In thalassemia major (β-

thalassemia, Cooley's anemia), it is generally thought that reduction of output of both loci governing β-chain synthesis is responsible for the hemoglobin disorder, and that one locus is involved in the instance of thalassemia minor.

Recently it has been proposed that there may exist two pairs of genetic loci in control of each globin chain type, a suggestion stemming from the observation that similar amino acid substitutions in identical loci of α- and β-chains in different mutant hemoglobins result in different percentages of abnormal hemoglobin. Differences in amount of messenger RNA could be an alternative to this hypothesis. It is of interest to note that 4 genes are known to be involved in the regulation of α-chain synthesis in horse and goat. Two pairs of controlling loci would help explain the broad variation in severity observed clinically, particularly in α-thalassemia and also in Hb H disease, which varies from the mildest cellular changes (occasional cells having Hb H) unaccompanied by clinical findings, to a clinical severity exceeding that of β-thalassemia minor. According to this 4-gene hypothesis, the degree of severity of Hb H disease would depend on homozygosity or heterozygosity of 2 of the 4 genes, and abnormalities of 3 or 4 genes would be lethal (hydrops fetalis).

Two mechanisms may be postulated to explain why peptide chain synthesis is defective in the thalassemias: (1) the total rate of messenger RNA production for the chain might be quantitatively defective; or (2) a qualitative defect in the chain-specific messenger RNA might result in a decrease in the rate at which normal globin chains are assembled on the m-RNA-ribosomal template. Apparently the ultimate defect is limited in that a qualitatively normal chain is produced, and it is only quantitatively altered.

In studies of incorporation of radioactively labeled amino acid into globin chains from nonthalassemic reticulocytes, it is clear that the total radioactivity incorporated into α-chains equals that in β-chains, indicating that the rate of α- and β-chain synthesis is equivalent during normal hemoglobin synthesis. From kinetic studies there is evidence that a small preformed pool of α-chains exists in the normal human reticulocyte, and it is suggested that α-chains, normally released into this pool, return to ribosomes where they combine with partially synthesized β-chains to form $\alpha\beta$ subunits.

In β-thalassemia, typically exhibiting high levels of Hb F, some A$_2$, and zero to 30% A, the in vitro rate of α-chain synthesis exceeds that of β-chains and also γ-chains. In cases in which only Hb F is synthesized, the number of α-chains still greatly exceeds γ-chains. Free α-chains are unstable, and after brief in vitro incubation of thalassemic reticulocytes, much of the synthesized α-chain becomes associated with the cell stroma, suggesting rapid precipitation of free α-chains. Such precipitates are recognized as Heinz bodies.

α-Thalassemia presents in two main hemoglobin varieties. Hb Barts, the

γ_4-tetramer, with smaller amounts of β_4-tetramer (Hb H) and traces of another uncharacterized γ-chain hemoglobin, are found in the clinical variety described as *hydrops fetalis*. It is of note that the γ-tetramer binds oxygen nearly irreversibly and thus is ineffective as an oxygen carrier. Hb H disease is characterized by the presence of 5 to 30% Hb H, with corresponding variation in the severity of hemolysis. In α-thalassemia, β-chains are produced at 2 to 3 times normal rate and the excess forms the β-tetramer. The β-tetramer is relatively more soluble than the α-chains and is apparently somewhat less liable to form insoluble precipitates. Hb H has been found as an acquired phenomenon in adult leukemia.

The anemia of the thalassemia syndromes results from the ineffective erythropoiesis typical of this disorder and from the accelerated destruction of Heinz body–containing cells in parts of the reticuloendothelial system, particularly the spleen. The poikilocytes resulting from loss of membrane due to fragmentation and Heinz bodies are vulnerable, probably due to membrane rigidity caused by irreversible distortion of membrane elements during the stresses of fragmentation and by membrane-associated, submicroscopic Heinz bodies, and they undergo early destruction. A second mechanism which may account for accelerated destruction of thalassemic cells is the low and often unstable ATP content of such cells. ATP, well known for its role as an energy source in active ion transport mechanisms of the erythrocyte, appears to be required for the maintenance of the normal biconcave disc shape and normal membrane flexibility of the cell. ATP protects the membrane from calcium-induced gelation of hemoglobin and soluble protein at the inner membrane surface and from possible calcium-induced contraction of actomyosin-like proteins of the membrane. Decrease of cellular deformability because of calcium-related membrane rigidity and sphering of the cell makes the cell liable to splenic trapping and destruction.

Hb Lepore is actually a family of hemoglobins containing normal α-chains and non-α-chains which consist of fusion products of portions of β- and Δ-chains. Lepore hemoglobin may account for approximately 10% of the hemoglobin and account for mild to severe hemolytic anemia on the basis of inclusion body–induced cellular destruction. Other disorders which combine a quantitative globin disorder with globin chain abnormalities— e.g., S-thalassemia, C-thalassemia—have shortened erythrocyte life-span because of the Heinz body mechanism and also show the mechanism typical of the second hemoglobin abnormality.

INDICATIONS FOR SPLENECTOMY IN THE HEINZ BODY DISORDERS

In the Heinz body anemias the major hemolytic mechanism, i.e., process leading to the shortened life-span of erythrocytes, is the fragmentation resulting from the pitting of the Heinz body–containing portion of the cell by the reticuloendothelial system. As already noted, the fragmentation process decreases the surface area to volume relationship as membrane is lost, tending toward a spherical shape in the "surviving" portion of the cell. Furthermore, local alterations of membrane plasticity at various points on the surface of cell which has undergone fragmentation may lead to the poikilocytic shape; the tendency toward the spherical shape or the altered plasticity, or both, render the cell less deformable and limit its potential for survival.

It is predictable that various portions of the reticuloendothelial system such as those in spleen, liver, bone marrow, or lung may trap and destroy such altered erythrocytes. The spleen, with its unique cord-sinus architecture, appears to be the severest threat to the cell that has lost its normal deformability, and thus splenectomy should be beneficial in disorders in which there is abnormal deformability. However, in the bone marrow, maturing erythrocytes at the reticulocyte stage must leave the hematopoietic cords and traverse apertures through the adventitial cell–basement membrane wall separating hematopoietic cords from the marrow sinuses in order to enter the peripheral circulation. If appreciable cell destruction occurs in the bone marrow itself or if erythrocytes are modified during bone marrow release, splenectomy would be expected to ameliorate accelerated destruction but not effect a complete restoration of normal erythrocyte life-span.

Splenectomy should be considered in chronic hemolytic states. The major criteria to be evaluated include the presence of splenomegaly, the appearance of spherocytes and poikilocytes on the blood smear, elevated reticulocyte index, increased levels of unconjugated bilirubin, and evidence of splenic sequestration indicated by progressive increase in splenic surface counts as compared to liver in a ^{51}Cr erythrocyte survival study. In addition, excessive transfusion requirement and thrombocytopenia due to splenic enlargement may be factors favoring splenectomy. In some instances splenectomy may prove effective in amelioration of the anemia despite lack of clear evidence by ^{51}Cr studies of splenic sequestration and accelerated destruction. Quite obviously, splenectomy may be essential in treatment of the chronic Heinz body disorder in which significant anemia is present. It should also be considered in the compensated states in which the bone marrow production is sufficient to maintain a normal hematocrit, in order to prevent the adverse effects of cholelithiasis and cholecystitis.

In thalassemia the magnitude of the imbalance of globin chain synthesis has been found to correlate well with decreased cell survival as shown by ^{51}Cr studies; hence, it is predictable that splenectomy may result in an increase in erythrocyte life-span, particularly in homozygous β-thalassemia. Splenectomy should be considered in the severe thalassemia disorders on the basis of chronic hemolysis, the presence of enlarged spleen, and red cell life-span shortening as shown by ^{51}Cr study, associated with an increasing

[51]Cr surface count over the splenic area. Thalassemia "intermedia," often a combination of G6PD deficiency and β-thalassemia, may require splenectomy, particularly in females whose hemolysis is notably worsened by pregnancy. In such cases in which significant anemia is present in the nonpregnant state, the placenta in the last half of pregnancy may be the site of considerable red cell destruction, leading to severe anemia which remits postpartum. In severe cases splenectomy during the later stages of pregnancy to remove the splenic contribution to hemolysis may be an essential part of management. Earlier suggestions that splenectomy adversely affects thalassemia patients in terms of resistance to infection or growth and development in children have not been substantiated. In light of the ineffective erythropoiesis typical of thalassemia, one should not anticipate normalization of erythrocyte life-span and reticulocyte count following splenectomy; however, some improvement in life-span and hence decrease in transfusion requirement would be expected.

Splenectomy should be performed in the unstable hemoglobin Heinz body disorders. In Hb Köln disease, definite clinical improvement was observed in 4 or 5 reported cases (in Glasgow, Windsor, Ube-I, and Fremantle families, but not in London), and the level of hemoglobin in each increased. Similar positive results have been observed in this medical center. Although only a limited number of splenectomies performed to date in these disorders has been reported, the clear decrease in hemolysis following the procedure is a positive indication for splenectomy in unstable hemoglobin Heinz body disorders.

The management of the acute hemolysis resulting from excessive oxidative stress in disorders involving defects in the pentose pathway generally does not require splenectomy, for the identification and removal of the offending drugs or chemicals will halt the induction of additional Heinz bodies. Cells already compromised will be destroyed, of course, but new erythrocytes will have a life-span typical of that in the individual in the unstressed state.

ACKNOWLEDGMENTS

Mrs. Linda Billingham prepared the illustrations and Miss Brigitte Ott prepared the manuscript; their assistance is gratefully acknowledged.

REFERENCES

Carrell, R. W., and Lehmann, H.   The unstable hemoglobin hemolytic anemias. *Seminars Hemat.* 6:116, 1969.
Heinz, R.   Morphologische Veränderungen der roten Blutkörperchen durch Gifte. *Virchow. Arch. Path. Anat.* 122:112, 1890.

Heller, P. Hemoglobinopathic dysfunction of the red cell. *Amer. J. Med.* 41:799, 1966.

Heuhns, E. R., and Bellingham, A. J. Diseases of function and stability of hemoglobin. *Brit. J. Haemat.* 17:1, 1969.

Jandl, J. H. The Heinz body hemolytic anemias. *Ann. Intern. Med.* 58:702, 1963.

Lehmann, H., and Huntsman, R. G. *Man's Hemoglobins.* Philadelphia: Lippincott, 1966.

Necheles, T. F., and Allen, D. M. Heinz-body anemias. *New Eng. J. Med.* 280:203, 1969.

Perutz, M. F., and Lehmann, H. Molecular pathology of human hemoglobin. *Nature* (London) 219:902, 1968.

Weatherall, D. J. The biochemical lesion in thalassaemia. *Brit. J. Haemat.* 15:1, 1968.

Weed, R. I. The Cell Membrane in Hemolytic Disorders. In E. R. Jaffé (Ed.), Proceedings of the XIIth Congress of the International Society of Hematology. New York, September, 1968.

Weed, R. I. The importance of erythrocyte deformability. *Amer. J. Med.* 49:147, 1970.

7. DISEASE STATES RESULTING FROM ABNORMALITIES IN HEMOGLOBIN SYNTHESIS

Robert I. Weed

DISORDERS OF hemoglobin synthesis provide superb examples of disease states in which the entire pathophysiology can be traced from the gene to mechanisms of red cell destruction. In recent years the rapid evolution of increasingly sophisticated techniques for the study of hemoglobin electrophoresis, peptide fingerprinting, and quantitative evaluation of normal and abnormal rates of globin chain synthesis combined with studies of oxygen association-dissociation have made it apparent that a wide range of pathophysiologic alterations may result from genetically determined abnormalities in hemoglobin synthesis. Quantitative alterations are illustrated by the thalassemia syndromes in which the rate of synthesis of either the α- or β-globin chain is pathologically diminished. In addition, however, more than a hundred structural variants of hemoglobin have been recognized as being attributable to specific qualitative amino acid substitutions in the globin chains.

Normal adult hemoglobin contains two α-chains, each having 141 amino acids, two β-chains, each with 145 amino acids, and 4 heme moieties. The hemoglobin molecule is composed of two dimers, each containing one α- and one β-chain which combine with an identical dimer in the presence of heme to form the hemoglobin tetramer. Synthesis of the α- and β-globin chains is under the control of separate genetic loci, as illustrated in Figure 7-1. The δ- and γ-loci which are responsible for hemoglobin A_2 and hemo-

This work was supported by U.S. Public Health Service Research Grant HE-06241 and the U.S. Atomic Energy Project at the University of Rochester. It has been assigned publication no. UR-49-1297.

101

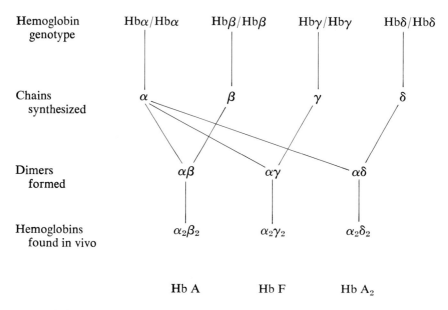

Figure 7-1. Formation of normal human hemoglobins. (From E. R. Huehns, *J. Med. Genet.* 2:48, 1965, with permission of the author and the Editor, *Journal of Medical Genetics.*)

globin F, respectively, are located in positions close to the β-locus. It is obvious that the complex structure of the hemoglobin molecule, with the opportunity for amino acid substitution at each of the normal sites in both globin chains, is potentially subject to a host of structural aberrations which may have functional significance for the hemoglobin molecule.

Table 7-1 is a summary of the aberrations which have been reported. Many of the abnormalities listed in the table are extremely rare; others, more common, may lead to a wide range of clinical consequences and implications. This chapter focuses primarily on the clinical picture in the major pathophysiologic abnormalities resulting from alterations in hemoglobin structure; it also deals with practical aspects of hemoglobinopathies which are encountered commonly in clinical practice in the United States.

Table 7-2 summarizes clinical and laboratory features underlying the various disease states which are attributable to abnormalities of hemoglobin synthesis. Although some structural alterations are not associated with any clinical symptomatology whatsoever, the majority result in abnormalities leading to shortened red cell life-span. Some substitutions may affect the function of heme, in addition to producing a defect leading to hemolysis, while others may affect only heme function and not red cell survival.

Table 7-1.   Hemoglobins with Distinctive Features

I. STRUCTURAL DISTORTION
   1. $S(\beta^{6\ \text{Glu} \to \text{Val}})$: sickling
   2. $C_{\text{Harlem}} \left(\begin{smallmatrix} \beta 6\ \text{Glu} \to \text{Val} \\ \beta 73\ \text{Asp} \to \text{Asn} \end{smallmatrix} \right)$: sickling
   3. $C(\beta^{6\ \text{Glu} \to \text{Lys}})$: cell rigidity

II. ABNORMAL FUNCTION
  Increased O_2 affinity
   1. Chesapeake
   2. Rainier
   3. Yakima
   4. Ypsi
   5. Kempsey
   6. J-Capetown
   7. Hiroshima
   8. Tacoma
   9. Zürich
   10. Köln
   11. St. Mary's
   12. Gun Hill
   13. Freiburg
   14. $H(\beta 4)$
   15. Barts $(\gamma 4)$
  Decreased O_2 affinity
   1. Kansas
   2. Hammersmith
   3. Bristol
   4. Seattle
   5. Torino
   6. Yoshizuka
   7. E
  Internal ligands
  Hemoglobins M
   1. M_{Boston}
   2. M_{Iwate}
   3. $M_{\text{Saskatoon}}$
   4. $M_{\text{Milwaukee1}}$
   5. $M_{\text{Hyde Park}}$

III. UNSTABLE
  Alpha mutants
   1. Hasharon
   2. Bibba
   3. Torino
   4. Ann Arbor
   5. Etiobicoke
   6. L-Ferrara
   7. Dakar

Beta mutants
   1. Zürich
   2. Köln
   3. Seattle
   4. St. Mary's
   5. Ube-I
   6. Genova
   7. Gun Hill
   8. Sabine
   9. Riverdale-Bronx
   10. Santa Ana
   11. Philly
   12. Wien
   13. Hammersmith
   14. Sydney
   15. Tacoma
   16. Borås
   17. Bristol
   18. Sogn
   19. Leiden
   20. Freiburg
   21. Toulouse
   22. Shepherd's Bush
   23. H

IV. DELETIONS
   1. Freiburg $(\beta^{23\ \text{Val} \to 0})$
   2. Gun Hill $(\beta^{91-95 \to 0})$
   3. Leiden $(\beta^{6\ \text{or}\ 7 \to 0})$

V. TWO SUBSTITUTIONS
   1. C_{Harlem}
   2. S_{Memphis}

VI. POLYMERIZATION (IN VITRO)
  Porto Alegre

VII. HOMOTETRAMERS
   1. $H\ (\beta_4)$
   2. Barts (γ_4)
   3. Gower-1 (ϵ_4)

VIII. LEPORE
   1. Boston (Washington, Augusta)
   2. Pylos
   3. Hollandia
   4. Cyprus

SOURCE: Courtesy of E. R. Simon.

103

Table 7-2. *Disorders of Hemoglobin Synthesis*

Disorders	Molecular Pathophysiology	Clinical Pathophysiology	Clinical Manifestations	Blood Smear	Laboratory Diagnosis
QUANTITATIVE Thalassemia syndromes T. major	Impaired synthesis of either α or β globin chains	Excess globin chains form intracellular gels or precipitates (Heinz bodies)	Homozygote: Severe anemia with intramedullary hemolysis (ineffective erythropoiesis) and splenic destruction (fragmentation)	Anisocytosis, poikilocytosis, hypochromia, microcytosis (fragments), targets, teardrops, polychromasia, normoblastemia, and basophilic stippling	Family studies: ↑ marrow iron and blasts ↑ Hb F (60%), A_2, normal Heinz bodies (phase or separated stain) ↓ osmotic fragility Direct study of globin chain synthesis[a]
T. minor			Heterozygote: (a) α-thalassemia, may be severe (homozygote lethal); (b) β-thalassemia, T. minor (or intermedia)	Similar but milder than homozygote, i.e., hypochromia, basophilic stippling, microcytosis—often with an increased number of RBC/cu mm	Family studies: (a) ↑ Hb H (α-Th) and normal F & A_2 (b) ↑ (>3%) Hb A_2 in most; normal or slightly increased Hb F and serum iron
QUALITATIVE Unstable hemoglobins (congenital Heinz body anemias)	Amino acid substitution (charged or nonpolar) Dominant trait	Physical instability of hemoglobin (may split off heme) with resultant intracellular precipitate (Heinz bodies)	Chronic, moderately severe hemolytic state with dark urine (dipyrroles) Some hemoglobins are predisposed to oxidant-drug hemolysis	Hypochromia, microcytosis, teardrops, basophilic stippling, occasional spheres	Family studies: Heat instability Abnormal electrophoresis for most but several uncharged substitutions have normal electrophoresis Peptide fingerprinting[a]

Aggregating hemoglobins (S and C)	β-chain Amino acid substitution (charged) Disease in homozygote but trait can be detected in the heterozygote	Homozygote Chronic hemolytic state with predisposition to multiple microthrombi and infarction	Homogeneous Intracellular crystallization of hemoglobin with resultant cellular rigidity and predisposition to fragmentation SS: low Po_2 CC: ↑ ionic strength Milder disease aggrevated by pregnancy (SS with high Hb)	SS-Anisocytosis and poikilocytosis (sickle cells) Fragmentation occasional sphere CC-target cells and occasional intracellular crystals seen on slowly dried smear	Hb SS-metabisulfite (sickle prep) Hb electrophoresis 80–99% abnormal Hb 2–20% Hb F 2–3% A_2 Hb CC-crystals in hypertonic medium and Hb electrophoresis
Hereditary methemoglobinemia	Charged amino acid substitution interacting with heme ring prevents Fe+++ → Fe++ Disease seen in heterozygote (homozygous state lethal)	Amino acid substitution in β chain: 50% Hb A, 30–40% Hb M plus 15–20% methemgb. M Substitution in α chain: 7–10% methemgb. M, 15–20% Hb M	Cyanosis; rarely symptoms of hypoxia under stress	Normal	Hb electrophoresis after conversion to methemoglobin Spectroscopic studies
Hemoglobins with ↑ O_2 affinity	Amino acid substitution Only heterozygotes reported	Altered α-β-chain interaction and diminished subunit interaction	Mild to moderate erythrocytosis without ↑ WBC or platelets Predisposition to hypoxic fetal injury and abortion	Normal	Hb electrophoresis or alkali denaturation Abnormal O_2 dissociation curve
Hemoglobins with ↓ O_2 affinity	Amino acid substitution Only heterozygotes reported	Cyanosis	Mild to moderate erythrocytosis without ↑ WBC or platelets Predisposition to hypoxic fetal injury and abortion		Hb electrophoresis or alkali denaturation Abnormal O_2 dissociation curve

Table 7-2 (Continued)

Disorders	Molecular Pathophysiology	Clinical Pathophysiology	Clinical Manifestations	Blood Smear	Laboratory Diagnosis
Hemoglobin Lepore	Normal α-chains plus chains that are part δ- and part β-chain	Physical instability of hemoglobin	Clinical picture of T. major or T. minor for homozygote and heterozygote, respectively	Like β-Thalassemia major and minor	Starch block electrophoresis
DOUBLE HETEROZYGOTE FOR QUANTITATIVE AND QUALITATIVE DEFECT S-T disease	β-chains may all be βS and no βA produced although only sickle trait present	Cellular rigidity and fragmentation High concentration of sickle Hb predisposes to aggregation (tactoids)	Milder than T. major; enlarged spleen in adults	Hypochromia, sickling, target cells, anisocytosis, and poikilocytosis	Electrophoresis and sickle prep Hb S: 65–85% A₂: 73% F: 15–35% A: 0 Family studies essential

a Generally available only in research centers.
KEY: ↑ = increased; ↓ = decreased.

HEMOLYTIC STATES

Defects in the rate of globin chain synthesis which give rise to the thalassemia syndromes, and the amino acid substitutions leading to the unstable hemoglobin syndromes, are both discussed in Chapter 6, the Heinz Body Disorders. An additional important clinical group is that of the aggregating hemoglobin disorders, primarily sickle cell and hemoglobin C disease. These disorders are characterized by changes in the entire hemoglobin content of affected cells rather than by precipitation of a portion of the contents, as in the Heinz body disorders.

SICKLE CELL DISEASE

Sickle cell trait is found in 8.5% of American Negroes, and sickle cell anemia, the homozygous state, is found in 0.3 to 1.3% of Negroes in the United States. Sickle cell disease does not become manifest until after the third or fourth month of life, when fetal homoglobin has been replaced by sickle hemoglobin, and it may not become symptomatic until months later. In certain individuals, persistence of relatively high (10 to 20%) fetal hemoglobin levels appears to offer protection to those cells in which it is found in highest concentration and thereby moderates the clinical picture. The varying composition of hemoglobin in sickle cell disease is illustrated in Figure 7-2.

The pathophysiology of sickle cell disease relates to the sickling of individual cells which occurs in regions of lowered oxygen tension (Po_2) or pH, or both, with a resultant increase of blood viscosity. This sequence of events results in sludging of the blood in regions of stasis, which in turn results in lower Po_2 at the site with the resultant further increase in viscosity predisposing to small vessel occlusion. The rigidity of the individual cells predisposes both to their removal from the circulation and to their fragmentation within the circulation. Since red cell membrane lipids are potentially thromboplastic, fragmentation of the membrane presumably contributes to the predisposition to development of small vessel thrombi which are the basis for the painful crises in this disorder.

THROMBOTIC COMPLICATIONS.   Painful crises may occur with acute joint symptomatology and also within the lung, where they result in pulmonary infarction with or without pneumonia. Painless occlusions may occur within the liver, giving rise to increased icterus and creating a problem of differential diagnosis with infectious hepatitis, especially if the patient has been transfused previously. Thrombotic crises, however, are not necessarily associated with any change in the hematocrit or rate of cell destruction. The thrombotic or painful crisis is a difficult and common problem in patients

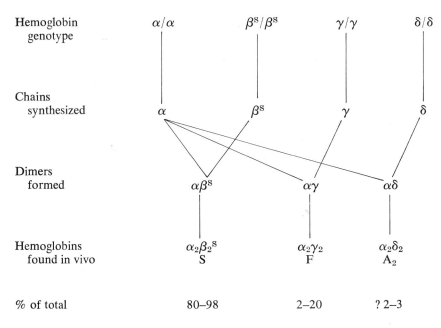

Figure 7-2. Formation of hemoglobin in sickle cell disease (Hb SS). (From E. R. Huehns, *J. Med. Genet.* 2:48, 1965, with permission of the author and the Editor, *Journal of Medical Genetics.*)

with sickle cell disease and may lead to death if massive generalized small vessel occlusion follows. In addition to occurring spontaneously, thrombotic episodes often complicate intercurrent infections such as pneumonia or occur during or after surgery and thereby interfere with healing. In the past, a variety of therapeutic approaches have been tried. Alkalinization with sodium bicarbonate may help in interrupting episodes of hematuria both in SS disease and in sickle trait but generally appears to be ineffective in painful crisis. Oxygen therapy by mask has been tried also, but breathing even 100% oxygen affects the dissolved oxygen in blood only slightly. Venous P_{O_2} is critical insofar as induction of sickling is concerned and is more closely related to cellular utilization of capillary oxygen than is the oxygen tension in the alveoli; therefore it is not hard to understand why oxygen by mask has not proved to be genuinely helpful. Recently, infusion of hypertonic urea in invert sugar has been recommended both for treatment of crisis and to improve red cell survival. This therapy is controversial and still under evaluation.

In many patients no specific therapy is necessary; rather, an initial period of observation for 24 to 36 hours is appropriate. Some patients in painful crisis will pass through this period and begin to improve spontaneously without any treatment except hydration and watchful waiting. However, for those who persist in their symptomatology or worsen over the

initial period of observation, in order to abort the painful crisis it is necessary to transfuse them to normal or near-normal hematocrit levels with
normal red cells. This form of therapy serves several purposes: (1) The
sickle cell blood is diluted with normal red cells so that the whole blood has
a significantly decreased tendency to undergo sickling at lowered Po_2. (2)
Even if some cells do sickle, their dilution in the whole blood minimizes the
tendency toward increased viscosity and further occlusion. (3) Restoration
of a normal hematocrit with transfused blood restores tissue oxygenation,
thereby decreasing erythropoietin production and the stimulus to increased
production of sickle cells. After the hematocrit is raised by transfusion, the
patient should be maintained at a hematocrit value from 37 to 42% until
the painful episode subsides.

Thrombotic problems are often encountered during or prior to major
surgery. Because such episodes may constitute significant complications
during the postoperative course and may retard healing, prophylactic transfusion to suppress sickle cell formation should be undertaken and maintained for at least 5 days prior to surgery in order to reduce the number of
sickle cells in the blood and to suppress further production. Suppressive
transfusion therapy should be maintained until wound healing is well under
way.

Pregnancy presents a special hazard for patients with homozygous sickle
disease or with any combination of sickle trait with other hemoglobinopathies. If one considers the physiology of the placenta, it is not difficult to
understand why pregnant patients may have aggravation of the hemolytic
process as well as increased predisposition to thrombotic episodes during
pregnancy. The Po_2 of the maternal venous side of the placental circulation
normally is between 13 and 30 mm Hg, low enough to produce very significant sickling in the homozygous individual and very close to oxygen tension
values that will produce sickling of blood in a patient with sickle trait. In
this regard the placenta may act as a temporary spleen and, following loss of
the placenta at the time of delivery, significant hematologic improvement
can be anticipated.

From the point of view of the fetus, pregnancy is a most serious problem
in sickle cell disease, with up to 12% stillbirths, 27% spontaneous abortions, and 42% premature deliveries. The abortion and prematurity figures
are 2 to 3 times those of appropriate control Negro populations. The severity of these complications is such as to justify sterilization, particularly if
the patient has been fortunate enough to carry one or two pregnancies
through to successful delivery.

Aplastic or hypoplastic crises may occur when some intercurrent illness
suppresses the hyperactive marrow which is attempting to compensate. This
type of episode, which unfortunately has often been designated a hemolytic
crisis because of a rapidly falling hematocrit, should be managed by a combination of attention to the primary illness or infection which is suppressing

the marrow and, second, to replacement transfusion as needed. An additional factor which may precipitate a hypoplastic crisis in patients with sickle cell disease is the tremendous demand of the hyperactive marrow for folic acid. Chronic hemolysis predisposes the patient to relative folic acid deficiency which may occur during periods of poor dietary intake or most especially during pregnancy, when the demands of the fetus for folic acid are great. Folic acid, 15 mg a day by mouth, should be given whenever a hypoplastic crisis is suspected, and during pregnancy 5 mg a day should be given as a routine prophylactic measure.

ANEMIA AND CONSIDERATION OF SPLENECTOMY. With the important exception of hypoplastic crises, most patients with SS disease can tolerate their relatively severe anemia remarkably well. It is not uncommon for adults to tolerate hematocrit levels of 17 to 20%. This is possible because of the right shift in the oxygen dissociation curve to favor oxygen release to the tissues at higher Po_2 values. As discussed in Chapter 10, this is largely due to the elevated DPG levels in these abnormal red cells as well as certain other factors not yet understood. Thus, except for hypoplastic crises or thrombotic crises, transfusions are usually not indicated for adults with SS disease.

In adult patients with sickle cell disease consideration of splenectomy is seldom necessary, because most patients will have undergone "autosplenectomy" by virtue of repeated infarction of their spleen during childhood and adolescence. This self-destruction of the spleen results in amelioration of the hemolytic process if the patients survive to adulthood. However, in some children the hemolytic process may be sufficiently severe to warrant splenectomy. The restrictive confines of the spleen combined with its lowered pH and stasis provide a severe hazard for sickle cells, and removal of this organ should be considered in children above the age of 4 years if they have a severe enough form of this disease to require transfusions and if the spleen is readily palpable. The hematologic evidence, however, should be balanced against the enhanced risk of infection in sickle cell disease, which may be increased after splenectomy in children. Some have advocated prophylactic penicillin for children after splenectomy, although gram-negative infection remains a threat. Homozygous sickle patients with persistence of fetal hemoglobin, because of the milder nature of their disease, may still have splenic enlargement persisting into adulthood; again, splenectomy should be considered in these individuals.

SICKLE CELL TRAIT

Sickle cell trait per se is usually a benign disorder. Such individuals, however, are predisposed to the same complications as homozygous patients if the blood anywhere within their circulation is exposed to a sufficiently low oxygen tension. Travel through the mountains or travel in unpressurized aircraft predisposes to splenic infarction. Exercise may cause marked decrease in local oxygen tension, and athletes with sickle trait have been known to develop splenic infarction after severe exertion. Occasional fatal episodes of this type have been reported in patients with sickle trait.

HEMOGLOBIN CC DISEASE

Hemoglobin C trait alone is completely benign and is usually detected incidentally upon careful examination of the blood smear, which reveals up to 50% target cells. The trait is found in 2 to 3% of American Negroes. Hemoglobin CC disease, the homozygous state, is therefore relatively rare and milder than sickle cell disease, but still potentially troublesome. CC patients have a moderate anemia with a hematocrit level of 25 to 35%, splenomegaly, and occasional complications which include aseptic necrosis of the femoral heads, hematuria, and occasional episodes of joint and abdominal pain, but usually much milder than with sickle cell anemia. Pregnancy may aggravate the anemia and, in fact, may be responsible for the establishment of the diagnosis, although the abnormality should be suggested by the finding of 60 to 90% target cells on the blood smear, with some evidence of fragmentation and occasional spherocytes which are the result of fragmentation. Hemoglobin electrophoresis establishes the diagnosis.

HEMOGLOBIN D

This trait occurs in 0.4% of American Negroes. The homozygous state is associated with a mild hemolytic anemia. The major practical reason for awareness of hemoglobin D is that it may be confused with hemoglobin S, since it has an identical electrophoretic mobility with that of S at pH 8.6, at which most hemoglobin electrophoretic studies are run. D can be distinguished from S, however, by running the electrophoresis at a pH of 6.2. This maneuver may also enable double heterozygote S-D cases to be distinguished when these patients might otherwise masquerade as mild homozygous S patients.

DOUBLE HETEROZYGOTE STATES

Patients inheriting genes for different hemoglobinopathies from each parent may manifest a disease which is less severe than homozygous SS disease but much more of a clinical problem than the trait alone. Sickle thalassemia presents many of the complicating features of sickle cell disease but should be suspected if splenomegaly persists into adulthood and the clinical course has been generally milder. The finding of significant targeting of the red cells in the peripheral blood in addition to sickling may be an important clue. Most ST patients will have some combination of hemoglobin S, hemoglobin A, and hemoglobin F, although some may have no hemoglobin A and therefore be very difficult to distinguish from a homozygous sickle patient. Family studies are essential in these cases. SC disease is also milder than SS disease but again may have many of the manifestations seen in SS disease. In both these groups of patients the complication rate increases significantly during pregnancy, and they may have a significant splenic component contributing to their hemolytic state which may warrant splenectomy to ameliorate the situation.

METHEMOGLOBIN

The methemoglobins are structural hemoglobin variants characterized by an amino acid substitution which predisposes the heme to remain in the Fe^{+++} and to resist reduction to Fe^{++}. In this state heme is incapable of transporting oxygen. The abnormality has been identified only in heterozygotes. Presumably the homozygous state is lethal. Normally only 1% of circulating hemoglobin exists as methemoglobin because the NAD-dependent diaphorase of the red cell normally reduces methemoglobin to ferrous hemoglobin.

Patients with the M hemoglobins indicated in Table 7-2 are normally asymptomatic except for persistent moderate cyanosis, which is seen when methemoglobin values are higher than 1.5 gm per 100 ml. Therapy with ascorbic acid or methylene blue, or both, which are used for acquired methemoglobin, is ineffective in this disorder; but generally the patients are asymptomatic and require no therapy.

The disorder appears to be related to amino acid substitutions which give rise to internal ligand formation, with the heme iron being stabilized in the trivalent state.

HEMOGLOBINS WITH ALTERED OXYGEN AFFINITY

Several of the unstable hemoglobin syndromes may also manifest altered affinity of the hemoglobin molecule for oxygen, but this fact is usually clinically less significant than the structural instability leading to shortened red cell life-span. Only in recent years, however, has another group of amino acid substitutions been recognized in which there is no physical instability or shortening of the red cell life-span, but only an altered oxygen affinity. To date, seven hemoglobins have been reported to have reduced oxygen affinity, while fifteen abnormal hemoglobins have been reported with increased oxygen affinity and a resultant erythrocytosis. The pathophysiology of the altered oxygen dissociation pattern in these disorders and the unstable hemoglobins are discussed in Chapter 10.

In the compensated state, patients having abnormal hemoglobins with high oxygen affinity have hematocrit values usually from 48 to 60%, but occasionally up as high as 65%. These patients are generally asymptomatic, but the elevated hematocrit poses an important problem in the differential diagnosis of polycythemia. Unlike patients with polycythemia vera, these patients do not have leukocytosis or thrombocytosis, but they must be distinguished from individuals having erythrocytosis secondary to pathologic secretion of erythropoietin by some type of tumor. An oxygen dissociation curve is critical for this distinction.

One potentially significant clinical problem is that associated with pregnancy. Since the normal supply of oxygen to the fetus across the placenta depends on the fact that fetal hemoglobin has a higher affinity than adult hemoglobin for oxygen, females with the hemoglobins having pathologically high oxygen affinities may be subject to frequent abortions because of fetal hypoxia. Whether this becomes a clinical problem or not obviously depends upon the magnitude of the shift in the oxygen dissociation curve. Since most patients with this abnormality do not have hematocrit values which rise above 60%, abnormal blood viscosity is not usually a problem. The fact that viscosity increases strikingly with hematocrit values above 60% suggests that patients who are predisposed to vascular occlusion for any reason should be maintained at a hematocrit level below 60% by phlebotomy. Similarly, since arteriography may often be part of the work-up of a patient with unexplained erythrocytosis, it is important to recognize that the contrast dye employed is by itself capable of inducing a significant increase in blood viscosity. For this reason it is desirable to phlebotomize polycythemia patients to near-normal hematocrit readings prior to undertaking contrast dye studies, since the additive viscosity effects of the dye and the high hematocrit value may predispose to an episode of vascular occlusion.

REFERENCES

Abel, H. E., Bradley, T. B., Jr., and Ranney, H. M.   Pathophysiology of the hemoglobinopathies. *Clin. Obstet. Gynec.* 12:15, 1969.

Bank, A., and Marks, P. A.   Genetic control of hemoglobin synthesis and the thalassemia syndromes. *Med. Clin. N. Amer.* 53:875, 1969.

Charache, S., Grisolia, S., Fiedler, A. J., and Hellegers, A. E.   Effect of 2,3-

diphosphoglycerate on oxygen affinity of blood in sickle cell anemia. *J. Clin. Invest.* 49:806, 1970.

Freeman, M. G., and Ruth, G. J.   SS disease, SC disease, and CC disease: Obstetric considerations and treatment. *Clin. Obstet. Gynec.* 12:134, 1969.

Heller, P.   Hemoglobinopathic dysfunction of the red cell. *Amer. J. Med.* 41:799, 1966.

Huehns, E. R., and Bellingham, A. J.   Diseases of function and stability of haemoglobin. *Brit. J. Haemat.* 17:1, 1969.

Jaffé, E. R., and Heller, P.   Methemoglobinemia in Man. In E. B. Brown and C. V. Moore (Eds.), *Progress in Hematology,* Vol. 4. New York: Grune & Stratton, 1964.

Lehmann, H., and Carrell, R. W.   Variations in the structure of human haemoglobin. *Brit. Med. Bull.* 25:14, 1969.

Rucknagel, D. L., and Laros, R. K., Jr.   Hemoglobinopathies: Genetics and implications for studies of human reproduction. *Clin. Obstet. Gynec.* 12:49, 1969.

Weatherall, D. J., and Clegg, J. B.   The Control of Human Hemoglobin Synthesis and Function in Health and Disease. In E. B. Brown and C. V. Moore (Eds.), *Progress in Hematology,* Vol. 6. New York: Grune & Stratton, 1969.

8. HEREDITARY SPHEROCYTOSIS

Lawrence E. Young

AMONG THE hereditary hemolytic disorders, hereditary spherocytosis and hereditary elliptocytosis are the best-known examples of defects in the red cell membrane. These disorders, with subtle abnormalities of the cell membrane, are to be contrasted with the recently but precisely identified deficiencies in enzyme activity of red cells and with the hemoglobinopathies. Although this chapter focuses attention on spherocytosis, it should be kept in mind that hereditary elliptocytosis is similar in many respects, including response to splenectomy.

About 100 patients with hereditary spherocytosis have been studied in our clinic during the last 25 years. These patients have been drawn from a region with a population currently listed at about 1,250,000. These figures and other estimates—as high as 200 to 300 cases per million—indicate that hereditary spherocytosis is not a major medical problem in terms of frequency, even among populations of predominantly northern European extraction. There are, nevertheless, two cogent reasons for devoting continuing attention to this disorder:

1. Much can be done for the propositus and his relatives, usually by splenectomy, once diagnosis is established.
2. Studies on this disorder are contributing steadily to our understanding of medical genetics, of red blood cell structure and metabolism, and of the splenic circulation and its effects upon red cell structure and metabolism.

Vanlair and Masius are credited with the first description of hereditary spherocytosis, in 1871. They described small, spherical red cells which were more deeply colored than normal and suggested that these cells were about to be destroyed and thus would contribute an excess of bile pigment.

It is humbling to realize that 100 years later we are still seeking a precise definition of the abnormality in the red cells of these patients.

Splenectomy was performed by Spencer Wells in England in 1887 on a 27-year-old woman who had had recurrent jaundice since age 9 and an abdominal tumor that proved at laparotomy to be an enlarged spleen. Wells seems to have reasoned that the enlarged spleen should be considered fair game for a surgeon. The patient's jaundice was promptly relieved. Osmotic fragility of her red blood cells was determined nearly 40 years later and found to be increased. Since she had a son with hemolytic icterus and increased osmotic fragility of the red cells that persisted after splenectomy, it seems likely that Wells's patient was suffering from hereditary spherocytosis. The efficacy of splenectomy in this disorder became well established during the second decade of this century.

CLINICAL FEATURES

Hereditary spherocytosis may be diagnosed at any age. Our youngest patient was diagnosed on the first day of life. Spherocytosis is in fact a more common cause of neonatal jaundice than generally appreciated. Our oldest patient, the grandmother of a propositus, was first shown to have spherocytosis at age 90.

Figure 8-1 illustrates the principal laboratory abnormalities in one of our patients whose splenectomy was delayed until age 13, by which time gallstones had developed. Cholecystectomy was performed at a separate operation. Like most patients with the disease, this young man appeared to be

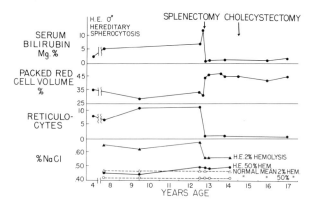

Figure 8-1. Changes in principal laboratory abnormalities after splenectomy in a representative patient.

healthy except for mild anemia, mild icterus, splenomegaly, and the complications of cholelithiasis. In our experience, skeletal abnormalities and leg ulcers are uncommon. Bilirubinemia, anemia, and reticulocytosis were terminated promptly by splenectomy in this case, but the "lateral" plot of osmotic fragility indicates that the median fragility, i.e., the percent NaCl at which 50% of the red cells were hemolyzed, remained considerably above normal after operation. There was reduction in the percent NaCl causing 2% hemolysis, an expression of the fact that red cells with the most marked increase in osmotic fragility were not evident after splenectomy.

A large share of patients with hereditary spherocytosis develop gallstones if not splenectomized before puberty. Delay in splenectomy, as in this case because of delay in parental consent, may thus have significant consequences. Another threat to these patients is the development of hyporegenerative crises which seem most apt to accompany infection. Since folate requirement is increased in this disorder, as in other hemolytic states, administration of folic acid may help to minimize failure of marrow response to increased demand. Impaired erythropoiesis is of little consequence in a person with red cells having a normal life-span of about 120 days. If the life-span is reduced to about 10 to 20 days or less, as in most patients with hereditary spherocytosis, a marked decrease in erythropoiesis associated with infection may become a serious matter. In the absence of infection or folate deficiency the bone marrow usually compensates sufficiently to maintain the hematocrit level above 30% and in some patients above 40%. Patients with hematocrit levels consistently below 25% are uncommon. Hemochromatosis, presumably resulting from increased iron absorption over a long period of time, has been described in patients with hereditary spherocytosis in whom splenectomy had not been performed or had been delayed until the third decade or later. The frequency of this complication has not been determined.

INHERITANCE

This disorder is inherited as an autosomal dominant trait. We have encountered 6 patients with probable hereditary spherocytosis whose parents were both normal, as determined by all available hematologic examinations. One patient had a maternal grandparent with spherocytosis, thus indicating strongly that the mother of the propositus carried the gene for spherocytosis but did not express it sufficiently to be recognized by available methods. Another propositus with hematologically normal parents had a sibling with spherocytosis, suggesting that spherocytosis in the propositus was not due to chance mutation and that one of the parents probably carried the mutant gene for this disorder. Similar findings have been reported by other observers. Studies aimed at detection of the genetic "carriers" of spherocytosis may help to elucidate the nature of the red cell membrane abnormality in its most feebly expressed state.

ALTERATIONS IN RED CELLS INCUBATED IN VITRO OR SEQUESTERED IN THE SPLEEN

Representative osmotic fragility curves are shown in Figure 8-2 with plots drawn to relate percent NaCl in the medium to the percent hemoglobin liberated from each sample of red cells from patients with hereditary spherocytosis prior to splenectomy. In some patients the fragility curve may be within or near the normal range, while in others a substantial portion of the red cell population has considerable increase in fragility as measured by this method. The most fragile cells in the circulation, i.e., those producing "tails" or "humps" in fragility curves such as illustrated in Figure 8-2, are thought to be cells "conditioned" by passage through the spleen. Griggs, Weisman, and Harris tagged with radioactive iron newly formed cells from patients with hereditary spherocytosis and showed that the new population of cells required about 10 days to reach the same degree of increase in osmotic fragility as the rest of the red cell population. This finding is in accord with the fact that the average life-span of red cells in this disorder is most frequently in the range of 10 to 20 days.

The effects of sterile in vitro incubation of red cells at body temperature were first studied systematically by Ham and Castle, who suggested that

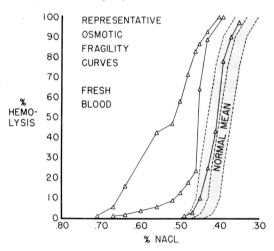

Figure 8-2. Representative osmotic fragility curves of fresh blood obtained prior to splenectomy in hereditary spherocytosis (see text). (From L. E. Young and G. Miller, *Amer. J. Med. Sci.* 226:664, 1953.)

changes taking place during in vitro incubation might be similar to those occurring when red cells are trapped within the spleen. Osmotic fragility curves obtained with red cells from patients with hereditary spherocytosis, after incubation of the cells at body temperature for 24 hours, are shifted much more toward the left than are curves obtained with normal red cells if results are plotted in graphs, as in Figure 8-2. Measurements of fragility of incubated red cells may thus be helpful in diagnosis when the fragility of freshly drawn red cells is in or near the normal range. It should be kept in mind that many changes occur in red cells during in vitro incubation. In general, changes found in hereditary spherocytes at 24 hours are found in normal red cells after incubation for periods of 36 to 48 hours.

Studies of osmotic fragility of hereditary spherocytes obtained at the time of splenectomy are of much interest. Samples of red cells from the spleen minced in a meat grinder immediately after removal from the patient invariably give results similar to those obtained after incubation of spherocytes from a peripheral vein. Red cells from the minced preparation are washed in autogenous serum to remove leukocytes and splenic tissue cells before the fragility measurements are made. Osmotic fragility curves thus obtained with red cells from the minced spleen are believed to show the effect of red cell stagnation within the splenic pulp. The lesser fragility of red cells in the splenic vein probably reflects mixing of red cells that have been sequestered in the splenic pulp with red cells that have passed from splenic arterioles to venous sinusoids by more direct routes. Samples of peripheral venous blood drawn at splenectomy for purposes of comparison represent still greater mixing of conditioned red cells with other red cells in the circulation.

The range of osmotic fragility curves obtained with red cells freshly drawn from a peripheral vein is illustrated in Figure 8-2. In any given patient the fragility is significantly greater in red cells from the splenic vein and still greater in red cells from the minced spleen.

In an effort to demonstrate a selective effect of the spleen on spherocytes as compared with normal-donor red cells, patients with hereditary spherocytosis have been transfused prior to splenectomy with normal red cells that could be differentiated serologically. Differential osmotic fragility curves for donor and autogenous cells have been plotted in such experiments by determining the proportion of the two types of cell remaining unhemolyzed in each tube of hypotonic saline solution. The results of such an experiment are illustrated in Figure 8-3, which shows (A) a blood smear prepared from peripheral capillary blood after transfusion of normal red cells and at the time of splenectomy, and (B) a blood smear prepared from red cells washed from the splenic pulp after mincing in the meat grinder. Spherocytes are scarce in the smear shown in (A), but numerous in the smear in (B). Differential studies showed clearly that the spherocytes were the patient's own cells. In the experiment illustrated, 61% of the red cells in the periph-

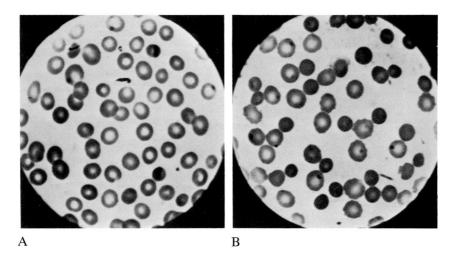

A   B

Figure 8-3. (A) Smear of capillary blood from transfused patient at time of splenectomy. (B) Smear of washed red cells from minced spleen of same patient. (From L. E. Young et al., *Blood* 6:1099, 1951.)

eral blood were autogenous, whereas 84% of the red cells in the splenic minced preparation were autogenous. The patient's own red cells were thus selectively trapped within the splenic pulp, and in that location they underwent a considerable increase in osmotic fragility. The normal donor cells, on the other hand, were found in smaller proportion in the splenic pulp than in the peripheral blood, and there was little or no increase in osmotic fragility of the normal donor cells within the spleen.

MECHANISM OF SPLENIC TRAPPING OF SPHEROCYTES

It has been believed for some time that there is nothing peculiar to the spleen in hereditary spherocytosis and that perhaps any human spleen will trap hereditary spherocytes. This belief was tested in a series of relatively crude experiments in which hereditary spherocytes of blood group O were mixed with normal group A red cells and perfused through spleens immediately after their removal from patients with idiopathic thrombocytopenic purpura. The perfusions were carried out for two hours at body temperature by pumping the two types of red cells into the splenic vein, collecting the blood escaping from the splenic artery, and pumping the red cell mixture back into the splenic vein again. In each of three such experiments the spherocytic group O cells were selectively removed from the mixture and predominated in the splenic pulp at the end of the perfusion. The donor of the spherocytes for each of these studies had been splenectomized, with the usual prompt relief of anemia and jaundice.

Weisman and associates obtained still more convincing results by transfusing group O spherocytes to a group A patient with thrombocytopenia. In their experiment 3% of the red cells in the peripheral blood were donor spherocytes, whereas 49% of the cells in the splenic minced preparation were group O spherocytes, thus showing highly selective retention of the abnormal cells.

The studies cited above are in accord with the demonstration that normal-donor red cells survive normally in patients with hereditary spherocytosis, whereas hereditary spherocytes drawn either before or after splenectomy undergo rapid destruction following transfusion to normal recipients. On the other hand, hereditary spherocytes survive almost normally when transfused into a recipient following splenectomy for traumatic rupture of the spleen. The capacity of various types of human spleens to trap and selectively condition and destroy hereditary spherocytes thus seems amply demonstrated. It is noteworthy that the patient's spherocytes may be destroyed less rapidly in his own circulation than in that of a normal recipient, perhaps because of reticuloendothelial blockade, accumulation of spherocytes within the splenic pulp, or arteriovenous shunting of blood within the patient's own spleen.

It has been recognized for many years that the splenic pulp in patients with hereditary spherocytosis is well packed with red cells, while the sinusoids appear relatively empty as seen in the customary tissue sections. Dacie has reported difficulty in washing red cells from the spleen of patients with hereditary spherocytosis when the spleen is perfused with saline solution. In the spleen of both the deer mouse and of man afflicted with spherocytosis, the red cell content per gram of spleen is about 3 to 5 times that of normal members of the same species. Studies by Anderson, Huestis, and Motulsky in the deer mouse, which provides an excellent animal model of hereditary spherocytosis, have shown that spherocytes are destroyed more rapidly in the normal mouse spleen than in the spleen of the spherocytic mouse. The spleen of the spherocytic mouse, like that of spherocytic man, is relatively packed with stagnating red cells and thus less able to trap additional spherocytes than a normal spleen containing few red cells prior to introduction of the spherocytes.

The proportion of red cells passing directly from splenic arterioles to venous sinusoids may vary from one individual to another and from time to time in the same individual. Red cells taking a more circuitous route through the cords of Billroth are required to pass through openings as narrow at 3 μ or less to enter the sinusoids from cordal tissue. There is probably more need for deformability of red blood cells to permit passage through the splenic pulp than through any other part of the body. The normally biconcave red cell, which is remarkably pliable, seems to manage well, but the spherocyte has difficulty.

Crosby and Conrad bled spherocytic patients until iron deficiency was produced with resultant thinning of the red cells and reduction in osmotic fragility to a nearly normal state. Hemolysis nevertheless continued at the usual rate, and the red cells were found trapped in the spleen much the same as though their thickness had not been reduced by iron deficiency. These experiments indicate that hereditary spherocytes probably are not trapped because of abnormal thickness. More recent studies suggest that trapping is related chiefly to inherent rigidity of the hereditary spherocyte.

ADDITIONAL STUDIES ON INCUBATED RED CELLS

When hereditary spherocytes are incubated in vitro for 48 hours at body temperature, they nearly always undergo much more lysis than do normal cells. Measurements of spontaneous autohemolysis at this interval may aid in case detection to about the same extent as measurements of osmotic fragility after incubation of the red cells for 24 hours. Addition of glucose to the incubating red cells usually reduces markedly the extent of autohemolysis. In a small proportion of cases such reduction in autohemolysis is not evident until after splenectomy. These patients have very marked spherocytosis, proportionately marked increase in osmotic fragility, and abnormally low lipid content of the red cell stroma, thus presumably reflecting marked conditioning of the red cells by the spleen. After splenectomy the red cells have normal lipid content, spherocytosis and increase in osmotic fragility are less marked, and the usual reduction in autohemolysis by glucose is observed. It seems likely that these patients do not represent a distinct, genetically determined variant of hereditary spherocytosis but are instead examples of the disease in which splenic conditioning of the red cells is strongly manifest.

Bertles measured the influx of radioactive sodium into the red cells from 10 of the splenectomized spherocytic patients in our clinic. The sodium transport rates ranged from high normal to considerably elevated values but did not correlate with osmotic fragility or rate of autohemolysis. Wiley recently reported a negative correlation between the rate of sodium influx and the survival time of hereditary spherocytes after transfusion to normal recipients. Jacob and Jandl demonstrated an increased rate of sodium efflux from red cells in hereditary spherocytosis and suggested that the increased energy requirement for active transport of sodium might be met within the active circulation but could not be provided within the spleen.

The rate of glycolysis in hereditary spherocytes is increased only slightly over normal, if measurements are made with physiologic concentrations of glucose and phosphate and with red cells from splenectomized patients in whom the contribution of immature red cells is largely eliminated. It is noteworthy, moreover, that the turnover rate of adenosine triphosphate in hereditary spherocytes is within normal limits. It seems unlikely that deficient energy production with consequent inability to prevent sodium accumulation is a significant part of the hemolytic mechanism in this disorder. Spherocytes increase in volume during about the first 16 hours of in vitro incubation but then shrink prior to hemolysis, the volume change becoming most pronounced during the second 24-hour period of incubation in the customary autohemolysis test. The role of glucose in maintaining the normal lipid and protein structure of the red cell membrane may be much more significant than its role in supplying energy to the sodium pump. Ouabain, which inhibits the sodium-potassium pump, does not interfere with the protective effect of glucose on autohemolysis. Spherocytosis reflects a decrease in the ratio between surface area of the red cell and its osmotically active constituents which in turn control the cell volume. If increased permeability of the hereditary spherocyte leads to sodium accumulation and increased volume, one would expect swelling of the cells prior to hemolysis; but in fact, the cells are known to decrease in volume. For reasons that follow, loss of cell membrane with consequent decrease in surface to volume ratio is quite likely of major importance in lysis.

When spherocytes are incubated in vitro, the loss of lipid during the first 24-hour period greatly exceeds that of incubated normal red cells. Since each lipid component is lost in proportion to its original content, data obtained from these studies support the growing conviction that fragmentation or loss of whole portions of the red cell membrane occurs during incubation in vitro as well as during splenic sequestration. Addition of glucose exerts a significant inhibitory effect on lipid loss as on autohemolysis. If ouabain is added in concentrations sufficient to inhibit the sodium-potassium pump, the effect of glucose on lipid loss continues.

Fragmentation of red cells in the circulation, within the splenic pulp, and in in vitro preparations has not been fully appreciated until recently. Preparations examined with the aid of phase microscopy, and in some instances with electron microscopy, reveal that fragmentation may be the final common pathway of red cell destruction in many hemolytic disorders. When hereditary spherocytes are incubated in platelet-free plasma, fragmentation becomes evident much sooner than in preparations of normal cells similarly incubated. Red cell fragments are also evident, if looked for, in the splenic pulp of both mice and men afflicted with hereditary spherocytosis. Red cell fragments can be identified within splenic macrophages, but erythrophagocytosis, i.e., phagocytosis of whole red cells, is not seen.

RED CELL RIGIDITY

LaCelle and Weed have applied the method of Rand and Burton to measure the negative pressure required to draw a portion of a red cell into or through a micropipette. When a portion of a red cell is removed by manipulation with the micropipette, the result is a greater loss of membrane than of cellular contents. The portion of the red cell remaining outside the pipette therefore becomes more nearly spherical and has increased rigidity as measured by the pressure required to draw the cell into or through the pipette. Whenever the portion of a red cell remaining outside the pipette is a perfect sphere, its rigidity is markedly increased. It seems likely that a similar increase in rigidity of hereditary spherocytes occurs as they lose portions of the cell membrane during repeated passages through the splenic pulp.

It is remarkable, moreover, that even prior to incubation hereditary spherocytes are shown to have much more rigidity or lack of deformability than normal red cells, as measured with the micropipette. With incubation, the rigidity of the spherocytes increases much more rapidly than that of normal red cells similarly incubated. The rigidity is a manifestation both of membrane abnormality and of cell shape rather than of cellular contents, since spherocytic ghosts and normal red cell ghosts show similar differences in deformability. The difference between the two types of cells, or their ghosts, increases as ATP concentration is reduced while calcium ion concentration remains constant.

LaCelle and Weed have recently shown that hereditary spherocytes manifest a marked increase in rigidity at oxygen tensions which are just slightly below that of the normal mixed venous Po_2. This effect has been attributed to the binding of adenosine triphosphate to deoxyhemoglobin. It seems likely that the low oxygen concentration within the splenic pulp as a consequence of red cell stagnation may limit the availability of ATP to a cell that is already somewhat rigid, and may thus make the cell still more rigid.

CURRENT CONCEPT OF HEMOLYTIC MECHANISM

A reasonable current concept of pathogenetic mechanisms in hereditary spherocytosis is presented in Figure 8-4. The mutant gene for this disorder is thought to determine an abnormality of the red cell membrane, the exact nature of which has not yet been elucidated. Increased permeability to sodium is an accepted feature of membrane abnormality but is thought not to be importantly involved in hemolysis. Of greater significance is the rigidity, or lack of deformability, of the hereditary spherocyte, which in turn seems largely responsible for its difficulty in passing through the splenic pulp.

When the spherocyte is trapped within the splenic pulp, the decreased availability of ATP because of increased binding to deoxyhemoglobin results in loss of cell surface, both lipid and protein, i.e., fragmentation. As a consequence of surface loss, the cell becomes more nearly spherical in shape and more rigid, and thus all the more liable to be trapped during its next circuit through the spleen if it takes the route through the splenic pulp rather than a more direct route from splenic arteriole to venous sinusoid. A vicious circle of conditioning of the hereditary spherocyte thus occurs with repeated passages through the spleen, until the cell disintegrates and the fragments are disposed of by splenic macrophages. It is noteworthy that neither erythrophagocytosis (of whole red cells) within the spleen nor accumulation of oxyhemoglobin or methemalbumin in the peripheral circulation can be demonstrated in patients with hereditary spherocytosis. Haptoglobin is nevertheless consistently depleted, presumably because of its binding to hemoglobin liberated from the cells destroyed within the spleen.

Once the splenic trap is removed, the membrane abnormality of the hereditary spherocyte is of little or no consequence. The inherent rigidity of the red cell is not such as to interfere with its negotiation of other circulatory pathways.

It seems unlikely that any treatment preferable to splenectomy will be found for this disorder. This condition is an excellent example of a medical problem for which adequate management has been found long before precise understanding of abnormalities of structure and metabolism could be achieved. Hereditary spherocytosis is also an excellent example of the interaction of hereditary and environmental factors in causing symptoms. In this instance the unfavorable environment is largely confined to the

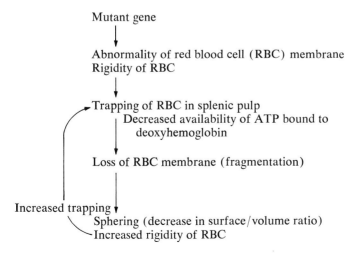

Figure 8-4.   Concept of pathogenic mechanisms in hereditary spherocytosis.

spleen, an organ that fortunately can be eliminated with relative ease and safety after the early years of childhood. Although the guidelines for clinical management of hereditary spherocytosis now seem clear, the precise nature of the red cell abnormality in this disorder presents a continuing challenge for further study.

REFERENCES

Anderson, R., Huestis, R. R., and Motulsky, A. G. Hereditary spherocytosis in the deer mouse: Its similarity to the human disease. *Blood* 15:491, 1960.

Barry, M., Scheuer, P. J., Sherlock, S., Ross, C. F., and Williams, R. Hereditary spherocytosis with secondary haemochromatosis. *Lancet* 2:481, 1968.

Bertles, J. F. Sodium transport across the surface membrane of red blood cells in hereditary spherocytosis. *J. Clin. Invest.* 36:816, 1957.

Crosby, W. H., and Conrad, M. E. Hereditary spherocytosis: Observations on hemolytic mechanisms and iron metabolism. *Blood* 15:662, 1960.

Dacie, J. V. *The Haemolytic Anaemias: Congenital and Acquired* (2d ed.). Part I, *The Congenital Anaemias*. New York: Grune & Stratton, 1960.

Dacie, J. V. Recent advances in knowledge of the hereditary haemolytic anaemias. *Schweiz. Med. Wschr.* 98:1624, 1968.

Dawson of Penn. The Hume lectures on haemolytic icterus. *Brit. Med. J.* 1:963, 1931.

Emerson, C. P., Jr., Shen, S. C., Ham, T. H., Fleming, E. M., and Castle, W. B. Studies on the destruction of red blood cells: IX. Quantitative methods for determining the osmotic and mechanical fragility of red cells in the peripheral blood and splenic pulp: The mechanism of increased hemolysis in hereditary spherocytosis (congenital hemolytic jaundice) as related to the functions of the spleen. *Arch. Intern. Med.* (Chicago) 97:1, 1956.

Griggs, R. C., Weisman, R. J., and Harris, J. W. Alterations in osmotic and mechanical fragility related to in vivo erythrocyte aging and splenic sequestration in hereditary spherocytosis. *J. Clin. Invest.* 39:89, 1960.

Ham, T. H., and Castle, W. B. Relation of increased hypotonic fragility and of erythrostasis to the mechanism of hemolysis in certain anemias. *Trans. Ass. Amer. Physicians* 55:127, 1940.

Jacob, H. W., and Jandl, J. W. Cell membrane permeability in the pathogenesis of hereditary spherocytosis. *J. Clin. Invest.* 43:1704, 1964.

Jandl, J. H. Hereditary Spherocytosis. In E. Beutler (Ed.), *Hereditary Disorders of Erythrocyte Metabolism*. New York: Grune & Stratton, 1968.

LaCelle, P. L., and Weed, R. I. Reversibility of abnormal deformability and permeability of the hereditary spherocyte. *Blood* 34:858, 1969.

LaCelle, P. L., and Weed, R. I. Low oxygen pressure: A cause of erythrocyte membrane rigidity. *J. Clin. Invest.* 49:54a, 1970.

Langley, G. R., and Felderhof, C. H. Atypical autohemolysis in hereditary spherocytosis as a reflection of two cell populations: Relationship of cell lipids to conditioning by the spleen. *Blood* 32:569, 1968.

Reed, C. F., and Swisher, S. M. Erythrocyte lipid loss in hereditary spherocytosis. *J. Clin. Invest.* 45:777, 1966.

Reed, C. F., and Young, L. E. Erythrocyte energy metabolism in hereditary spherocytosis. *J. Clin. Invest.* 46:1196, 1967.

Selwyn, J. G., and Dacie, J. V.   Autohemolysis and other changes resulting from the incubation in vitro of red cells from patients with congenital hemolytic anemia. *Blood* 9:414, 1954.

Weed, R. I.   The importance of erythrocyte deformability. *Amer. J. Med.* 49:147, 1970.

Weed, R. I., and Bowdler, A. J.   Metabolic dependence of the critical hemolytic volume of human erythrocytes: Relationship to osmotic fragility and autohemolysis in hereditary spherocytosis and normal red cells. *J. Clin. Invest.* 45:1137, 1966.

Weed, R. I., LaCelle, P. L., and Merrill, E. W.   Metabolic dependence of red cell deformability. *J. Clin. Invest.* 48:795, 1969.

Weisman, R. J., Ham, T. H., Hinz, C. F., Jr., and Harris, J. W.   Studies of the role of the spleen in the destruction of erythrocytes. *Trans. Ass. Amer. Physicians* 68:131, 1955.

Wiley, J. S.   Red cell survival studies in hereditary spherocytosis. *J. Clin. Invest.* 49:666, 1970.

Wiley, J. S., and Firkin, B. G.   An unusual variant of hereditary spherocytosis. *Amer. J. Med.* 48:63, 1970.

Williams, J. D., Scott, P. J., and North, J. D. K.   Hemochromatosis in association with hereditary spherocytosis. *Arch. Intern. Med.* (Chicago) 120:701, 1967.

Young, L. E., Izzo, M. J., Altman, K. I., and Swisher, S. N.   Studies on spontaneous in vitro autohemolysis in hemolytic disorders. *Blood* 11:977, 1956.

Young, L. E., and Miller, G.   Differentiation between congenital and acquired forms of hemolytic anemia: Observations on 47 cases of hereditary spherocytosis and 24 cases of autoimmune hemolytic disease. *Amer. J. Med. Sci.* 226:664, 1953.

Young, L. E., Platzer, R. F., Ervin, D. M., and Izzo, M. J.   Hereditary spherocytosis: II. Observations on the role of the spleen. *Blood* 6:1099, 1951.

9. ACQUIRED IMMUNE HEMOLYTIC DISORDERS: CLINICAL ASPECTS AND LABORATORY EVALUATION

Richard F. Bakemeier
John P. Leddy

ACQUIRED IMMUNE HEMOLYTIC DISORDERS (AIHD) are characterized by shortened red cell life-span in vivo mediated by one or more components of the immune system. The red cells of patients with these disorders often demonstrate a positive direct antiglobulin or Coombs' test, and antibodies reactive with the patient's own red cells may be found in the serum.

Such disorders can be classified as either *idiopathic* or *secondary* (symptomatic) (Table 9-1). In the former category, comprising half to two-thirds of cases, no associated disease can be detected. Associated with the secondary cases are (a) underlying malignant proliferative disorders of the lymphoreticular tissues, such as malignant lymphoma or chronic lymphocytic leukemia; (b) connective tissue disorders, particularly systemic lupus erythematosus; (c) certain infections including *Mycoplasma* pneumonia and infectious mononucleosis; (d) exposure to certain drugs; and less commonly (e) nonlymphoid tumors such as ovarian teratoma and (f) chronic inflammatory states such as ulcerative colitis.

AIHD may also be classified according to the serologic characteristics of the antibodies involved, particularly relating to the reactivity of the antibodies at different temperatures. In general, two major categories can be identified: those with *warm-active* autoantibodies, reacting best at about 37°C, and those with *cold-active* autoantibodies with optimal activity at lower temperatures, often below 10°C. The latter autoantibodies are associated with two clinical syndromes, cold agglutinin disease and paroxysmal cold hemoglobinuria. Idiopathic and secondary forms occur in association with both warm-active and cold-active autoantibodies.

Supported in part by U.S. Public Health Service Grants AI-04841 and AM-09810. Dr. Bakemeier is recipient of U.S. Public Health Service Research Career Development Award AM-14902. Dr. Leddy is a recipient of the Senior Investigator Award of the Arthritis Foundation.

Table 9-1.   Classification of Acquired Immune Hemolytic Disorders

---

With warm-active autoantibodies
  Idiopathic
  Secondary
    Associated with lymphoreticular malignancies, systemic lupus
      erythematosus, infections, ovarian teratoma

With cold-active autoantibodies
  Idiopathic (cold agglutinin disease)
  Secondary
    Associated with *Mycoplasma* pneumonia, infectious mononucleosis,
      lymphomas
  Paroxysmal cold hemoglobinuria
    Idiopathic
    Secondary
      Associated with viral infections or syphilis

Drug-related
  Haptene mechanism (penicillin)
  Immune complex mechanism (quinidine, quinine, stibophen)
  Anti-RBC antibodies (α-methyldopa, mefenamic acid)

HEMOLYTIC DISEASE WITH WARM-ACTIVE AUTOANTIBODIES

AIHD with warm-active antibodies occurs at all ages but is most common in older adults, when the incidence of lymphoid neoplasia also increases. Because the severity varies considerably, with many patients having no anemia despite positive direct antiglobulin tests, the actual incidence is difficult to assess. For example, serologic evidence of red cell autoantibodies has been found in up to 20% of patients with chronic lymphocytic leukemia (CLL), although the incidence of associated overt hemolytic anemia in CLL is probably only 5% or less.

CLINICAL FINDINGS.   The clinical manifestations range from those of a mild anemia slowly progressive over several months to a fulminating hemolytic anemia with jaundice and prostration. Stress such as surgery, infection, or pregnancy may precipitate such an acute episode. The onset of hemolysis has been observed to occur not long after alkylation therapy for an associated lymphoma. Physical signs include variable pallor, icterus, and splenomegaly of moderate degree. Massive splenic enlargement in AIHD may be associated with lymphoid malignancy.

LABORATORY FINDINGS.   An elevated reticulocyte count is regularly present although anemia may be slight or absent, depending on the ability of the bone marrow to compensate for the degree of shortening of red cell life-span in a particular patient. The bone marrow is normally able to compensate for decreases in red cell life-span with a sixfold maximal increase in erythropoiesis. Anemia usually develops when the half-life of ^{51}Cr-labeled cells is below 5 days. During highly active hemolysis, spherocytosis, fragmented red cells, normoblastemia, and punctate basophilia are seen in the peripheral blood smear. Indeed, acquired spherocytosis should alert the physician to the possibility of AIHD. A positive direct antiglobulin test should serve to distinguish AIHD from hereditary spherocytosis. White blood cell counts often are moderately elevated with neutrophilia unless an associated neoplastic lymphocytosis is present. Blood monocytes may occasionally show erythrophagocytosis, and this process, particularly in the form of partial phagocytosis of red cells in the spleen, is thought to contribute to red cell fragmentation. Platelets may be normal, elevated, or decreased; occasionally thrombocytopenia is marked and the patient appears to have both idiopathic thrombocytopenic purpura and AIHD.

The urine may contain mildly increased urobilinogen. The bone marrow usually shows normoblastic erythroid hyperplasia, although occasionally megaloblastic changes may reflect associated folic acid deficiency caused by the greatly accelerated cell production in the marrow. Red blood cell osmotic fragility is increased in the presence of spherocytosis. However, autohemolysis tests show no correction of lysis by glucose, unlike the results in hereditary spherocytosis. Red cell life-span determinations usually are not required to diagnose AIHD but may be useful, in conjunction with organ scanning, to evaluate splenic sequestration in patients being considered for splenectomy.

SEROLOGIC ASPECTS. The serologic aspects of AIHD have received much attention in recent years. Antiglobulin tests employing rabbit antisera to human serum have been further refined by employing antisera against single immunoglobulin classes and against individual components of serum complement. Three major patterns of positive antiglobulin reaction are seen in AIHD with warm-active autoantibodies (Table 9-2): those with anti-IgG sera, those with both anti-IgG and anticomplement, and those with anticomplement only. Anticomplement was formerly called "anti-non-γ-globulin." In our experience the "anti-non-γ" reagents and broad-spectrum antisera ("γ + non-γ") obtained from commercial sources have often been weak in respect to anticomplement antibodies, so that complement ("non-γ") coating of red cells could be missed. No direct antiglobulin reactions with anti-IgA or anti-IgM sera have been seen at Rochester, although they have been observed elsewhere on isolated occasions. In those cases in which only complement can be detected on the red cells by the standard antiglobulin test, special techniques, such as antiglobulin consumption tests

Table 9-2. Patterns of Antiglobulin Tests in Acquired Immune Hemolytic Disorders

Antibody Characteristics	Direct Antiglobulin Test Positive with Antibody to:	Antibody Specificity
1. Warm-active	IgG	Often "Rh-related"* In some cases undefined
2. Warm-active	IgG + complement	Often undefined
3. Warm-active	Complement alone (subthreshold IgG)	Often undefined
4. Cold-active Cold agglutinins Donath-Landsteiner	Complement alone	Anti-I, -i; other Anti-P

* "Rh-related" signifies autoantibodies reactive with all human red cells except phenotype Rh_{null} (see text), in the presence or absence of additional autoantibodies having specificity for known Rh antigens (anti-e, anti-C, anti-c, or anti-D).

and the use of highly concentrated eluates, have detected small amounts of IgG autoantibody in the majority of such cases (see Gilliland et al.). This pattern has frequently been associated with systemic lupus erythematosus and often is not associated with significant hemolysis.

IgG warm-active autoantibodies may demonstrate definite specificities within the Rh system such as anti-e or anti-c, in which case the corresponding antigens are present in the patient's own red cells. More commonly the IgG antibodies react strongly with *all* common human red cell types and thus seem "nonspecific." However, in a substantial proportion of these cases the autoantibodies fail to react with red cells of the rare human phenotype Rh_{null} which lack all known Rh determinants. Such antibodies may have specificity for some fundamental structural unit or precursor substance of the Rh system and, in our experience, are usually found in patients exhibiting negative direct antiglobulin tests with anticomplement sera (pattern 1, Table 9-2). There remain a large number of cases in which the autoantibodies react strongly with Rh_{null} red cells and therefore may have specificity (or specificities) unrelated to Rh but so far undefined. It is of interest that these patients are particularly prone to give positive direct antiglobulin tests with both anti-IgG and anticomplement (pattern 2, Table 9-2). Additional aspects of serology in AIHD are discussed in the references by Leddy and Swisher, Dacie and Worlledge, and Leddy and Bakemeier.

CLINICAL COURSE. The clinical course of AIHD with warm autoantibodies is quite variable. Active hemolysis may subside after one episode. More commonly the disease is chronic, with periods of increased hemolysis, sometimes associated with stresses such as infections or trauma.

In a given patient's course, the intensity of direct antiglobulin reactions and hemolytic severity tend to be correlated. The severity of the hemolytic process cannot be predicted by the strength of the direct antiglobulin reactions. Some patients may demonstrate little or no anemia despite strongly positive antiglobulin tests. Other patients with overt hemolyic anemia show surprisingly modest direct antiglobulin reactions. Rarely, a patient is seen with active hemolytic anemia with so little red cell–bound IgG antibody that it escapes detection by antiglobulin tests but can be measured by special assays (see Gilliland et al.).

THERAPY.   Therapy of AIHD with warm-active autoantibodies is based primarily on the use of corticosteroids. At least three-quarters of patients benefit from such therapy, although only about one-fifth have a complete remission which persists after corticosteroids are discontinued. Ten percent or less have no appreciable benefit from such therapy. We recommend doses of 40 to 80 mg of prednisone daily for adults until the hemolytic process is clearly under control. This should be evident in 2 to 3 weeks if the patient is responsive to steroids. A very gradual decrease in dosage is then begun, over a period of months, with each step in reduction weighed against the patient's progress. It cannot be overemphasized that too rapid tapering is regularly followed by relapse. Severely ill patients with active hemolysis may benefit from large doses of intravenous hydrocortisone, e.g., 300 to 400 mg per day. ACTH has been used in steroid-unresponsive patients, occasionally with apparent success.

In steroid-responsive patients clinical improvement typically precedes any detectable change in the direct antiglobulin reactions. Then as steroid therapy continues, responsive patients show a gradual diminution in the strength of antiglobulin reaction and may, in the most favorable cases, become antiglobulin-negative. Our experience suggests that it is unwise in most cases to attempt complete withdrawal of steroids before the antiglobulin test has become negative. However, administering steroids every other day in roughly the same total weekly dose has recently been found effective in our clinic for maintaining clinical remission in those patients already brought under good control with daily steroids, and the side effects are far less troublesome.

Splenectomy has been performed on selected patients not responding to steroid therapy or who require excessive doses for prolonged periods to maintain remission. Splenectomy may also provide a source of diagnostic tissue in AIHD secondary to malignant lymphoma. Approximately 40% of patients reported from several centers have had "complete" or "good" remissions following splenectomy for AIHD. The spleen acts both as an effective filter for pathologic red cells such as spherocytes and as one likely source of antibody. Particularly affected are red cells which have become sensitized by moderate amounts of nonagglutinating IgG antibodies. Other reticuloendothelial tissues, especially in the liver, play a major role in removing red cells heavily sensitized by IgG antibodies or by complement-fixing or agglutinating antibodies. The utilization of chromium-labeled red cells and surface scanning has afforded certain predictive criteria which may be useful in selecting patients for splenectomy. A ratio of splenic uptake to liver uptake of greater than 2.3:1.0 was associated with a favorable response to splenectomy in the series of 15 patients reported by Allgood and Chaplin. Further discussion of this diagnostic procedure is contained in Chapter 4. Although reports of postoperative mortality have made some centers cautious in their use of splenectomy, the careful selection of patients for elective splenectomy during partial remission and close cooperation between members of a joint surgical-hematologic team make splenectomy an acceptable alternative (or adjunct) to long-term corticosteroid therapy.

Antimetabolites, especially azathioprine (Imuran), 6-mercaptopurine, and thioguanine, have been used as immunosuppressive agents with some success, especially in patients refractory to tolerable doses of corticosteroids and to splenectomy. Schwartz and Dameshek reported good responses in 4 of 9 patients treated with antimetabolites after an unsatisfactory response to corticosteroids. The usefulness of azathioprine in decreasing or eliminating the need for corticosteroids in childhood AIHD was demonstrated by Hitzig and Massimo. The use of other potent immunosuppressive agents such as cyclophosphamide deserves further study. This is particularly pertinent in those patients with an associated malignant lymphoma, in whose management therapy should be primarily directed toward the neoplastic disease. However, the erythropoiesis-suppressing effect of these cytotoxic agents must be weighed against the potential benefit of decreasing autoantibody synthesis.

Transfusions should be reserved for life-threatening situations and used with the recognition that they are usually temporary in their effect because of destruction of the transfused red cells. Since most autoantibody populations do not represent single, identifiable specificities, the transfusion usually involves serologically incompatible red cells. Increased jaundice, hemoglobinemia, fever, and general deterioration may occur owing to destruction of donor red cells. If a response to corticosteroids cannot be awaited, the choice of donor red cells which react no more strongly with the patient's serum than do the patient's own red cells is a reasonable compromise; but meticulous observation of the patient for complications is important.

Discussion of other therapeutic approaches to AIHD-associated warm-active autoantibodies such as heparin, thymectomy, and splenic irradiation are found in references by Dacie and by Pirofsky. More satisfactory management of AIHD must await further understanding of its pathogenesis and of normal mechanisms of immune tolerance.

HEMOLYTIC DISEASE WITH COLD-ACTIVE AUTOANTIBODIES

AIHD with cold-active antibodies manifests itself as several different clinical syndromes determined in part by the serologic characteristics of the associated autoantibodies (Table 9-1). Cold agglutinin–mediated AIHD may occur acutely in association with *Mycoplasma* pneumonia or infectious mononucleosis, or as chronic cold agglutinin disease, either idiopathic or associated with lymphoid neoplasia. Paroxysmal cold hemoglobinuria (PCH), characterized by intermittent intravascular hemolysis, may be idiopathic or associated with various viral disease or with syphilis.

COLD AGGLUTININ DISEASE

Cold agglutinin disease refers to a group of relatively uncommon disorders characterized by cold sensitivity, hemolytic anemia with positive antiglobulin tests of the anticomplement type, and high titers of anti–red cell antibodies causing maximal agglutination at low temperatures (0° to 5°C). The *acute form* may be a rare complication of *Mycoplasma* pneumonia, when pallor, jaundice, and weakness may develop following recovery from the pulmonary symptoms. Peripheral blood smears usually show polychromasia, spherocytosis, and erythrophagocytosis. Autoagglutination, hyperbilirubinemia, and decreased serum haptoglobins are characteristically seen. Cold agglutinins in this condition are IgM antibodies, usually with anti-I specificity. The I antigen is thought to be related to the ABH blood group system and is present on almost all adult red cells. Neonatal (cord) red cells have weak representation of the I antigen, and one in about 5000 individuals has no representation of I antigen (phenotype i). Occasionally an acute hemolytic anemia occurs following infectious mononucleosis, and the associated cold agglutinins generally demonstrate anti-i specificity, reacting more strongly with cord red cells than with adult. At times, such patients may have major hemolytic episodes. Similar autoantibodies may be associated with a cold agglutinin syndrome in cases of Hodgkin's disease or other malignant lymphomas.

The cold agglutinins appear to react, perhaps only transiently, with red cells in cooler peripheral blood vessels and to mediate complement fixation. Although the cold agglutinins typically dissociate from the red cells on return to the warmer central circulation, complement components remain bound to the red cell membrane. Such red cells may undergo outright (intravascular) lysis by complement or, more commonly, may be left as complement-coated red cells, as detected by antiglobulin tests with anti-complement serum.

The acute forms associated with *Mycoplasma* pneumonia or infectious mononucleosis generally subside spontaneously within a short period, up to a few weeks. Therapy may include only maintaining a warm environment. With severe, life-threatening hemolysis, transfusions with *washed* * red cells can be employed, although transfused cells may be more agglutinable than those of the patient and survive less well in vivo. Corticosteroids are generally disappointing in this setting.

Chronic cold agglutinin disease is seen most often in elderly patients and usually presents as a chronic anemia with exacerbations in cold weather. Occasionally there may be episodes of hemoglobinuria. There may be an associated acrocyanosis with ulcerations. Splenomegaly may be seen. The peripheral blood shows autoagglutination, microspherocytosis, and polychromasia. As in the acute form, the direct antiglobulin test is positive because of red cell coating with complement components. The cold agglutinin titer may be as high as 1,000,000 at 4°C, but titers of 2000 to 20,000 are more usual. Cold agglutinin disease may be associated with overt malignant lymphomas, and the clinical picture is generally that of the malignancy. Furthermore, Schubothe and others have suggested that even the "idiopathic" forms may belong to the category of lymphoproliferative disorders because of marrow lymphocytosis, a tendency to progressive increase in serum macroglobulins, and occasionally termination in a frank malignant lymphoma. Just as antibody specificity, such as rheumatoid factor activity, has recently been identified in the "monoclonal" IgM of Waldenström's macroglobulinemia, the cold agglutinins of this chronic disease also have monoclonal characteristics and may reflect a neoplastic proliferation related to Waldenström's macroglobulinemia.

THERAPY. The treatment of those patients with an associated malignant lymphoma is primarily directed toward the neoplastic disease. In idiopathic cases of chronic cold agglutinin disease, bed rest alone, especially in a warm environment, may decrease hemolysis. Protection of the extremities with warm gloves and footwear should be emphasized in those with acrocyanosis. Blood transfusions often are not very effective and should be used only when the anemia threatens life. Corticosteroids and splenectomy have not been nearly as effective as in the warm-active antibody cases. Immunosup-

---

* Washed red cells are employed to avoid replenishing depleted complement components by giving donor plasma. The depletion of complement components during intravascular lysis appears to be a rate-limiting, life-sparing factor in certain patients with intravascular hemolysis.

pressive agents, including chlorambucil and cyclophosphamide, have led to decreases in cold agglutinin titers in several reported cases, although hemolysis may persist. Dacie reports that of 9 patients, 3 had a good clinical response. Treatment with disulfide-reducing agents such as pencillamine, designed to dissociate chemically the cold agglutinin, has occasionally led to improvement but has generally been disappointing, and the side effects are considerable. In our judgment, the alkylating drugs (cyclophosphamide or chlorambucil) deserve a trial when symptoms are disabling.

PAROXYSMAL COLD HEMOGLOBINURIA

Paroxysmal cold hemoglobinuria (PCH) is a very uncommon acquired hemolytic disease characterized by episodes of massive hemolysis following exposure to the cold. Donath and Landsteiner described in 1904 the complement-dependent autoantibody (D-L antibody) causing the hemolytic disease, which may be chronic and idiopathic or may be acute and transient in association with viral diseases such as measles, chickenpox, mumps, infectious mononucleosis, or "flulike" illness or, much more rarely nowadays, with latent or congenital syphilis.

PCH may have its onset at any age, usually during cold weather. Shortly after being chilled the patient passes dark red urine, and there may be accompanying fever and back and abdominal pains. Raynaud's phenomenon and cold urticaria may occur.

Laboratory findings include a rapid drop in hematocrit of variable degree with reticulocytosis, microspherocytosis, erythrophagocytosis, leukopenia followed by leukocytosis, and depressed serum complement titers. The direct antiglobulin test (anticomplement) may be positive during acute attacks but becomes negative at other times.

The D-L antibody is an IgG globulin generally showing anti-P blood group specificity. In vitro, attachment of antibody and certain complement components occurs in the cold (generally below $20°C$). When the temperature is raised the antibody dissociates from the red cells, but the (early-acting) complement components remain cell-bound and can react with other (late-acting) complement components, leading to cell lysis. In vivo, binding of D-L antibody to red cells apparently can occur only in superficial vessels during severe chilling, with completion of hemolysis presumably occurring mainly on return to the warmer general circulation.

THERAPY.   The most effective therapy for paroxysmal cold hemoglobinuria is preventive, by avoidance of cold. Treatment of associated syphilis is usually effective in curing the hemolytic disease, while cases associated with virus infections clear spontaneously. The chronic idiopathic form may persist for years. Corticosteroids and splenectomy are not effective.

General Comment

It may be helpful to the practicing internist to have some appreciation of the prevalence of these various forms of AIHD. During 7 years of actively searching out patients in these categories in the Rochester, New York, area, we have seen over 40 cases of warm-antibody AIHD; 3 patients with chronic cold agglutinin disease; 2 with acute, self-limited intravascular hemolysis associated with cold agglutinins (anti-i); and 1 definite case of PCH in a child following viral infection.

DRUG-RELATED IMMUNE HEMOLYTIC DISORDERS

Positive direct antiglobulin tests and hemolytic anemia can result from the administration of certain drugs. These include (1) penicillin, which binds to the red cell membrane and acts as a chemical hapten, (2) quinidine, quinine, and stibophen, apparently through formation of immune complexes with antibody which, in turn, are adsorbed to the red cell surface, and (3) α-methyldopa and mefenamic acid, which are associated with the formation of anti-RBC antibodies without apparent specificity for the drugs themselves. The importance of distinguishing these drug-related disorders from "spontaneous" AIHD is clear, since the former are curable by eliminating the offending drug. Furthermore, understanding these drug-related mechanisms may permit clarification of the etiology of idiopathic AIHD.

PENICILLIN

The haptene mechanism is best illustrated by patients developing a positive direct anti-IgG antiglobulin test while receiving large doses (10 to 30 million units per day) of penicillin or, in patients on lesser dosage, in the presence of renal failure. In some patients with these very high blood levels of penicillin, IgG antipenicillin antibodies are formed which then can react with penicillin already bound to the patient's red cells. These IgG antibodies, after elution from the patient's red cells, react only with penicillin-coated red cells, and not with normal red cells. They are therefore drug-specific antibodies, not red cell autoantibodies. Occasionally IgM, IgA, or IgD has been detected on such penicillin-coated red cells. IgM antipenicillin antibodies actually are found very commonly in the serum of penicillin-treated patients, but in general these do not appear related to immune red cell injury. Furthermore, lower doses of penicillin, even in the presence of IgG antipenicillin antibodies, do not appear capable of coating red cells sufficiently to contribute to hemolysis.

Treatment for this form of AIHD consists of stopping penicillin. Transfusions are useful in critically ill patients. Based on limited observations, corticosteroids appear to be ineffective in the presence of continued penicillin therapy.

QUININE, QUINIDINE, AND STIBOPHEN

The immune complex mechanism is involved in immune hemolytic disease associated with quinine, quinidine, and the antiparasitic drug stibophen. These drugs apparently do not have a high affinity for the cell membrane, as does penicillin. They do stimulate the production of IgM antidrug antibodies, however, which are thought to react with the drug in the circulation, forming complexes. These complexes may then be adsorbed to the surface of red cells. The resulting reaction causes activation and binding of complement at the membrane, and the positive antiglobulin test is the complement type. These drugs also stimulate IgG antibodies, which may mediate platelet damage by the same mechanism. The hemolytic anemia or thrombocytopenia subsides at a variable rate when the drug is discontinued.

α-METHYLDOPA AND MEFENAMIC ACID

Anti-red cell antibodies associated with α-methyldopa (α-MD) or mefenamic acid therapy may cause a hemolytic anemia indistinguishable from idiopathic AIHD with warm-active IgG autoantibodies. A relatively large number (10 to 20%) of patients taking the antihypertensive drug α-MD (Aldomet) for more than 5 months develop positive antiglobulin tests, especially those taking large doses. Few of these develop overt hemolytic anemia. The anticomplement antiglobulin test is negative as a rule.

The immunologic mechanisms involved are distinct from those of penicillin-associated hemolytic anemia and from the immune complex mechanism seen with quinidine. The IgG antibodies react not with α-MD but with antigens on autologous or homologous human red cells, usually exhibiting specificity within the Rh system. Therefore they appear to qualify as true red cell autoantibodies. Like autoantibodies from idiopathic cases, they show maximal activity at 37°C. They are not inhibited by α-MD or known related derivatives, and such chemicals do not appear to be bound to red cell membranes as penicillin is. The antibodies causing positive antiglobulin tests in patients receiving L-dopa for Parkinson's disease and in arthritic patients receiving the antiinflammatory drug mefenamic acid appear to have similar characteristics. The mechanism for such autoantibody production is obscure.

Withdrawal of α-MD is followed by return of the hematocrit level to normal within a few weeks, even without corticosteroid therapy. The strength of the direct and indirect antiglobulin tests progressively diminishes and becomes negative within 4 to 18 months. Resolution after drug withdrawal is considered crucial in implicating α-MD, because no other tests are available to establish a drug-related etiology in a given patient. A patient showing continued hemolytic anemia or undiminished persistence of a positive antiglobulin test would currently be considered an idiopathic ("spontaneous") case.

REFERENCES

Allgood, J. W., and Chaplin, H., Jr. Idiopathic acquired autoimmune hemolytic anemia. *Amer. J. Med.* 43:254, 1967.

Bakemeier, R. F., and Leddy, J. P. Erythrocyte autoantibody associated with alpha-methyldopa: Heterogeneity of structure and specificity. *Blood* 32:1, 1968.

Croft, J. D., Swisher, S. N., Gilliland, B. C., Bakemeier, R. F., Leddy, J. P., and Weed, R. I. Coombs'-test positivity induced by drugs. *Ann. Intern. Med.* 68:176, 1968.

Dacie, J. V. *The Haemolytic Anaemias: Congenital and Acquired* (2d ed.). Part II, *The Auto-Immune Haemolytic Anaemias.* New York: Grune & Stratton, 1962.

Dacie, J. V., and Worlledge, S. M. Auto-Immune Hemolytic Anemias. In E. B. Brown and C. V. Moore (Eds.), *Progress in Hematology.* New York: Grune & Stratton, 1969. Vol. 6, p. 82.

Gilliland, B. C., Leddy, J. P., and Vaughan, J. H. Measurement by a new method of previously undetected cell-bound antibody on complement-coated human red cells. *J. Clin. Invest.* 49:898, 1970.

Hitzig, W. H., and Massimo, L. Treatment of autoimmune hemolytic anemia in children with azathioprine (Imuran). *Blood* 28:840, 1966.

Leddy, J. P., and Bakemeier, R. F. Structural aspects of human erythrocyte autoantibodies. *J. Exp. Med.* 121:1, 1965.

Leddy, J. P., and Swisher, S. N. Acquired Immune Hemolytic Disorders. In M. Samter (Ed.). *Immunological Diseases* (2d ed.). Boston: Little, Brown, 1971.

Pirofsky, B. *Autoimmunization and the Autoimmune Hemolytic Anemias.* Baltimore: Williams & Wilkins, 1969.

Schubothe, H. The cold hemagglutinin disease. *Seminars Hemat.* 3:27, 1966.

Schwartz, R. S., and Dameshek, W. The treatment of autoimmune hemolytic anemia with 6-mercaptopurine and thioguanine. *Blood* 19:483, 1962.

10. CLINICAL IMPLICATIONS OF ALTERED AFFINITY OF HEMOGLOBIN FOR OXYGEN

Denis R. Miller
Marshall A. Lichtman

THE PRIMARY FUNCTION of the erythrocyte is the delivery of oxygen to and the removal of carbon dioxide from the tissues. The determinants of oxygen delivery include (1) the functional capacity of the cardiovascular and pulmonary systems, (2) the quantity and functional characteristics of hemoglobin, and (3) intraerythrocytic environmental factors that influence the affinity of hemoglobin for oxygen.

Two recent advances have furthered our understanding of the pathophysiology of anemia and are highlighted in this chapter. The first is the influence of globin chain variation on the function of hemoglobin, and the second is the role of intracellular phosphate compounds, principally 2,3-diphosphoglycerate (2,3-DPG) and adenosine triphosphate (ATP), as regulators of the affinity of hemoglobin for oxygen.

PHYSIOLOGY OF OXYGEN DELIVERY

The interrelated factors affecting oxygen delivery to the tissues are presented schematically in Figure 10-1. Hemoglobin becomes fully saturated with oxygen at the pulmonary capillary Po_2 of 100 mm Hg. Oxygen deliv-

Dr. Lichtman is a Scholar of the Leukemia Society of America.

This work was supported in part by U.S. Public Health Service Grants AM 13947, CA 11174, and HE-06241-09; General Research Support Grant; the Clinical Research Center, Division of Research Facilities and Resources (RR-44); the Monroe County Cancer and Leukemia Society; U.S. Army Medical Research and Development Command, Department of the Army, D.O.D. Contract DA 49-193 MD-2656; and the U.S. Atomic Energy Project at the University of Rochester. It has been assigned publication no. UR-49-1299.

141

ery to the tissues can be represented by the differences between the saturation of arterial (Sa) and venous (Sv) blood. This difference is determined by the amount of oxygen released by hemoglobin during tissue perfusion, which in the case of normally structured hemoglobin is influenced by the P_{CO_2} and pH of the blood, and the concentration of erythrocyte organic phosphate compounds, primarily 2,3-DPG and secondarily ATP. These two compounds comprise 95% of the organic phosphates in the erythrocyte.

The influence of pH on the oxygen dissociation curve (Bohr effect) is due to the reciprocal binding of oxygen and hydrogen ion by deoxyhemoglobin. Acidosis decreases and alkalosis increases the affinity of hemoglobin for oxygen. In addition to the effect of pH on oxyhemoglobin concentration, a marked decrease in blood pH can reduce erythrocyte glycolysis,

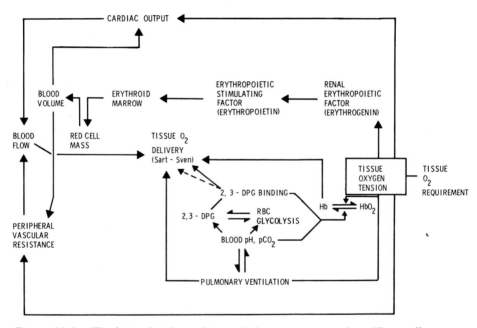

Figure 10-1. The interrelated regulators of tissue oxygen tension. The cardiovascular compensatory mechanisms for anemia include an increase in cardiac output and alterations in peripheral resistance, resulting in a redistribution of blood flow to vital organs. This form of compensation has been studied most thoroughly in animal models made acutely hypovolemic by reduction in blood volume. Generalizations cannot be made from these observations to subacute and chronic anemias. Compensatory adjustments in red cell mass are relatively slow in attaining maximum effectiveness (days to weeks) and are inadequate when marrow hypofunction is present and when blood loss or destruction exceeds the maximum limit of erythroid marrow expansion. (Modified from C. H. deVerdier, L. Garby, and M. Hjelm, 1969.)

ATP, and 2,3-DPG synthesis and thereby affect the affinity of hemoglobin for oxygen.

The appreciation of the effect of 2,3-DPG and ATP on the binding of oxygen with hemoglobin constitutes one of the important recent advances in medical science. Although several details remain to be clarified, studies have confirmed that oxygen dissociation from hemoglobin is facilitated by increased intraerythrocytic 2,3-DPG and ATP concentrations as a result of their preferential binding to deoxyhemoglobin. Therefore, in the absence of a change in the red cell mass or blood flow rate, oxygen delivery by a normal hemoglobin molecule can be altered by changes in blood hydrogen ion concentration, PCO_2, or red cell organic phosphate concentration.

Cardiovascular compensation can result in increased blood flow in response to a decreased oxygen flow to tissues as a result of a reduction in blood volume. This sequence of events is usually a manifestation of acute blood loss. In mild to moderate anemia of gradual development, cardiac output does not increase. With severe anemias or severe hypoxia, blood flow to certain organs such as brain, heart, and liver is increased because of a reduction in peripheral resistance to those organs and a redistribution of blood.

In addition, in the absence of renal disease and in the presence of a normally responsive marrow, renal chemoreceptors respond to a decreased oxygen flow by elaborating renal erythropoietic factor (erythrogenin) which, after interacting with a plasma globulin, results in the formation of an active erythropoietic principle, erythropoietic-stimulating factor, or erythropoietin. Erythropoietin increases erythroid differentiation and leads to eventual restoration of red cell mass. The recruitment of cardiovascular and erythropoietic compensatory mechanisms varies depending on the circumstances. In a gradually developing anemia due to decreased red cell production, neither mechanism is evoked. Instead the primary compensation for anemia and hypoxemia in such situations is a reduction in the affinity of hemoglobin for oxygen due to an increase in red cell organic phosphate compounds.

ASSOCIATION OF HEMOGLOBIN WITH OXYGEN

The oxygen dissociation curve is constructed by plotting the proportion of hemoglobin saturated with oxygen (HbO_2) at various partial pressures of oxygen (PO_2). A family of curves exists in relation to the additional effect of PCO_2 and pH.

A normal oxygen dissociation curve is shown in Figure 10-2. In the pulmonary capillary, the PO_2 is approximately 100 mm Hg and the blood contains nearly 100% oxyhemoglobin. At a PO_2 of a peripheral artery, 90

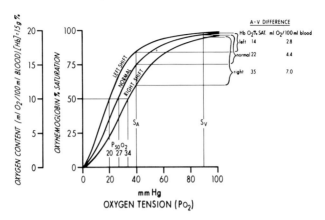

Figure 10-2. The oxygen dissociation curve of whole blood. A gram of hemo-globin carries about 1.34 ml of oxygen. If blood contains 15 gm of hemoglobin per 100 ml that is 97% saturated with oxygen, arterial oxygen content will be 19.4 ml per 100 ml, disregarding the negligible amount of oxygen in physical solution in plasma. If hemoglobin-oxygen affinity is normal ($P_{50} = 27$ mm Hg), 4.4 ml of oxygen per 100 ml of blood will be released to the tissues as blood passes from artery (Sa = 97%) to vein (Sv = 75%). With a shift of the curve to the left, less oxygen is removed from hemoglobin at the Po_2 observed in tissue capillaries, and hence delivery would be reduced if other factors remained constant. A shift to the right increases the amount of oxygen removed from hemoglobin.

mm Hg, approximately 97% of hemoglobin is oxygenated, whereas in venous blood the Po_2 is 40 mm Hg and Hbo_2 is 75%.

A practical way of expressing the affinity of hemoglobin for oxygen is by determining the partial pressure of oxygen at which 50% of hemoglobin is in the form of oxyhemoglobin ($P_{50}O_2$). Normally, $P_{50}O_2$ is approximately 27 mm Hg, the difference in Hbo_2 saturation from artery to vein is 22% (97% vs 75%), and the oxygen donated is 4.4 ml per 100 ml of blood, as shown in Fig 10-2. A displacement, or shift, of the oxygen dissociation curve to the right ($P_{50}O_2 = 34$ mm Hg) results in decreased oxygen affinity. Fifty percent of hemoglobin has been deoxygenated at a higher Po_2 (34 mm Hg vs 27 mm Hg); therefore, at a given Po_2 an increased delivery of oxygen may occur. In the example shown in Figure 10-2, the decrease in oxygen affinity would provide about 60% more oxygen (4.4 vs 7.0 ml per 100 ml of blood) to the tissues at a hemoglobin concentration of 15 gm per 100 ml and a given blood flow. Conversely, a shift of the curve to the left ($P_{50}O_2 = $ 20 mm Hg) indicates increased oxygen affinity and decreased oxygen delivery to the tissues (2.8 ml per 100 ml of blood).

The sigmoid shape of the oxygen dissociation curve is determined primarily by cooperative interaction of the heme moieties, i.e., the oxygenation and deoxygenation of one heme facilitates the oxygenation and deoxygenation of the second, and so on until all four heme groups are oxygenated or deoxygenated. The sigmoid shape of the curve permits significant compensation for hypoxemia by a change in hemoglobin's oxygen affinity, since a shift of the curve to the right results in a greater increase in oxygen release at tissue capillary O_2 tensions ($Po_2 = 40$ mm Hg) than it does a decrease in oxygen binding by hemoglobin at pulmonary capillary oxygen tensions ($Po_2 = 100$ mm Hg).

ROLE OF 2,3-DPG IN OXYGEN DISSOCIATION

2,3-DPG is the most abundant of the glycolytic intermediates within the erythrocyte; however, its function in regulating oxygen dissociation did not become apparent for 40 years after its isolation from red cells. Since 1921 it has been known that the oxygen affinity of intact erythrocytes is lower than that of hemoglobin solutions. At that time it was postulated that some other substance or substances present in the red cell interacted with hemoglobin, thereby decreasing its affinity for oxygen. Recently the studies of Chanutin and Curnish and of Benesch and Benesch established that 2,3-DPG binds to the β-chain of hemoglobin and that the binding of either oxygen to heme or 2,3-DPG to the β-chain of hemoglobin inhibits the affinity of hemoglobin for the other (allosteric inhibition). The oxygen dissociation curve of hemoglobin is shifted progressively to the right as the molar ratio of added 2,3-DPG to hemoglobin approaches unity. Maximal values for heme interaction and oxygen affinity are reached at concentrations of 2,3-DPG which exist within the red cell. The role of 2,3-DPG is complex in that a small portion ($< 30\%$) of the effect of 2,3-DPG on oxygen affinity is probably due to its effect on red cell pH.

The possible physiologic implications of these important observations soon became apparent, and a series of clinical studies further strengthened the association of anemia and hypoxemia with increased red cell 2,3-DPG and a resultant decrease in the oxygen affinity of hemoglobin. Evidence now strongly supports the conclusion that this physiologic system operates to compensate for the inability to replete a reduced red cell mass or for an inadequacy in oxygenation by a normal red cell mass.

RAPOPORT-LUEBERING CYCLE

In 1951 an important metabolic pathway in the erythrocyte, the Rapoport-Luebering cycle, was elucidated. The cycle, illustrated in Figure 10-3, provides for the conversion of 1,3-DPG to 2,3-DPG by 2,3-DPG mutase and the hydrolysis of 2,3-DPG by a phosphatase. Several inorganic and organic compounds in the red cell influence the rates of reaction of the two enzymes in this cycle.

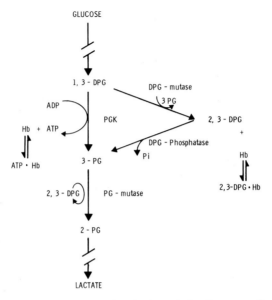

Figure 10-3. Red cell anaerobic glycolysis and the Rapoport-Luebering shunt. The rate of 1,3-DPG formation during glycolysis, the regulation of the entrance of 1,3-DPG into the shunt pathway, the binding of 2,3-DPG to hemoglobin, thereby reducing free 2,3-DPG concentrations, and the conversion of 2,3-DPG to 3-PG determine the total 2,3-DPG concentration.

The rate of glucose utilization as well as the proportion of 1,3-DPG that enters the Rapoport-Luebering pathway influences the resultant concentration of red cell ATP and 2,3-DPG. 2,3-DPG accumulation limits glycolysis and limits its own synthesis. Thus the Rapoport-Luebering shunt can influence ATP and 2,3-DPG concentrations rapidly. In turn, their binding to hemoglobin influences oxygen affinity and thereby relates glycolysis to oxygen delivery.

ALTERED OXYGEN DISSOCIATION: THE HEMOGLOBIN MOLECULE

During the past several years human hemoglobin variants with abnormalities of (1) oxygen affinity, (2) cooperative heme-heme interaction, or (3) the absence of the Bohr effect have been recognized. Such abnormal hemoglobins result from a mutation which codes for a difference in hemoglobin structure of a single amino acid. Some of these uncommon mutants are listed in Table 10-1.

Patients with variants of hemoglobin structure associated with increased oxygen affinity such as hemoglobin Chesapeake are polycythemic because of the reduced release of oxygen to the tissues at normal blood hemoglobin

Table 10-1. Hemoglobin Variants Associated with Altered Oxygen Affinity[a]

Hemoglobin	Amino Acid Substitution or Structure	2,3-DPG (μmoles/ml RBC)	Clinical Findings
Hb A	$\alpha_2\beta_2$	4.19 ± 0.13	Normal adult
High O_2 affinity			Erythrocytosis
Chesapeake	$\alpha^{92\ Arg \to Leu}$		
Yakima	$\beta^{99\ Asp \to His}$		
Ranier	$\beta^{145\ Tyr \to Asp}$		
Hb F	$\alpha^2\gamma^2$	Increased	Normal neonate; thalassemia major
Hb H	β_4	Low normal	Thalassemia syndrome
Hb Barts	γ_4		Severe hemolytic anemia
Unstable Hb			
Köln	$\beta^{98\ Val \to Met}$	Increased	Compensated hemolysis
Zürich	$\beta^{63\ His \to Arg}$		Hemolysis with sulfa
Tacoma	$\beta^{30\ Arg \to Ser}$		No symptoms
Low O_2 affinity			
M Hemoglobins			Cyanosis, methemoglobin
M_{Boston}	$\alpha^{58\ His \to Tyr}$		Mild hemolytic anemia
M_{Iwate}	$\alpha^{87\ His \to Tyr}$		
$M_{Milwaukee}$	$\beta^{67\ Val \to Glu}$		
$M_{Saskatoon}$	$\beta^{63\ His \to Tyr}$		
$M_{Hyde\ Park}$	$\beta^{92\ His \to Tyr}$		
Kansas	$\beta^{102\ Asn \to Thr}$		Cyanosis
Seattle	$\beta^{76\ Ala \to Glu}$	Normal	Reduced hemoglobin concentration (new steady state)
Other hemoglobinopathies			
C	$\beta^{6\ Glu \to Lys}$	Increased	Moderate hemolytic anemia
D	$\beta^{121\ Glu \to Gln}$		Mild hemolytic anemia
E	$\beta^{26\ Glu \to Lys}$		Mild hemolytic anemia
S	$\beta^{6\ Glu \to Val}$	Increased	Severe hemolytic anemia

[a] Only representative examples are given for each group. See Table 7-1 for more complete listing.

concentrations. This results in increased excretion of renal erythropoietic factor and an increase in the circulating red cell mass. In patients with unexplained erythrocytosis, particularly those with a family history of polycythemia, hemoglobin electrophoresis on starch gel and studies of the affinity of hemoglobin for oxygen ($P_{50}O_2$) should be performed in order to identify a hemoglobinopathy which could result in polycythemia.

Intraerythrocytic Heinz body formation and hemolytic anemia are associated with the unstable hemoglobins such as Köln and Zürich. Oxygen dissociation curves have been found to be shifted to the left, resulting in tissue hypoxia greater than would be expected from the degree of anemia. The resultant stimulation of red cell production eventuates in a compensated hemolytic anemia (i.e., despite a shortened red cell life-span, the red cell mass is nearly normal because of marrow erythroid hyperplasia). Hence in these patients expanded erythropoiesis represents the major compensatory mechanism to improve oxygen delivery, since the abnormal hemoglobin cannot reduce its oxygen affinity. Presumptive evidence of the presence of such a hemoglobinopathy is obtained by testing the heat precipitability of a hemoglobin solution.

The α-thalassemias, hemoglobin H disease with tetramers of β-chains (β_4), and hemoglobin Barts with tetramers of γ-chains (γ_4) are associated with very high oxygen affinities. Whereas the unstable hemoglobins (Köln and Zürich) shift the oxygen dissociation curve to the left throughout the physiologic range of Po_2, perhaps by an interaction of the mutant hemoglobin chains with normal hemoglobin chains within individual red cells, β_4 and γ_4, lacking α-chains, do not interact with the normal hemoglobin. It has been suggested that the absence of α-chains prevents a significant alteration of the oxygen dissociation curve in the physiologic range of Po_2. Oxygen delivery by hemoglobin A, which makes up 85 to 90% of the red cell hemoglobin, is not affected, and therefore there is little alteration in the $P_{50}O_2$. Hence in these α-thalassemia syndromes the additional erythropoietic stimulus induced by a leftward shift of the oxygen dissociation curve is absent, and the compensatory increase in red cell mass is less prominent. Although compensation as traditionally judged in terms of hemoglobin concentration is incomplete (a now obsolete way of determining compensation), compensation in terms of oxygen delivery is probably similar in the α-thalassemia and unstable hemoglobin syndromes as a result of the differences in oxygen affinity.

Hemoglobinopathies characterized by reduced oxygen affinity include the M hemoglobins and hemoglobins Seattle and Kansas. M hemoglobin has its heme iron in the oxidized or ferric form (methemoglobin) and cannot transport oxygen. This is a result of either a single amino acid substitution involving one of the two histidines between which the heme group is suspended, or an amino acid substitution in the pocket of globin in which the heme moiety is inserted. The homozygous state is lethal. The disorder is seen in heterozygotes who have about 25% of their hemoglobin as methemoglobin. Cyanosis may be present and, interestingly, erythrocytosis is rare. A mild hemolytic anemia has been observed in patients with M hemoglobins, probably due to molecular instability of the hemoglobin molecule. Some M hemoglobins are α-chain mutants and others, β-chain mutants (Table 10-1). The α-chain mutation can be associated with cyanosis at birth, whereas the β-chain mutations are associated with cyanosis only after several months of age, when β-chain synthesis replaces γ-chain (fetal) synthesis.

Other abnormal hemoglobins with decreased oxygen affinity are not associated with methemoglobin formation. Cyanosis in hemoglobin Kansas is caused by a markedly increased dissociation of oxygen from hemoglobin and the high proportion (40%) of deoxyhemoglobin in the circulation. This form of cyanosis is not associated with tissue hypoxia and is of only cosmetic consequence. With hemoglobin Seattle the decreased oxygen affinity is accompanied by anemia, although oxygen supply is normal since the reduced red cell mass provides normal oxygenation and allows erythropoiesis to be maintained at a reduced new steady state. This does not occur with hemoglobin Kansas because the oxygen dissociation curve is altered so severely as to reduce oxygen affinity even at the high Po_2 of pulmonary capillaries. This arterial unsaturation maintains the hemoglobin mass at near-normal levels, and under these conditions normal oxygen delivery results.

The oxygen affinity of normal human fetal hemoglobin (Hb F, $\alpha_2\gamma_2$) is greater than that of normal adult hemoglobin (Hb A, $\alpha_2\beta_2$). This may be related to the finding that deoxyhemoglobin A binds more 2,3-DPG and ATP than does deoxyhemoglobin F. The differences in oxygen affinity of intraerythrocytic hemoglobin A and hemoglobin F are not related to erythrocyte 2,3-DPG since the red cells of full-term newborns have the same 2,3-DPG concentration as those of normal adults. The increased oxygen affinity of hemoglobin F facilitates oxygen transport across the placenta from mother to fetus and also provides an explanation for the erythrocytosis of the newborn.

In pathological states in which anemia and a high concentration of hemoglobin F are present, such as thalassemia major, hemoglobin oxygen affinity is not reduced despite an increase in red cell 2,3-DPG. In the presence of large proportions of hemoglobin F in the red cell, a compensatory shift of the oxygen dissociation curve does not occur due to the failure of 2,3-DPG to interact with the γ-chain of hemoglobin F as it does with the β-chain of hemoglobin A.

Recent observations have indicated that the concentration of hemoglobin per volume of red cells (MCHC) can influence the oxygen affinity of normal hemoglobin, independent of 2,3-DPG concentration. The correlation of MCHC with $P_{50}O_2$ is such that a decrease of 1.0 gm per 100 ml in MCHC results in a decrease in $P_{50}O_2$ of 0.5 mm Hg. This effect is brought about as a result of the dependence of the deoxyhemoglobin–2,3-DPG complex on the concentration of hemoglobin as well as 2,3-DPG.

ALTERED OXYGEN AFFINITY:
INTRAERYTHROCYTIC ENVIRONMENT

PRIMARY HYPOXEMIA

Several recent studies have demonstrated a significant relationship between hypoxemia, increased red cell 2,3-DPG content, and decreased oxygen affinity of hemoglobin. Patients with arterial hypoxemia due to cardiac and pulmonary disease and after ascent to high altitude have an elevated concentration of red cell 2,3-DPG and decreased oxygen affinity of hemoglobin.

At present the pathogenesis of the changes is seen to proceed as follows: With hypoxia, as after ascent to high altitude, the amount of deoxyhemoglobin is increased. This results in greater 2,3-DPG binding and decreased free (unbound) 2,3-DPG. The decreased concentration of free 2,3-DPG relieves the 2,3-DPG–mediated inhibition of hexokinase, and glucose utilization increases. Furthermore, 2,3-DPG inhibition of 2,3-DPG mutase is then relieved and metabolism of 1,3-DPG through the Rapoport-Luebering cycle enhanced (Fig. 10-3). This continues until free 2,3-DPG reaches concentrations which reduce the rate of glycolysis. Increased 2,3-DPG binding to hemoglobin occurs. This favors enhanced dissociation of oxygen at capillary Po_2. When hypoxia is removed, as when mountain residents descend to sea level, deoxyhemoglobin content is decreased and 2,3-DPG is released from hemoglobin. With greater quantities of free 2,3-DPG, hexokinase activity, glucose utilization, and 2,3-DPG mutase activity are reduced and 2,3-DPG synthesis is retarded. Dissociation of the hemoglobin–2,3-DPG complex is favored, and the affinity of hemoglobin for oxygen returns to normal. These adaptations are rapid, unrelated to the hemoglobin concentration, and not dependent upon changes in erythropoiesis.

SECONDARY HYPOXEMIA

Although it had been appreciated that hemoglobin has reduced affinity for oxygen in anemic subjects, it was only recently that studies have confirmed that the change is related to the increase in 2,3-DPG that occurs with reduction in blood hemoglobin concentration. In addition to the extent of anemia, blood pH, proportion of reticulocytes, plasma phosphate concentration and the adequacy of red cell metabolism can influence the concentration of erythrocyte organic phosphates. As demonstrated in Table 10-2, the erythrocytes of patients with renal failure, hyporegenerative anemias (iron deficiency anemia, leukemia, aplastic anemia), hemoglobinopathies, and congenital hemolytic anemias have significantly elevated concen-

Table 10-2. Erythrocyte 2,3-DPG Concentration in Anemia

Disease	Number of Patients	2,3-DPG (μmoles/ml RBC, mean $\pm$ S.E.)
Normal subjects	13	4.19 $\pm$ 0.03
Anemia of chronic renal disease	15	5.56 $\pm$ 0.33
Hyporegenerative anemia	17	7.28 $\pm$ 0.61
Hemoglobinopathy	15	7.02 $\pm$ 0.48
Hemolytic anemia	12	6.97 $\pm$ 0.54

trations of 2,3-DPG. Furthermore, as shown in Figure 10-4, the red cell 2,3-DPG concentration of anemic patients studied in our clinic is correlated with severity of anemia as represented by the hematocrit.

Blood of patients with hemoglobin S or C has been shown to have decreased oxygen affinity. Markedly increased 2,3-DPG concentrations have been observed in patients we have studied with hemoglobin S or C disease. The increase in intracellular organic phosphate compounds is related to the anemia and to the presence of a high proportion of reticulocytes which have an increased concentration of 2,3-DPG and ATP. The increased red cell organic phosphate compounds are probably primary factors in the decreased oxygen affinity of hemoglobin S and C. Evidence for abnormal oxygen affinity due to the structural alteration in these globin chains has not been demonstrated. Further studies are needed on this subject, however. The crystallization of hemoglobin S during sickling may alter oxygen affinity. The result of the rightward shift of the oxygen dissociation curve is to facilitate oxygen delivery to the tissues. Thus, although the anemia is incompletely compensated, the available red cell mass in sickle cell anemia is capable of providing more oxygen to the tissues than an equivalent mass of erythrocytes not possessing a decreased affinity of oxygen for hemoglobin. However, the high levels of erythropoietic-stimulating factor and the marked marrow erythroid hyperplasia that exist in these hemolytic anemias indicate that tissue oxygenation is not completely compensated by the shift in the oxygen dissociation curve. Furthermore, the increased deoxyhemoglobin at capillary Po_2 may enhance sickling. This is a potentially important determinant in sickle cell crises which needs further investigation.

The erythrocytes of patients suffering with renal failure with hyperphosphatemia have significantly elevated glycolytic rate and an increased concentration of 2,3-DPG and ATP. The increase in red cell ATP is greater and the proportional increase in 2,3-DPG less than in nonuremic anemic subjects. These changes have been shown to be related primarily to the stimulating effect of elevated extracellular phosphate concentrations on red

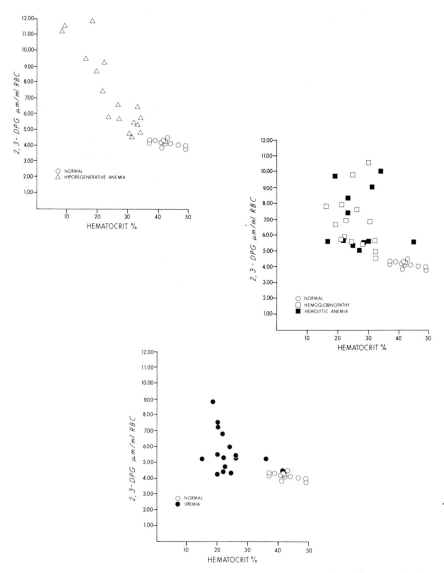

Figure 10-4. Correlation of erythrocyte 2,3-DPG concentration and anemia. In the case of hyporegenerative (reticulocytopenic) anemias, a near-linear relationship between 2,3-DPG and severity of anemia exists. In hemolytic anemias and hemoglobinopathies 2,3-DPG concentration is elevated with more modest hematocrit reductions due to younger-aged cell populations and peculiarities in O_2 affinity of individual hemoglobinopathic states. In severe chronic renal disease some subjects have relatively little increase in 2,3-DPG, perhaps related to the accompanying acidosis and to the more marked increase in red cell ATP present in such subjects, with the result that the total of ATP and 2,3-DPG is often as high as in other anemic subjects.

cell glycolysis. Oxygen dissociation curves are shifted to the right and the $P_{50}O_2$ is elevated. Oxygen delivery to the tissues is facilitated by the increased levels of 2,3-DPG and ATP and should compensate, in part, for the decreased red cell mass. Hence hyperphosphatemia results in an intracellular adaptation to anemia which facilitates oxygen delivery. In the less common situation of sustained severe hypophosphatemia, intracellular organic phosphate compounds are decreased, oxygen affinity increases, and, in an anemic subject, tissue hypoxia could ensue.

It is likely that the ability to tolerate severe chronic anemia is in large part explained by an increase in red cell 2,3-DPG, as well as in ATP in those cases with hyperphosphatemia or reticulocytosis. The resultant facilitation of oxygen delivery partially compensates for a reduced red cell mass, as shown in Figure 10-5.

DEFECTS OF ERYTHROCYTE METABOLISM

Enzymatic deficiencies of erythrocyte glycolysis associated with high or low concentrations of 2,3-DPG can fortuitously influence the affinity of

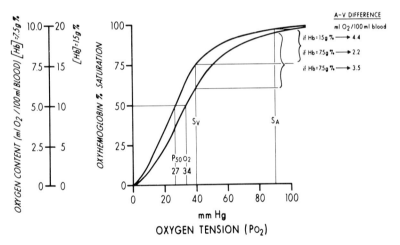

Figure 10-5. Compensatory effect of reduced affinity of hemoglobin for oxygen in an anemic subject. When hemoglobin concentration is halved, the arterial blood oxygen content is 10 rather than 20 ml per 100 ml. Oxygen delivery, assuming unchanged blood flow, will be 2.2 ml per 100 ml if hemoglobin affinity remains unchanged ($P_{50} = 27$ mm Hg). If increased 2,3-DPG synthesis results in a decreased hemoglobin-oxygen affinity ($P_{50} = 34$ mm Hg), the oxygen delivery could be increased 60%. Tissue blood flow rate and oxygen requirements are variables which are difficult to assess. Inferences regarding tissue oxygen supply can be made by the measurement of erythropoietin, which would be increased if tissue hypoxia is present.

hemoglobin for oxygen. In pyruvate kinase (PK) deficiency hereditary hemolytic anemia, the concentration of 2,3-DPG is markedly elevated and in hexokinase deficiency, markedly decreased, because of the location of the respective enzymatic deficiencies. As expected, the oxygen dissociation curve in PK deficiency is shifted to the right, and in hexokinase deficiency it is displaced to the left. The rightward shift in the oxygen dissociation curve in PK deficiency allows the delivery of as much oxygen from 9 gm of hemoglobin per 100 ml of blood as would normally be delivered by 15 gm per 100 ml at a similar rate of blood flow. In hexokinase deficiency, in spite of the decreased 2,3-DPG content a compensatory increase in red cell mass does not occur because of the rapid hemolytic rate. Other rare enzymatic anomalies of the Rapoport-Luebering cycle and glycolysis shown in Table 10-3 may also be associated with changes in oxygen affinity of hemoglobin for similar reasons.

Change in the concentration of 2,3-DPG allows the erythrocyte to adjust the supply of oxygen to tissues in response to hypoxia. Like hemoglobin concentration, oxygen affinity is inversely correlated with 2,3-DPG concentration. A change in 2,3-DPG concentration of 1 mM per liter of RBC causes a shift of the $P_{50}O_2$ value of 3.8 mm Hg. Alternate compensatory mechanisms for hypoxemia depend upon an increase in red cell mass as a result of the increased secretion of renal erythropoietic factor. This takes several days and cannot be invoked when anemia is due to a primary decrease in red cell production, or when accelerated destruction is too rapid for compensation to be achieved even by maximal marrow hyperplasia. Cardiovascular compensation involves an increased cardiac output and decreased peripheral resistance so as to increase oxygen flow through tissues. The latter mechanism is primarily evoked in response to decreased blood volume, which is usually near normal in chronic anemias.

STORED BLOOD

In 1954 Valtis and Kennedy demonstrated that the oxygen dissociation curve of blood stored over 7 days was shifted to the left and did not return

Table 10-3. Intrinsic Defects of Erythrocyte Metabolism Associated with Altered Organic Phosphate Content

Metabolic Defect	2,3-DPG	ATP	Oxygen Affinity
Pyruvate kinase deficiency	Increased	Decreased	Decreased
Hexokinase deficiency	Decreased	Normal	Increased
2,3-DPG mutase deficiency	Decreased	?	?
High ATP syndrome	Decreased	Increased	?

to normal for 24 hours after infusion in a recipient. The cause of the increased oxygen affinity of stored blood was unknown, but the physiologic implication was that an anemic recipient might receive red cells which were unable to release oxygen normally for hours. The increased oxygen affinity of blood with increased duration of storage appears causally related to the depletion of erythrocyte 2,3-DPG. Whereas red cell ATP concentration falls gradually in acid-citrate-dextrose over 3 weeks, 2,3-DPG phosphatase activity is stimulated and 2,3-DPG degradation is enhanced by conversion to 3-phosphoglycerate (Fig. 10-3). A rapid decrease in 2,3-DPG ensues. The practical implications of these storage changes are discussed further in Chapter 11.

OTHER METABOLIC ABNORMALITIES

Alterations in oxygen delivery and erythrocyte 2,3-DPG have been observed recently in other nonhematologic diseases associated with abnormal metabolism. In diabetic ketoacidosis, erythrocyte 2,3-DPG is decreased, $P_{50}O_2$ is increased, and tissue oxygen delivery is decreased. The decreased 2,3-DPG concentration results from decreased erythrocyte glycolysis and from decreased 2,3-DPG synthesis and increased 2,3-DPG catabolism, both produced by acidosis. Although acidosis through the Bohr effect shifts the oxygen dissociation curve to the right, prolonged acidosis results in decreased 2,3-DPG levels and decreased $P_{50}O_2$. Abrupt correction of acidosis at this point results in a further shift in the oxygen dissociation curve to the left and may produce tissue hypoxia.

Decreased erythrocyte 2,3-DPG, a shift of the oxygen dissociation curve to the left, and reduced oxygen consumption have been found recently in patients with septic shock and in patients with severe hypophosphatemia. Conversely, in thyrotoxicosis red cell 2,3-DPG levels are increased. This may be related to a direct effect of thyroxine on enzymes involved in erythrocyte 2,3-DPG synthesis. Along with increased blood flow, these alterations may contribute to the increased delivery of oxygen for the increased tissue need of thyrotoxic patients.

In summary, adequate oxygen delivery requires (1) normal cardiovascular and pulmonary function, (2) normally structured hemoglobin in adequate concentration, and (3) normal erythrocyte metabolism. The physiology of maintenance and regulation of tissue oxygen flow and the normal hemoglobin–oxygen relationship have been outlined. Red cell metabolism as it relates to the oxygen-carrying capacity of hemoglobin is discussed.

The role of cardiovascular, pulmonary, and erythropoietic compensatory mechanisms in response to hypoxemia is reviewed. Emphasis has been placed on the influence of structural abnormalities of hemoglobin and of red cell 2,3-DPG and ATP concentration on the affinity of hemoglobin for oxygen and the efficiency of oxygen delivery. Changes in red cell 2,3-DPG and ATP as a result of primary and secondary hypoxemia, alterations in erythrocyte metabolism, and blood storage have been described. The clinical implications of such changes are emphasized.

Recently acquired knowledge has permitted a greater understanding of the interrelationships of erythrocyte metabolism and hemoglobin function. 2,3-DPG as a modulator of glucose utilization—and thereby energy production and its own synthesis—and as a ligand with hemoglobin—thereby altering hemoglobin oxygen affinity and oxygen delivery during tissue perfusion—has a central physiologic role in satisfying tissue oxygen requirements in health and disease.

The future development of pharmacologic means of decreasing the affinity of hemoglobin for oxygen would be a major advance in the medical therapy of localized (e.g., heart, brain) or generalized hypoxia.

REFERENCES

Adamson, J. W. Oxygen Delivery by Abnormal Hemoglobins. In F. Stohlman, Jr. (Ed.), *Hematopoietic Cellular Proliferation.* New York: Grune & Stratton, 1970.

Bellingham, A. J., and Huehns, E. R. Compensation in haemolytic anaemias caused by abnormal haemoglobins. *Nature* (London) 218:924, 1968.

Benesch, R. How do small molecules do great things? *New Eng. J. Med.* 280:1179, 1969.

Benesch, R., and Benesch, R. E. Intracellular organic phosphates as regulators of oxygen release by hemoglobin. *Nature* (London) 221:618, 1969.

Beutler, E. A "shift to the left" or a "shift to the right" in the regulation of erythropoiesis. *Blood* 33:496, 1969.

Bunn, H. F., and Jandl, J. H. Control of hemoglobin function within the red cell. *New Eng. J. Med.* 282:1414, 1970.

Chanutin, A., and Curnish, R. R. Effect of organic and inorganic phosphates on the oxygen equilibrium of human erythrocytes. *Arch. Biochem. Biophys.* 121:96, 1967.

deVerdier, C. H., Garby, L., and Hjelm, M. Intraerythrocytic regulation of tissue oxygen tension. *Acta Soc. Med. Upsal.* 74:209, 1969.

Edwards, M. J., Novy, M. H., Walters, C. L., and Metcalfe, J. Improved oxygen release: An adaptation of mature red cells to hypoxia. *J. Clin. Invest.* 47:1851, 1968.

Keitt, A. S. Pyruvate kinase deficiency and related disorders of red cell glycolysis. *Amer. J. Med.* 41:762, 1966.

Lenfant, C., Torrance, J., English, E., Finch, C. A., Reynafarje, C., Ramos, J., and Faura, J. Effect of altitude on oxygen binding by hemoglobin and on organic phosphate levels. *J. Clin. Invest.* 47:2652, 1968.

Lichtman, M. A., and Miller, D. R.   Erythrocyte glycolysis, 2,3-diphosphogly-cerate and adenosine triphosphate concentration in uremic subjects: Rela-tionship to extracellular phosphate concentration. *J. Lab. Clin. Med.* 76:267, 1970.

Oski, F. A., Gottlieb, A. J., and Miller, L.   The influence of heredity and environment on the red cells' function of oxygen transport. *Med. Clin. N. Amer.* 54:731, 1970.

Ranney, H. M.   Clinically important variants of human hemoglobin. *New Eng. J. Med.* 282:144, 1970.

Weatherall, D. J.   Polycythemia resulting from abnormal hemoglobins. *New Eng. J. Med.* 280:604, 1969.

11. RECENT ADVANCES IN TRANSFUSION THERAPY

Leon W. Hoyer
Marshall A. Lichtman

Advances in transfusion therapy have expanded the internist's ability to treat a wide range of conditions. The resources available for optimal patient care depend upon the facilities of the regional blood bank. The internist's awareness of progress in this field permits the appropriate use of such facilities.

Preparation of blood components, the availability of frozen blood, and the identification of changes in the erythrocyte during blood storage that may alter its survival and oxygen-carrying capacity are three major areas of development in blood transfusion which are summarized in this chapter. Details of blood bank methods and blood group immunology are not considered. Mollison's comprehensive monograph *Blood Transfusion in Clinical Medicine* provides a reference source of great value.

COMPONENT THERAPY

Efficient separation of blood components became possible with the introduction of plastic collection equipment. It is now possible to provide the patient with one or more of the following specific components: erythrocytes, platelets, albumin, fibrinogen, specific clotting factors, and gamma globulin. Blood transfusion is no longer synonymous with the infusion of

Dr. Lichtman is a Scholar of the Leukemia Society of America.

This work was supported in part by U.S. Public Health Service Research Grant HE-11841; General Research Support Grant; a research grant from the Monroe County Cancer and Leukemia Society; in part by the U.S. Army Medical Research and Development Command, Department of the Army, under D.O.D. Contract DA-49-193-MD2656; and by the U.S. Atomic Energy Project at the University of Rochester. It has been assigned publication no. UR-49-1295.

whole blood. It should be rare, indeed, for the internist to order whole blood for one of his patients.

RED CELLS

Chronic anemia is associated with a compensatory increase in plasma volume, and infusion of plasma (as a part of whole blood) only contributes to vascular volume overload. Whole blood is necessary only if there is rapid massive blood loss due to acute hemorrhage. It has become apparent that even moderate blood loss, for example during surgery, does not always require whole-blood transfusion. Limited erythrocyte replacement (2 to 4 units) can be given in the form of packed cells with buffered saline solution. Plasma protein loss is rapidly repaired in patients who have adequate hepatic function.

PLATELETS

Until multiple transfer packs were available, thrombocytopenic bleeding required transfusions of fresh whole blood. The large number of platelets required made this an impractical and inefficient means for sustaining platelet counts, however. Platelet-rich plasma prepared from whole blood by low-speed centrifugation may also cause excessive volume expansion and may not provide the large number of platelets in short enough time to induce hemostasis. Platelet concentrates prepared from the platelet-rich plasma recover nearly half the platelets in a unit of blood in a very small volume. Platelets from 10 to 20 donors may, therefore, be provided for a single patient in a small volume which can be administered rapidly. Biologic products stored for later use are usually held at low temperatures. This strategy limited platelet transfusion for many years, as it was widely accepted that rapid loss of platelet viability was inevitable with storage. Recent studies have demonstrated that chilling the platelets reduces posttransfusion viability and that room temperature (22°C) storage is optimal for in vitro platelet maintenance. Surprisingly, survival of platelets stored at 22°C is very similar to fresh platelet life-span (T½ of approximately 4 days). Room temperature storage of platelet-rich plasma has been adopted by many Centers; satisfactory platelet infusions are possible for at least 48 hours of storage. This has reduced the need for "walk-in" donors of fresh blood and increased the effectiveness of each unit collected under routine conditions. Multiple platelet packs can be prepared from routine donors and held at room temperature if the need for platelets is anticipated.

The indications for platelet transfusion are considered in detail in Chapter 13. Patients with reduced platelet production—whether due to intrinsic bone marrow disease or to drug- or irradiation-induced bone marrow suppression—are most likely to be helped by these infusions. Ideally, the platelet count of such thrombocytopenic adults should increase 5,000 to 10,000 per cubic millimeter for each unit of fresh platelet concentrate transfused. The number of platelet packs needed for a given patient depends upon the initial platelet count, the amount of active bleeding, the patient's blood volume, and the storage period of the infused platelets. The posttransfusion platelet count is less than expected in patients with splenomegaly, those who are febrile or bleeding actively, and patients who have become isosensitized by previous transfusions. The isosensitivity is a result of histocompatibility antigens which are a part of the platelet membrane; patients who are apparently refractory to platelet infusion may be benefited by transfusion of histocompatible platelets if these are available. Close relatives are the most likely source of compatible platelets.

The infusion of platelets in patients with accelerated platelet destruction, such as in idiopathic thrombocytopenic purpura, is usually futile because of their rapid sequestration and destruction in vivo.

Blood stored at 4°C for longer than 24 hours lacks viable platelets, and it is not unexpected that thrombocytopenia may be caused by massive replacement with stored blood during profound hemorrhage. Significant reduction in platelet count is usually recognized when more than 15 units of stored blood are administered over a 48-hour period. Viable platelets must be provided for these patients if bleeding continues. Under such relatively infrequent circumstances administration of fresh whole blood or platelet concentrates or both may be required.

In general, when treating deficiencies in soluble clotting factor and platelet deficiencies, rapid infusion of quantities sufficient to raise the circulating concentration to at least 25% of normal is a good goal. The ability to do this without volume overload is now possible with the use of concentrates. However, because infused platelets are rapidly removed from the circulation and utilized in hemostasis in patients with active bleeding, cessation of bleeding is a better indicator of the effectiveness of platelet transfusion than the platelet count.

Platelet transfusion is best not used in the absence of bleeding or in the presence of trivial bleeding which can be managed with local measures. This is particularly important if platelets from random donors (histoincompatible) are used; for transfusion of these platelets will eventually engender antiplatelet antibodies which will reduce the usefulness of later platelet transfusions when needs may be critical due to serious bleeding.

LEUKOCYTES

White cell transfusion has proved thus far to be a more difficult problem than platelet replacement. Even with plasmaphoresis or leukophoresis, it is not yet practical to use normal donors. Patients with chronic granulocytic leukemia have been used as a source of white cells in experimental treatment of overwhelming infections in patients with granulocytopenia and acute leukemia. The results of such treatment have been disappointing. Further research in this area is needed. The ability to harvest normal mature granulocytes in large quantities and to use them in compatible donors is urgently needed in the treatment of patients with quantitative and qualitative deficiencies of granulocytes.

Advances in typing of leukocytes and administration of compatible cells so that they are not rapidly destroyed in recipients because of acquired isosensitization will further enhance the usefulness of transfusion of these cellular elements.

PLASMA AND PLASMA PROTEINS

Transfusion of whole plasma is rarely necessary. Albumin is an excellent volume expander, and the risk of hepatitis is minimal. Whole plasma is not optimal therapy for patients with bleeding disorders who require replacement of specific factors. Coagulation factors now available for specific therapy include fibrinogen, factor VIII (cryoprecipitates or concentrates prepared by Hyland and Cortland Laboratories), and the proteins of the prothrombin complex—factors II, VII, IX, and X (Konȳne, Cutter Laboratories). Fresh-frozen plasma remains the only practical source of factor V, reduced in rare individuals with a specific hereditary deficiency and often low in patients with severe liver disease. Whole plasma has some advantages for therapy of individuals with von Willebrand's disease (see Chap. 15).

One of the major advantages of component therapy is the attendent reduction in the risk of serum (transfusion-mediated) hepatitis. Those fractions which are rich in fibrinogen are the most dangerous in this regard; donor selection and optimal separatory methods provide the only protection. Albumin and heat-stable plasma fractions (Plasmanate, Cutter Laboratories) are hepatitis-free plasma expanders which should replace single-unit or pooled whole plasma for emergency use.

Fully one-third of cases of transfusion-related hepatitis are in patients who have received 1 or 2 units of whole blood. Recent reports indicate that posttransfusion hepatitis is less frequent when packed cells have been administered; this strengthens the case against the indiscriminate use of whole blood. At the present time carefully interviewed voluntary donors are the safest source of blood, for posttransfusion hepatitis is much more common if paid donors of whole blood are used. Nevertheless, hepatitis will result from transfusion therapy until a means is developed for the identification of the asymptomatic carrier. Studies using antibodies to the Australia antigen provide encouraging progress toward this goal. The Australia antigen is either a virus or a portion of a virus which is a causative agent of serum hepatitis. Rapid screening of blood for the presence of hepatitis virus antigen would allow the elimination of donors capable of transmitting hepatitis. Recently devised sensitive and practical immunologic techniques will allow identification of a major fraction, although not all, of donors with circulating hepatitis-associated viral antigen.

AUTOTRANSFUSION

The patient's own stored blood provides the safest form of transfusion, but the limited blood storage period prevents frequent use of autotransfusion. However, selected patients with isoantibodies may be managed by this strategy, and as many as 4 units can be obtained from healthy individuals during the 3 weeks prior to surgery. The patient may be mildly anemic, but the blood volume will be maintained and oxygen transport will be satisfactory. Increased availability of frozen blood will permit more frequent use of autotransfusion.

FROZEN BLOOD

Red cell preservation at $-80°C$ permits satisfactory transfusion after storage for at least 2 and possibly more than 5 years. This is in contrast to the present 21-day limit on blood stored at $4°C$. Unfortunately, irreparable membrane damage is associated with the freeze-thaw cycle in the absence of cryoprotective additives. The most extensive experience has been obtained using glycerol, an agent that penetrates the red cells. Red cells must be washed free of glycerol after thawing, and this requirement presents the major technical limitation to widespread use of low-temperature preservation. The cell washing can be done by batch or continuous-flow centrifugation or by agglomeration. Equipment to deglycerolate red cells by agglomeration is commercially available (Huggins Cytoagglomerator, International Equipment Company) and is being used by civilian and military blood banks.

Red cells stored at $-80°C$ have several specific therapeutic indications. Red cells lacking specific antigens can be stored by this technique, and a true "bank" on a regional or national basis could become available for the treatment of individuals who have developed isosensitivities. Multiple isosensitivities present a very difficult problem, and local sources may not be able to screen the necessary number of donors to detect the rare individual whose cells lack the specific antigens in question. The likelihood of obtaining sufficient compatible units is very small in these instances, and only a nationwide bank could provide enough units of a rare blood type.

Frozen blood is also useful for transfusion of patients with chronic renal disease who are candidates for renal transplantation. Histocompatibility antigens are present on white cell and platelet membranes, and they can sensitize potential recipients transfused with whole blood. Washing red cells removes a proportion of these cellular elements, but the freeze-thaw cycle followed by washing more effectively removes the histocompatibility antigens.

An additional benefit of the red cell washing necessary for frozen blood is the complete removal of plasma. All the undesirable properties of banked blood are in the plasma, and reconstituted frozen blood is free of isoantibodies, accumulated ammonia and potassium, citrate, platelets, white cells, plasma proteins, and the hepatitis virus. Febrile and allergic tranfusion reactions associated with white cell, platelet, or plasma protein sensitivities are avoided, therefore, by the use of frozen blood. Patients with paroxysmal nocturnal hemoglobinuria present a special instance in which transfusion of washed red cells is indicated because of the enhancement of hemolysis frequently observed after the transfusion of compatible whole blood. Even the small volume of plasma contained in red cell packs may prove deleterious to these patients.

Unfortunately the cost in time and equipment makes frozen blood an impractical method for routine red cell transfusion, and there is an associated in vitro loss of 20 to 30% of the red cells. It should be remembered that the advantages of single-component administration are outweighed if massive blood replacement is required, since frozen blood does not contain platelets and the coagulation proteins. Careful monitoring of the platelet count and coagulation assays is necessary if large amounts of frozen blood are used to replace rapid blood loss.

RED CELL PRESERVATION

Erythrocyte adenosine triphosphate (ATP) and 2,3-diphosphoglycerate (2,3-DPG) fall to low levels in blood stored at refrigerator temperatures. ATP is converted by a sequence of dephosphorylations to adenosine monophosphate (AMP), and the adenine moiety of AMP is irreversibly converted to inosine. Although further degradation of inosine ensues, it is the irreversible deamination of adenine to inosine that deprives the erythrocyte of the ability to restore ATP levels (from adenine, ribose, and phosphate) unless an exogenous source of adenine is provided.

ATP is the primary high-energy compound in the red cell, and adequate quantities are essential for the survival of the transfused erythrocyte. The maintenance of membrane integrity (surface area and deformability), the maintenance of cell shape, the active efflux of sodium and calcium, the active influx of potassium, and the maintenance of glycolytic metabolism are each dependent on the presence of adequate quantities of ATP.

Several studies have shown that red cell ATP content is closely correlated with posttransfusion survival. It is the level of ATP (and the other residual adenine-containing compounds capable of being regenerated quickly to ATP) that governs the period of time blood may be stored before use. In general, at the currently allowable 21-day period of storage at 4°C, greater than 70% of cells show a normal viability after transfusion. Studies have indicated that addition of adenine (with or without inosine) and phosphate can maintain acceptable levels of posttransfusion red cell viability after 6 weeks of storage. These additives are not yet approved for routine use, however.

2,3-DPG is the organic phosphate present in highest concentration in the human red cell. This compound has been thought to function as an intracellular buffer and a source of potential energy for the cell during periods of substrate deprivation. More recently, it has been shown that 2,3-DPG and ATP bind with deoxyhemoglobin and in so doing reduce the affinity of hemoglobin for oxygen. 2,3-DPG is more important in this regard principally because it is present in a quantity about 3 times greater than ATP in the red cell. Several clinical studies have confirmed the role of these red cell organic phosphate compounds as an important modulating factor in the association of oxygen with hemoglobin. This subject is reviewed in detail in Chapter 10. The increased affinity of hemoglobin for oxygen in red cells stored at 4°C is primarily related to the progressive reduction in red cell 2,3-DPG and ATP. Recent studies suggest that 2,3-DPG is rapidly regenerated in vivo so that 30 to 50% of normal levels are obtained within 4 hours after infusion, and complete restoration occurs within 24 hours. These considerations suggest that oxygen delivery might be less than that expected from the restored red cell mass for several hours after rapid administration of stored blood. Although oxygen-hemoglobin dissociation curves have not been measured in patients who have been transfused with large quantities of stored blood over a short period of time, the in vitro data indicate that in such situations it is prudent to use blood stored for less than 24 hours. In patients with severe anemia, such as advanced pernicious anemia, and the additional complications of congestive heart failure or angina pectoris, the use of fresh red cells if needed would insure an immediate increase in oxygen delivery.

Recent studies have indicated that addition of inosine, phosphate, and pyruvate to 3- or 4-week-old blood can rapidly increase 2,3-DPG concentrations. Such an effect should enhance the oxygen-carrying capacity at the time of transfusion. Although the use of additives remains an experimental procedure, these studies suggest their potential usefulness in prolonging the shelf-life of stored blood and in improving its immediate oxygen-carrying capacity in situations in which this could be a crucial factor in the patient's improvement.

REFERENCES

Benesch, R., and Benesch, R. E.   Intracellular organic phosphates as regulators of oxygen release by hemoglobin. *Nature* (London) 221:618, 1969.

Bunn, H. F., May, M. H., Kocholaty, W. F., and Shields, C. E.   Hemoglobin function in stored blood. *J. Clin. Invest.* 48:311, 1969.

Greenwalt, T. J., and Perry, S.   Preservation and utilization of the components of human blood. *Progr. Hemat.* 6:148, 1969.

Mollison, P. L.   *Blood Transfusion in Clinical Medicine* (4th ed.). Philadelphia: Davis, 1967.

Murphy, S., and Gardner, F. H.   Platelet preservation: Effects of storage temperature on maintenance of platelet viability—deleterious effect of refrigerated storage. *New Eng. J. Med.* 280:1094, 1969.

Murphy, S., Sayar, S. N., and Gardner, F. H.   Storage of platelet concentrates at 22°C. *Blood* 35:549, 1970.

Schmidt, P. J., and Grindon, A. J.   Blood and blood components in prevention and control of bleeding. *J.A.M.A.* 202:967, 1967.

Schwarzenberg, L., Mathé, G., Amiel, J. L., Cattan, A., Schneider, M., and Schlumberger, J. R.   Study of factors determining the usefulness and complications of leukocyte transfusions. *Amer. J. Med.* 43:206, 1967.

Simon, E. R.   Adenine and purine nucleosides in human red cell preservation: A review. *Transfusion* 7:395, 1967.

Sutnick, A. I., London, W. T., Millman, I., Coyne, V. E., and Blumberg, B. S.   Viral hepatitis: Revised concepts as a result of the study of Australia antigen. *Med. Clin. N. Amer.* 54:805, 1970.

Tullis, J. L., and Pennel, R. B.   Transfusion of specific plasma components. *Ann. Rev. Med.* 19:233, 1968.

Valeri, C. R.   Frozen blood. *New Eng. J. Med.* 275:365, 425, 1966.

Valtis, D. J., and Kennedy, A. C.   Defective gas-transport function of stored red blood cells. *Lancet* 1:119, 1954.

12. MANAGEMENT OF BONE MARROW FAILURE

Arthur W. Bauman

BONE MARROW FAILURE is defined as the combination of findings of a significant reduction in one or more of the cellular elements of the peripheral blood accompanied by a reduction in the precursor cells in the bone marrow. Splenomegaly and lymph node enlargement are not present. The cause of marrow failure is usually apparent when leukopenia is present and tends to be reversible if the causal agent is removed (Table 12-1). Erythroid aplasia has been associated with thymic tumors, drugs (Table 12-2), and autoimmune mechanisms. Megakaryocytic aplasia is rare as a single entity but has been reported in association with drug therapy, particularly chloramphenicol. Megakaryocytic failure but not necessarily aplasia has also become a recognized entity secondary to the ingestion of alcohol. Aplastic anemia is unexplained in about 50% of the cases and chemotherapeutic agents are implicated in the rest (Table 12-3). Aplastic anemia has also been reported to occur following infectious hepatitis, and its association with paroxysmal nocturnal hemoglobinuria has received recent attention.

Pancytopenia associated with a cellular marrow is not uncommon. In the absence of evidence of a deficiency state, we view most patients with these findings as being in a preleukemic state.

EVALUATION OF THE PATIENT

Each patient should have a careful history taken with particular attention to the use of all drugs and combinations of them. Patients with erythroid aplasia and aplastic anemia by definition will have a reticulocytopenia, and examination of the peripheral blood smear in all these situations usually shows normal morphology of the remaining cells. A bone marrow aspira-

Table 12-1. Drugs Associated with the Development of Leukopenia

Phenothiazines
  Chlorpromazine (Thorazine)
  Promazine (Sparine)
  Imipramine (Tofrānil)
  Prochlorperazine (Compazine)

Analgesics
  Aminopyrine
  Phenylbutazone

Chloroquine

Chloramphenicol

Sulfonamides
  Sulfanilamide
  Sulfisoxazole (Gantrisin)
  Salicylazosulfapyridine (Azulfidine)

Sulfonamide derivatives
  Chlorothiazide (Diuril)
  Tolbutamide (Orinase)

Antithyroids
  Thiouracil and propylthiouracil
  Methimazole (Tapazole)

Miscellaneous
  Diphenylhydantoin sodium (Dilantin)
  Meprobamate (Miltown, Equanil)

tion should be carried out in all patients and usually demonstrates, in patients with aplastic anemia, a predominance of lymphocytes, plasma cells, and occasionally mast cells. In all patients in whom a hypocellular marrow is found it is advisable to obtain a marrow biopsy also, preferably from a site different from where the aspirate is taken; this measure is for the occasional patient in whom the aspirate constitutes a "dry tap" because of re-

Table 12-2. Drugs Associated with the Development of Erythroid Aplasia

Chloramphenicol
Sulfonamides
Benzene
Diphenylhydantoin sodium (Dilantin)
Isoniazid
Para-aminosalicylic acid

placement of marrow by tumor or fibrosis. Occasionally, acute leukemia with a "packed marrow" is also diagnosed on the basis of the marrow biopsy.

Table 12-3.   Drugs Associated with the Development of Aplastic Anemia

Chloramphenicol
Phenylbutazone (Butazolidin)
Methylphenylethylhydantoin (Mesantoin)
Diphenylhydantoin sodium (Dilantin)
Sulfonamides and their derivatives
Benzene

Paroxysmal nocturnal hemoglobinuria should be considered in the initial evaluation of all patients with aplastic anemia, and an acid hemolysis test (Ham test) or sugar water test should be carried out. The sugar water test is quite sensitive and specific and is relatively simple to perform. (For details, see Hartmann et al. in the Appendix.)

All patients found to have evidence of pure erythroid aplasia should be carefully evaluated for the presence of thymoma with appropriate x-ray studies and consideration of mediastinoscopy.

MANAGEMENT

Patients with the isolated finding of leukopenia, particularly those with acute granulocytopenia which is clearly drug induced, usually respond within a few days after removal of the offending agent. Apart from the diligent treatment of infection if present in these patients, little else needs to be done except to avoid subsequent use of the implicated drugs. A similar approach with withdrawal of all suspected drugs should be employed in the patient who seems to have a more chronic form of leukopenia. Little else can be done for these patients except to be vigilant for infection and to treat it early if it should develop.

The management of patients with isolated erythroid aplasia and megakaryocytic aplasia generally follows the same approaches used in the treatment of aplastic anemia, i.e., with specific attention to treatment of anemia in patients with erythroid aplasia and to treatment of bleeding complications in patients with megakaryocytic aplasia.

All patients with erythroid aplasia who are found to have thymic tumors should have the tumor removed if possible. Unfortunately, only about 30% of these patients respond to removal of the thymic tumor with a good hematologic remission. The mechanism by which the thymus induces red cell aplasia is not clear, but it has been suggested that these tumors release a specific inhibitor of erythropoietin response by the bone marrow rather than a general inhibitor of erythropoietin release.

It is too early to say what role immunosuppressive therapy may have in the treatment of erythroid aplasia, but the possibility that some patients with this disorder may have an autoimmune inhibitor of erythropoiesis may provide us with another mode of therapy for certain patients.

TRANSFUSIONS

All patients who are chronically anemic as a result of bone marrow failure should be given transfusions of packed red cells as often as is necessary either to keep the hematocrit level at 25% or better, or to keep the patient relatively free of symptoms. In a patient whose marrow has stopped making red cells one can anticipate a fall in hematocrit of approximately 3 points a week, equivalent to the red cells in 1 unit of blood. The average patient who is not losing blood and who is not making red cells, starting with a hematocrit reading of 25%, will therefore require 2 units of packed cells every 2 weeks as long as his marrow is not making red cells. The administration of whole blood is not necessary and may be dangerous in some patients who have significant cardiac disease.

In anticipation of the requirement for long-term transfusion therapy, it is wise to type the patient's red cells as extensively as possible prior to any transfusions. Should isoantibodies develop at some later date, identification of these antibodies will be much simpler if the patient's original cell type has been determined.

About 50% of patients receiving red blood cells are likely to develop buffy coat reactions secondary to isoantibodies against the transfused white cells and occasionally the transfused platelets. These reactions, usually consisting of fever and occasionally chills, can sometimes be counteracted by prior or concomitant administration of acetaminophen (Tylenol) and possibly antihistaminics. Steroids (e.g., cortisone, prednisone) are generally not useful in counteracting buffy coat reactions. Salicylates should be avoided because of their interference with platelet function and the consequent possible development of further bleeding tendencies in any patient who is thrombocytopenic. Occasionally, severe buffy coat reactions which do not respond to the above measures will develop. Such reactions can be minimized if these patients are given either washed red cells or frozen red blood cells, the latter having been washed during their preparation.

Administration of platelets to patients with megakaryocytic aplasia or with aplastic anemia should be considered only after careful evaluation of the patient's overall status. It is not wise to treat the platelet count and, generally speaking, dependent petechiae and occasional bruises are not sufficient indications to give platelet transfusions. Platelet transfusions at the present time must be used sparingly because of the likelihood that iso-antibodies will develop in time, thereby negating the usefulness of the plate-lets. Likewise, the preparation of large quantities of platelets still is an expensive and arduous task. Overt bleeding from mucous membranes or into the gastrointestinal or genitourinary tract usually are indications for the administration of platelets. On the other hand, if bleeding is sufficient to cause overt blood loss, administration of fresh "walk-in" donor blood in lieu of or in conjunction with the use of platelets should also be considered. Local bleeding, as from one nostril, in the absence of a generalized tendency for bleeding, even in the face of severe thrombocytopenia, should be investigated for possible local treatment.

The techniques for concentrating platelets and indeed even for storing them overnight while retaining their viability have recently been developed to the point where the administration of large quantities of platelets is feasible in many centers. Theoretically, the platelets from a single unit of whole blood should raise the platelet count by about 40,000 per cubic millimeter. In actual practice the rise is usually in the range of 6000 to 10,000 per cubic millimeter. These observations should be kept in mind when assessing the need for platelets in any patient with aplastic anemia. It is readily apparent that a unit or two of concentrated platelets is of little value in the patient with a very low platelet count who is actively bleeding. Often 10 to 20 units daily is required for 2 to 4 days before control of bleeding can be achieved. Additional limitations to the use of platelets is their short survival ($T\frac{1}{2}$ of 2 to 4 days) and our inability to do practical platelet typing at this time. As noted above, eventual development of antibodies by the recipient is inevitable, limiting subsequent use of platelets. Antibody production is markedly reduced when platelets obtained from compatible donors on the basis of histocompatibility antigen (HL-A) lymphocyte typing are given. Unfortunately, few laboratories are equipped to do lymphocyte typing at this time.

In summary, platelets, even though they are available, should be used infrequently and then usually vigorously in the management of patients with thrombocytopenia due to marrow failure. More liberal use of platelets is probably indicated also during the first 4 months of the illness, during which time remission is more likely to occur if it is going to. The use of HL-A compatible donors will markedly reduce platelet requirements in the future.

The administration of white cells to patients with severe granulocytopenia and with aplastic anemia is not usually practical. The best source of large quantities of white cells is an untreated patient with chronic myelogenous leukemia (see Chap. 27), and there have been reports to suggest that these cells may be of value in controlling infection in severely neutropenic patients. Pooling blood from normal patients in order to obtain an adequate quantity of white cells on a daily basis simply cannot be done at the present time.

Hormonal Therapy .

Various preparations of male hormone or cortisone derivatives have been reported to be effective in stimulating return of marrow function in patients with erythroid aplasia and with aplastic anemia. The male hormones mediate their action through enhancement of release of erythropoietin, which in turn stimulates production of an increased number of marrow red cell precursor cells and accelerates their maturation. The male hormones consequently have their most marked effect on erythroid activity but may also improve the production of myeloid cells for reasons that are not well understood at the present time. The corticosteroids mediate their action through release of the "marginal pool" of marrow leukocytes but probably also have a direct effect on leukopoiesis, which is also not well understood at the present time. Neither of these hormones has much direct effect that is known on megakaryocytic function.

Prolonged use of male hormones and corticosteroids is advisable in all patients with aplastic anemia; several months of intensive therapy may be required before marrow function returns. In general, these drugs are somewhat more effective in myeloid metaplasia than they are in aplastic anemia or erythroid aplasia. Our practice is to give fluoxymesterone (Halotestin), 20 to 30 mg per day by mouth, or testosterone enanthate (Delatestryl), 600 mg intramuscularly every week, plus prednisone, 45 to 60 mg per day by mouth for 3 to 4 months before deciding that remission will not occur.

In general, responsiveness to hormones tends to be proportional to the original cellularity of the marrow. The first evidence of response is usually reticulocytosis, and this is followed by variable increases in the white cells and platelets. The platelets are the least likely to return. The white cells and the platelets almost never return in the absence of reticulocytosis. Sustained improvement on this type of regimen has been observed in 20 to 30% of patients with aplastic anemia. The hormone dose is gradually tapered after apparent maximal response has been achieved with complete cessation of therapy after about a year. About two-thirds of the patients who respond to hormones have a prolonged remission after cessation of hormonal therapy. In a recent report Sanchez-Medal and co-workers suggested that oxymetholone may produce remission in up to 50% of all patients with aplastic anemia who are treated for more than 3 months.

Side effects with prolonged use of high doses of male hormones and corticosteroids are likely to occur. The most troublesome of these is hepatotoxicity, usually cholestatic in nature. The incidence of chemical hepatic dysfunction may range as high as 80% associated with oxymetholone. Serious hepatotoxicity is much less, at 10%. Although the 17-alkylated steroids are associated with the highest incidence of hepatotoxicity, as discussed in Chapter 26, it is our impression that the route of administration is also important in the production of liver toxicity. Because there is a lesser incidence of hepatotoxicity when male hormone is given parenterally as opposed to the oral preparations, it may be that presentation of relatively high concentrations to hepatic parenchymatous cells after direct passage through the portal bed is as important as the chemical preparation itself. It is also noteworthy that the parenteral preparations of male hormones are usually much less expensive than the oral preparations and, as a result, we favor parenterally administered male hormones almost exclusively, unless the patient is thrombocytopenic and predisposed to hemorrhage at the injection site.

Other side effects which can be anticipated are hoarseness in most women who are treated for more than a month, hirsutism, acne, amenorrhea, and increase in libido. Cushingoid changes and fluid retention are likely to be secondary to the administration of cortisone derivatives. For patients treated with corticosteroids it is also our practice to add supplemental potassium to the diet and to advise most patients to take antacids or milk between meals and at bedtime. A tuberculin test should be carried out and isoniazid, 300 mg per day, should be given to patients with a positive tuberculin reaction if they are to receive corticosteroids.

INFECTIOUS COMPLICATIONS

Infection and bleeding are the cause of death in nearly all patients with aplastic anemia who neither respond to therapy nor recover spontaneously. The offending infectious agents are usually gram-negative colonic organisms which are almost impossible for the patient to avoid. For this reason we take no precautions except to advise the patient to avoid contact with others who obviously have staphylococcal infections. Isolation and sterilization techniques are generally impractical and increase the anxiety of the patient and his family. Indeed, patients with these disorders, particularly aplastic anemia, should be encouraged to lead as normal a life as possible but to report immediately any symptoms of infection. Symptoms of infection are of course viewed with considerable alarm, and aggressive therapy —following appropriate cultures—is initiated immediately, prior to isolation of a specific organism. Usually in the first 48 hours a combination of sodium cephalothin (Keflin) and kanamycin sulfate (Kantrex), or these two antibiotics plus colistin, is utilized at high doses. After the identification of the specific offending organism, the therapy can be tailored accordingly.

Various "gut sterilization" regimens have been introduced, particularly in the management of acute leukemia, and these may have some promise in the future management of patients with aplastic anemia. They are discussed in considerable detail in Chapter 22.

OTHER MEASURES

As noted, patients with aplastic anemia and thrombocytopenia due to isolated megakaryocytic aplasia should be advised to avoid salicylates in any form. Drugs which may cause marrow suppression probably should be avoided, but they are not absolutely contraindicated if they are not implicated as the original offending agent and are clearly needed. This specifically applies to the use of chloramphenicol in the occasional patient who might develop *Salmonella* infection. Hematinics such as iron, folic acid, vitamin B_{12}, and vitamin B_6 are of no value. Indeed, iron may be detrimental, as these patients have increased iron stores secondary both to increased iron absorption and to breakdown of the transfused red cells. Splenectomy rarely has been beneficial in the treatment of aplastic anemia or of isolated marrow precursor cell failure, and it is not advocated.

REFERENCES

Grumet, F. C., and Yankee, R. A.   Long term platelet support of patients with aplastic anemia. *Ann. Intern. Med.* 73:1, 1970.

Hirst, E., and Robertson, T. I.   Syndrome of thymoma and erythroblastopenic anemia: Review of 56 cases including 3 case reports. *Medicine* (Balt.) 46:225, 1967.

Huguley, C. M., Jr., Lea, J. W., Jr., and Butts, J. A.   Adverse Hematologic Reactions to Drugs. In E. B. Brown and C. V. Moore (Eds.), *Progress in Hematology,* Vol. V. New York: Grune & Stratton, 1966.

Krantz, S. B., and Kao, V.   Studies on red cell aplasia: I. Demonstration of a plasma inhibitor to heme synthesis and an antibody to erythroblast nuclei. *Proc. Nat. Acad. Sci. U.S.A.* 58:493, 1967.

Publications of the Registry on Adverse Reactions, Vol. 1. Chicago: Council on Drugs. American Medical Association, 1964–1965.

Rubin, E., Gottlieb, C., and Vogel, P.   Syndrome of hepatitis and aplastic anemia. *Amer. J. Med.* 45:88, 1968.

Sanchez-Medal, L., Gomez-Leal, A., Duarte, L., and Rico, M. G.   Anabolic androgenic steroids in the treatment of acquired aplastic anemia. *Blood* 34:283, 1969.

Vincent, P. C., and deGruchy, G. C.   Complications and treatment of acquired aplastic anaemia. *Brit. J. Haemat.* 13:236, 1967.

II
PROBLEMS OF
HEMOSTASIS

13. NORMAL HEMOSTASIS AND EVALUATION OF THE BLEEDING PATIENT

Stanley B. Troup

THE BIOLOGY OF NORMAL HEMOSTASIS

During its evolution the human organism has developed many complex systems for achieving homeostasis. A central requirement in most of these is the maintenance of an intact vascular system. A major responsibility for the integrity of the vascular system is the hemostatic process. The multi-dependent phenomenon which we call hemostasis occurs as a consequence of many related events. The ultimate goal can be taken as the simplest definition: the cessation of blood flow from an injured vessel.

Blood coagulation is one of the important events in the hemostatic process but should not be equated, as has been done in the past, with the entire series of events. A patient may have a major defect in blood coagulation—the heparinized patient, for example, or the patient with congenital afibrinogenemia—and still retain relatively good hemostasis. The maintenance of normal hemostasis, then, depends on a variety of factors. These include the patient's general clinical status, the nature of the hemostatic stress or insult, the type of blood vessel or vessels injured, the anatomic site of injury, the coagulation mechanism, and occasionally the fibrinolytic activity. Should any of these factors be sorely stressed, hemostasis may prove defective.

Frequently, when a fault in hemostasis appears, more than a single factor may prove contributory. For example, the abnormal bleeding noted in a patient with severe liver disease may be a combined consequence of thrombocytopenia, defective synthesis of several blood clotting factors, and a variety of defects related to increased fibrinolytic activity. Similarly, the bleeding tendency in a patient with severe renal insufficiency may prove to be a

This work was supported in part by U.S. Public Health Service Grant HE-04167-11.

cumulative consequence of poor tissue turgor, thrombocytopenia, qualitative as well as quantitative platelet abnormalities, and deficiencies in certain blood clotting factors.

A practical therapeutic principle emerges from the recognition that many failures in hemostasis derive from multiple causes: namely, one need not correct all abnormalities in order to achieve effective hemostasis. Significant improvement in one aspect of the impaired hemostatic mechanism may suffice to correct the cumulative defect. The patient with severe liver disease and pathologic bleeding need not have all defects corrected in order to achieve normal hemostasis. Vitamin K administration to the patient who has had significant exclusion of bile from the intestine may raise the level of the vitamin K–dependent factors (factors II, VII, IX, and X) to levels at which the bleeding tendency may diminish significantly even though the patient may still be thrombocytopenic or have deficiency of factor V not corrected by the vitamin K administration.

Not all breaches in hemostasis are necessarily due to multiple causes. The patient with severe classic hemophilia (factor VIII deficiency) will bleed because of that unique deficiency. The patient with thrombocytopenia secondary to bone marrow aplasia may bleed solely because of the quantitative platelet deficiency.

MECHANISM OF HEMOSTASIS

The earliest recognized response to vascular injury, although inconstant, is vasoconstriction. This seemingly simple response may, by itself, achieve hemostasis at the microscopic level. Whether such vasoconstriction occurs secondary to neural or humoral mechanisms is not firmly established. Human platelets contain vasoactive amines which may be liberated at the site of injury, but this earliest vasoconstriction may occur prior to recognizable platelet accumulation. Patients with a mild bleeding disorder have been described in whom the only laboratory abnormality noted has been a prolonged bleeding time. Microscopic study of the capillary loops in the nailfolds of such patients occasionally reveals that these capillary loops do not constrict following injury. Failure of such capillary constriction may be significant but is not thought to be a frequent cause of bleeding.

COLLAGEN-PLATELET REACTION.   Within a few seconds following vascular injury, platelets begin to adhere to the margin of the injured vessel. This earliest platelet adherence is to subendothelial collagen fibrils. The attraction of the collagen for the platelets has not been characterized. The importance of this affinity in normal hemostasis is inferential but rather suggestive.

Aspirin (acetylsalicylic acid) ingestion interferes with platelet function in at least two ways. The collagen-platelet attraction is diminished and the release of adenosine diphosphate (ADP) from the platelet following the collagen reaction is inhibited. Since the bleeding time in normal individuals may be lengthened following aspirin ingestion and the bleeding time in some patients with coagulation disorders similarly may be lengthened, the inference is drawn that the platelet-collagen reaction is of physiologic importance.

PLATELET-TO-PLATELET ADHERENCE. Seconds following the normal adherence of platelets to collagen, platelets loosely adhere to one another at the point of vascular injury. This platelet-to-platelet aggregation occurs, it is believed, because of a platelet-ADP-platelet interaction. The ADP may be provided by release of this substance from the platelets following the collagen-platelet reaction. The significance of this loose aggregation in normal hemostasis again is inferential. Patients with the rare qualitative platelet abnormality known as thrombasthenia of Glanzmann have a prolonged bleeding time. The platelets from such patients fail to aggregate when ADP is added in vitro to their platelet-rich plasma. These same platelets lack fibrinogen, a necessary component for the ADP reaction, and also fail to support clot retraction. Which of these functional failures is the most important in these patients is not certain. Further, the ADP-platelet interaction may be important in maintaining hemostasis in the patient who has been treated with heparin. The reaction works well in the presence of heparin. Quite possibly, the maintenance of hemostasis is accomplished in the heparinized patient by the ability of the platelets to aggregate in the presence of ADP.

FORMATION OF HEMOSTATIC PLUG. The next phase of platelet function probably is the most important. The loose aggregate of platelets that has accumulated, presumably in response to ADP release, is converted into a compact platelet mass, the "hemostatic plug." While the loose platelet aggregate formed by the platelet-ADP interaction results in some degree of hemostasis, it is evident from animal studies that this can be breached by blood issuing from small arterioles. The more compact platelet mass is a much more effective device. The formation of the hemostatic plug corresponds in time to what we measure as the bleeding time.

The event that normally triggers the transformation of the loose platelet aggregate to the compact platelet plug is not known with certainty. Again by inference, it is believed that the appearance of trace amounts of thrombin at the surface of the platelet initiates this dramatic change. The appearance of thrombin in this short a time, some 2 to 3 minutes, is explained by the presence of "tissue thromboplastin" released from damaged cells and the presence of the normal plasma coagulation factors at the surface of the platelet. In vitro effects that seem comparable can be demonstrated by the addition of trace amounts of thrombin to platelet-rich plasma. The platelets promptly aggregate then fuse, compact, and manifest the morphologic and biochemical changes characterized as viscous metamorphosis.

Biochemical Basis of Platelet Function

The biochemical events that parallel the morphologic events occurring in these early stages of hemostasis have been studied in detail. The platelet, normally rich in adenosine triphosphate (ATP), also contains a contractile protein, thrombosthenin. This material has ATPase activity and resembles actomyosin in its function. During viscous metamorphosis, platelet ATP is hydrolyzed and ADP released. The liberated ADP theoretically then participates in further platelet aggregation, thus expanding the hemostatic process.

Substances liberated during the interaction of platelets and collagen and of platelets and ADP include serotonin and various platelet enzymes. Platelet factor 3 also is made available during these early events. This clot-accelerating substance is a phospholipid, possibly a phospholipid-protein complex. The platelet membrane is the site of this activity, as are certain of the platelet granules. Which is the physiologic source of clotting activity is not established with certainty.

Although microscopic strands of fibrin are found within the compact platelet hemostatic plug, suggesting that trace amounts of thrombin indeed have been present, much of hemostasis is accomplished without gross blood coagulation. When large vessels are disrupted, the platelet plug alone is not enough to stanch the flow of blood, so that the clotting process assumes a more major role.

Blood Coagulation

The importance of blood coagulation in hemostasis is most dramatically expressed in such disorders as hemophilia. The failure of blood clotting here represents a failure in what has been called intrinsic blood coagulation. Intrinsic blood coagulation describes clotting that involves factors native to the blood alone. Extrinsic blood coagulation is clotting that relies for its initiation on tissue thromboplastin, a product not native to the blood.

The importance of the extrinsic system was implied earlier in speaking of the trace amounts of thrombin on the platelet surface which are required to induce the formation of the hemostatic platelet plug. The importance of the intrinsic system of coagulation is manifested by the hemophilic patient, whose hemostatic failure results from a deficiency of factor VIII, an essential part of the intrinsic clotting system.

FACTOR XII.   The initial step in the intrinsic coagulation process involves the activation of a plasma protein known as Hageman factor (factor

XII). The absence of factor XII activity from plasma, strangely enough, results in no clinical hemostatic defect. The laboratory abnormality, quixotically, is rather dramatic. Individuals with factor XII deficiency have long blood clotting times. Despite this frightening finding, the patients do not bleed spontaneously or excessively following trauma. Hageman, the original patient described, underwent gastrectomy without bleeding complications and, in fact, died many years later of thromboembolic disease.

Factor XII normally circulates in an inactive state. The transformation of factor XII from this state to the active form occurs by contact with virtually any nonendothelial surface. The activated form of factor XII has enzymatic activity. This property, which may have greater biologic importance outside the coagulation system than within it, is responsible for the next step in the intrinsic clotting mechanism.

FACTOR XI. Factor XI (plasma thromboplastin antecedent, or PTA) is a protein whose absence results in the clinically mild bleeding disorder known variously as Rosenthal's syndrome, hemophilia C, PTA deficiency, or more uniformly as factor XI deficiency. The enzymatically active form of factor XII is thought to use factor XI as a substrate. This initial sequence heralds the graphically described "waterfall" or "cascade" sequence of blood coagulation.

Factor XI deficiency, inherited as an autosomal trait, usually is a mild disease. This defect is not often associated with spontaneous bleeding but rather with bleeding following surgery, trauma, or childbirth.

The peculiar discrepancy between the severe laboratory expression of factor XII deficiency and its virtual lack of clinical abnormalities is best explained at present in terms of certain features of factor XI. While factor XI normally depends upon activated factor XII for its conversion to an active form, in vitro studies suggest that factor XI can be activated without the presence of factor XII. This seeming "autoactivation" could account for the failure of factor XII deficiency to result in clinical problems.

FACTOR IX. The third step in the intrinsic clotting sequence is the conversion of factor IX (Christmas factor; plasma thromboplastin component, or PTC) from an inert plasma precursor to an active procoagulant substance. This is the first step of the coagulation process that requires ionized calcium. The deficiency of factor IX activity expresses itself clinically in the disorder known variously as Christmas disease, hemophilia B, or PTC deficiency. This disease, a sex-linked recessive disorder, is indistinguishable clinically from true hemophilia, factor VIII deficiency.

FACTOR VIII. Activated factor IX appears to interact with factor VIII, probably not as an enzyme-substrate reaction. The nature of the interaction is not known. Phospholipid (platelet factor 3) and ionized calcium both are necessary. If factor VIII has been exposed to trace amounts of thrombin, the reaction is enhanced.

Inherited deficiency of factor VIII is expressed clinically as classic hemophilia. Factor VIII deficiency also has been demonstrated to be due to circulating anticoagulants directed against this activity. Hemophilia is discussed in greater detail in Chapter 14.

The events of blood coagulation described to this point are collectively referred to as the first phase of blood coagulation. These are the most time-consuming steps and represent some 95% of the time required for blood to clot in vitro. Deficiencies of activity within this phase of blood clotting, when severe, characteristically prolong the whole-blood clotting time. The phases to be described subsequent to this are much more rapid and are measured in seconds rather than in minutes. Accordingly, deficiencies in these later stages do not usually prolong the whole-blood clotting time to any measurable extent.

FACTOR X.   The second phase of blood coagulation arbitrarily begins with the activation of factor X (Stuart-Prower factor). The activation seemingly is accomplished by activated factor VIII, but possibly by a complex of factors IX and VIII, phospholipid, and calcium. Factor X (as also factor IX) requires vitamin K for its synthesis in the liver. Interfacing with the first phase of blood coagulation as it does, deficiency of factor X activity may reflect itself in the laboratory as a defect in the first phase of blood coagulation when severe (prolonged whole-blood clotting time) or in defects of tests measuring the second phase (prolonged prothrombin time) or tests that do not distinguish between the two phases (partial thromboplastin time).

THROMBIN.   Activated factor X combines with factor V and, as with the factor IX-VIII interaction, requires ionized calcium and phospholipid. The resultant product (prothrombinase, prothrombin converting activity) acts enzymatically to split the prothrombin molecule (factor II) and form thrombin. Deficiency of factor V activity, found rarely as an inherited defect and more commonly in patients with severe liver disease, also prolongs the prothrombin time and partial thromboplastin time. Factor V is not dependent on vitamin K for its synthesis by the liver.

Thrombin, quite rightfully, may be viewed as the central enzyme in the hemostatic process. While other important roles are ascribed to it, the prime function appears to be its effect on fibrinogen. Thrombin splits pairs of polypeptides from the fibrinogen molecule so that the fibrin monomers thus formed are able to link up, forming the fibrin polymer clot. The role of thrombin is to cleave the two pairs of polypeptide chains. The polymer formation is not related to thrombin activity but occurs through chemical bonding attraction. These events occur quickly in normal plasma. In vitro, some 10 or 11 seconds transpire between the addition of thrombin to normal plasma and the appearance of the fibrin polymer clot.

Thrombin, as noted previously, plays a role early in the hemostatic process as well. The compaction of the platelets, with resultant formation of the hemostatic plug, is thought to be triggered by the formation of trace amounts of thrombin at the surface of the loosely aggregated platelets. The postulate is that this thrombin is not formed through the intrinsic coagulation process just described, but rather evolves via the extrinsic pathway of coagulation. A tissue source of lipoprotein is thought to combine with factor VII and ionized calcium to then play the same role that the complex of activated factor IX, factor VIII, phospholipid, and ionized calcium play in the intrinsic system. Participation with phospholipid and calcium in the formation of this complex is the only known role of factor VII in coagulation. The evolution of thrombin then similarly follows via the pathway of activation which includes factor X and factor V.

This shortcut, evading the time-consuming activation of factors XII, XI, IX, and VIII, is what occurs in vitro when the one-stage prothrombin time is determined. A tissue source of lipoprotein (tissue thromboplastin) is added with calcium to citrated plasma. The clotting time of the plasma then is recorded. Normally this will vary between 11 and 15 seconds, depending upon the tissue thromboplastin employed. The time is lengthened if deficiencies of factors II (prothrombin), VII, V, X, or fibrinogen exist.

Since the conversion of prothrombin to thrombin and the clotting of fibrinogen normally require less than 15 seconds, it is clear that the largest proportion of time consumed in intrinsic coagulation relates to the earlier phases of activation of factors XII, XI, IX, and VIII. Accordingly, it is more easily understood that clinical defects involving the latter factors would result, when severe, in prolonged whole-blood clotting times. Equally logically it can follow that defects in factors immediately involved in the activation of thrombin or the effect of thrombin on fibrinogen are not likely to reflect themselves in a prolonged whole-blood clotting time amounting to minutes when prolongation of clotting time in these defects is a matter of seconds.

The importance of thrombin in blood clotting is reflected by our approach to clinical anticoagulation. Coumarin drugs impair the synthesis of prothrombin and the related activating factors VII and X, as well as factor IX. Heparin, on the other hand, interferes chiefly with the interaction of thrombin and fibrinogen.

In addition to its central effect on fibrinogen, thrombin triggers the viscous metamorphosis of the platelets and appears to enhance the activation of factors VIII and V and the final phase of blood coagulation, the activation of factor XIII.

FACTOR XIII.   This plasma protein is better known as fibrin-stabilizing factor. When activated by thrombin, it serves as an enzyme to convert the fibrin polymer from a loosely bonded substance into an insoluble internally disulfide linked protein. Rare patients with absence of factor XIII activity have been identified. The clinical expression of this uncommon illness is a relatively mild bleeding disorder and, even more interestingly, deficiencies in wound healing. Severe liver disease also has been associated with diminished factor XIII activity.

CLINICAL EVALUATION OF THE PATIENT

While our understanding of hemostasis remains incomplete, sufficient knowledge has accumulated so that a patient's problem usually can be logically solved and rationally treated. More often than not, the patient's history provides information that is most meaningful. The physical examination, as always, is helpful; finally, the laboratory can be confirmatory and specific although its value often is overestimated.

HISTORY

Bleeding following circumcision is a fairly common occurrence in males with inherited hemostatic disorders. The history of circumcision thus should be sought.

The dental history may be of some importance. Interestingly, many patients do not view dental extractions as surgery. Bleeding after surgery may be denied, and yet subsequent information may develop that serious bleeding followed dental procedures. The dental history thus must be sought specifically.

When patients report that they bled significantly following dental extraction, some judgments must be made about this. My experience has been that if the patient has postextraction bleeding from a significant hemostatic defect, it usually requires more than a simple trip back to the dentist. Dental bleeding lasting less than 24 to 48 hours is not likely to be terribly significant. As dental skills increase, one must bear in mind that a skilled oral surgeon may extract a tooth from a person having severe hemophilia without difficulty, and without prior transfusion therapy. If the site is fastidiously packed, bleeding may be minimal.

Tonsillectomy also is often viewed lightly by the patient. History of tonsillectomy should be sought specifically. In my experience, posttonsillectomy bleeding in patients with significant hemostatic defects usually is profound. The patient who reports that he or his parents recall that he had to be taken back to the operating room so that suturing could be done following tonsillectomy does not necessarily represent a suspicious case. The patient with a significant hemostatic defect usually will bleed for 3 or 4 days following tonsillectomy if not treated, and more often than not will require transfusion.

The menstrual history is particularly important in women who prove to have thrombocytopenia. Thrombocytopenia does not often cause intermenstrual bleeding but commonly causes menorrhagia.

The importance of ingestion of medications in patients with hemostatic failure has become increasingly evident. Again, it is not sufficient to inquire what drugs a patient may have taken recently; rather one should inquire specifically after agents known to be related to abnormal bleeding. Perhaps foremost on the list is aspirin. We now know that acetylsalicylic acid interferes with the platelet-collagen interaction and also interferes with the secondary release of ADP from the platelet. Further, the effect of aspirin on platelets may be noted for as long as a week following the ingestion of modest amounts of aspirin. In the patient taking a coumarin drug who begins to bleed seemingly spontaneously, aspirin will occasionally be discovered to be the villain that tipped the hemostatic balance. Products such as quinidine and quinine should be inquired for and the ingestion of phenylbutazone also noted.

The dietary history is of particular interest in the patient who may be thrombocytopenic. Thrombocytopenia of consequence may accompany severe folic acid deficiency. I have seen several patients in whom massive colonic hemorrhage occurred in the setting of a megaloblastic state secondary to folate deficiency. If the patient consumes a generous amount of alcohol and the folate deficiency is related to poor dietary intake, then the patient may be in double jeopardy. We now know that alcohol by itself may diminish the platelet production significantly.

A particular point should be made of the patient's family history. Inquiry about the health of siblings and parents is not enough. Since some of the most serious inherited clotting disorders are transmitted in a sex-linked recessive fashion, appreciation of genetic principles requires that one delve into the health of grandparents, occasionally great-grandparents, and certainly uncles and cousins. This takes but a moment and can yield important data.

PHYSICAL EXAMINATION

Several points about the physical examination also merit emphasis. The patient must be thoroughly examined for petechiae and ecchymoses. This is emphasized because frequently the internist will see a patient referred from a surgical specialist who may have performed a less than complete physical examination. Petechiae, for example, are likely to appear where tight straps are worn. While brassieres are apparently being discarded by the more liberated feminists, a number of our patients still wear them, and petechiae frequently appear beneath the straps and supports of such devices.

The lesions of hereditary hemorrhagic telangiectasia often are found beneath the fingernails or on the lips. Women are particularly offended by these cosmetic defects and may wear heavy nail lacquer or use lipstick in greater amounts than fashionable. When suspicious of such a possibility, I have occasionally found it worthwhile to ask the patient to remove the lipstick and even the nail polish for a subsequent visit.

Spider nevi suggest the possibility of liver disease, as in the male do gynecomastia and loss of chest and axillary hair. When the skin is being inspected, sites of recent venipunctures must be evaluated for the presence of unusual bleeding. An enlarged liver or spleen and widespread lymph node enlargement suggest the possibility of reticuloendothelial disease. The finding of any of these signs should alert us to the possibility that the hemostatic problem may be secondary to some other illness.

Evaluation of the patient with possible hemostatic failure is not a complicated affair. The importance of a thorough history and complete physical examination requires no further stress. If the history suggests a familial problem, a serious effort must be made to gain cooperation of the family members so that they also can be examined. Hospital records may yield valuable information, and frequently the pharmacy with which the patient does business may be of help in identifying specific drugs that the patient has taken, the nature of which the patient may not be able to recall.

LABORATORY TESTS

The ideal laboratory test to identify the problem of pathologic bleeding has not yet been designed. The least effective test is, regrettably, in popular use. The whole-blood clotting time performed in glass is of precious little value in the diagnosis of actual or potential hemostatic failure. If he is suffering from a gross abnormality, the patient has had so much trouble of such a characteristic sort that the diagnosis usually has been made before the test is ordered.

The single most valuable laboratory procedure remains the examination of the peripheral blood smear. Because thrombocytopenia is the most common cause of abnormal bleeding, this test is essential. In addition to the possible identification of thrombocytopenia in the well-stained blood smear, other valuable information may be forthcoming. The presence of abnormally sized and shaped or nucleated red blood cells may suggest the presence of some disorder of the bone marrow. Striking rouleaux formation may raise the question of a dysproteinemic state, and, of course, the presence of pathologic white blood cells may lead to diagnosis of a serious underlying disease.

The partial thromboplastin time (PTT) will detect not only those abnormalities that are identified by the whole-blood clotting time and some that might be missed by the whole-blood clotting time, but also will reveal abnormalities characterized by defects in the second stage of the coagulation mechanism. When this test is performed with care, employing suitable controls, it is a worthwhile screening test. When performed together with the one-stage prothrombin time, it permits further characterization of a possible coagulation defect. With a normal one-stage prothrombin time and an abnormal partial thromboplastin time, it is apparent that the defect lies within the first stage of the clotting mechanism.

Measurement of the bleeding time can be of considerable value but, as frequently performed, may be an imperfect test. Its principal use today is in the diagnosis of von Willebrand's disease, in which PTT is usually prolonged and the factor VIII level is consistently diminished. It is established that aspirin may cause bleeding in certain normal individuals, but the bleeding time has not proved of consistent value in identifying such persons. While the bleeding time classically has been recognized as prolonged in the thrombocytopenic patient, it is a needlessly indirect method of identifying that problem. Careful examination of the blood smear and a direct platelet count are much more effective in confirming the diagnosis of thrombocytopenia.

When a hemostatic defect has been identified as due to a problem in coagulation, and that in turn is suspected of being in the first stage of the clotting mechanism, specific clotting factor assays provide the most reliable and precise method of establishing an accurate diagnosis. While not difficult to perform, these should be done in laboratories accustomed to carrying them out. Where the clinical history suggests that fibrinolysis may be responsible for abnormal bleeding, several simple and effective laboratory tests are available. In this area of study we have laboratory tests that are more sensitive, rather than less sensitive, than needed. The euglobulin clot lysis test normally will detect physiologic amounts of fibrinolytic activity. The dilute whole-blood clot lysis is comparable in its sensitivity. The whole-blood clot lysis will identify pathologic fibrinolysis when severe, but this can be a difficult test to evaluate. Red cells may fall off the poorly retracted clot from the thrombocytopenic patient, falsely suggesting some degree of fibrinolysis. Also, the small clot that forms quickly in blood from the thrombocytopenic and hypofibrinogenemic patient with intravascular coagulation may be mistaken for rapid clot lysis when the whole-blood clot lysis test is used. These problems usually are circumvented by the previously mentioned tests.

Diagnosis of the patient with a bleeding disorder thus is usually accomplished without elaborate laboratory effort. For more specific diagnostic procedures—for example, identifying the drug responsible for what appears to be an immunologic form of thrombocytopenia or looking for circulating anticoagulants—other laboratory tests are necessary. For detailed information the reader is referred to the references provided at the end of the chapter.

BLEEDING ASSOCIATED WITH SURGERY

The physician summoned to see a patient who begins to bleed excessively during or following surgery faces special problems. The diagnostic and therapeutic responses to this uncomfortable summons must be brisk and well organized.

Excessive bleeding at the time of surgery usually can be related to one of several problems. The most common is that of ineffective local hemostasis, primarily a surgical problem. Bleeding from a single site alone, such as the surgical wound, usually is not due to a generalized hemostatic problem. The patient who bleeds excessively from the operative wound but not, for example, from a wound where a drain has been placed, or the patient bleeding excessively from a chest tube following thoracotomy but not at all from his tracheostomy wound, probably has a local problem rather than generalized hemostatic failure. Exceptions to these generalizations occur. Excessive bleeding from the prostatic bed occasionally follows prostatic surgery and may be the only site of significant bleeding. In this circumstance local increased fibrinolysis may be occurring. The hemostatic failure locally is thought due to activation of the plasminogen activator present in prostatic tissue when the urokinase in the urine washes over the operative prostatic bed. This local failure may be corrected by administering epsilon-aminocaproic acid to interrupt plasminogen activation.

Although it may be clinically likely that surgical bleeding is related in a given instance to local problems, laboratory investigation must confirm this. Examination of a blood smear can be done promptly to determine if platelets are present, and an actual platelet count can be done if the blood smear is not perfectly clear. The one-stage prothrombin determination, a partial thromboplastin time, and thrombin times also can be obtained within a few minutes. Normal or near-normal results would tend to confirm the clinical impression. One can then suggest to the surgeon with some confidence that the area be reexamined surgically if bleeding is severe.

Blood transfusions also may play a role in the genesis of abnormal bleeding during or following surgery. Thrombocytopenia is known to occur when transfusion has been massive and banked blood has been used. Patients who receive 15 units or more of bank blood in a period of less than 24 hours usually will be measurably thrombocytopenic, and some will have significant bleeding. As a general rule, one may assume that bleeding is due to thrombocytopenia in the patient in whom evidence of hemostatic failure develops during or following surgery when enormous quantities of bank blood have been transfused. This assumption must be confirmed by further evaluation, but until demonstrated otherwise, the bleeding accompanying massive transfusion is assumed to be thrombocytopenic. Examining the blood smear and counting the platelets can quickly provide the answer. The therapeutic approach would involve transfusion of fresh blood if the patient continues to require volume correction, or the use of platelet-rich plasma or platelet concentrates if the red cells and blood volume no longer require correction.

Hemolytic transfusion reactions also represent a potential cause of hemostatic failure in the surgical patient. The pathogenesis of the abnormal bleeding is not securely established. Several possible factors may play a role. The release of ADP from the hemolyzed red cells may be sufficient to cause platelet aggregation and removal of the platelets from the circulation. The release of phospholipid from hemolyzed red cells, leading to intravascular clotting, also has been suggested as a triggering mechanism. Further, the fibrinolytic mechanism may be stimulated secondarily by the intravascular clotting. Evidence of both defibrination and fibrinolysis has been documented following hemolytic transfusion reactions.

The patient who has been transfused and who begins to bleed during or following surgery also should have prompt inspection of a plasma sample to determine if hemoglobin is present. Examination of the urine for hemoglobin is not adequate since the level of hemoglobin in the plasma may not exceed the level of the binding capacity.

The bleeding that may accompany or follow surgery employing cardiopulmonary bypass raises yet other problems. Many pathogenetic mechanisms may be at play. The most common problem, in my experience, has proved due to excess heparin activity in the circulation. Although protamine usually is administered in excess of heparin, we have seen many examples in which the pathologic bleeding nonetheless seemed associated with excess heparin activity. This may be related to dissociation of heparin-protamine complexes or possible return of heparin from lymph. Prolonged thrombin time is the abnormality most commonly found in these patients. Prolongation of thrombin time may be related to the presence of fibrin split products from secondary fibrinolysis, but addition of more protamine would not correct the latter abnormality.

POTENTIAL BLEEDING PROBLEMS

The patient suspected of having an increased risk of hemostatic failure but who is not actually bleeding is best identified, not unexpectedly, by his history. This usually is in the form of a personal history suggesting excessive bleeding from minor trauma or previous surgery on the one hand, or because of a family history suggesting the possibility of hemostatic failure on the other. The evaluation of such a patient to a large extent has been dealt with earlier in this chapter. Points deserving reemphasis are the family history, the degree of bleeding accompanying past trauma or surgery, and a careful history of drug ingestion.

Evaluation of Surgery

The patient being evaluated prior to surgery must have similar consideration. It is important to note that certain illnesses enhance the possibility of pathologic bleeding during surgery. This is particularly true in the case of polycythemia vera or myeloid metaplasia. While the danger of excessive bleeding is diminished when the polycythemia and thrombocytosis have been corrected, these patients still carry an increased risk. We have seen dangerous bleeding following arterial needle puncture for angiographic studies in patients whose hematocrit level and platelet count were normal. Fatal bleeding is known to occur following simple hernia repair in such patients. The mechanism of the bleeding varies, and the reader is referred to the reference by Wasserman and Gilbert for a more complete discussion of this problem.

REFERENCES

Hardisty, R. M., and Ingram, G. I. C.   *Bleeding Disorders.* Philadelphia: Davis, 1965. Chap. 1, The Diagnostic Approach to Bleeding Disorders.

Lüscher, E. F.   Platelets in haemostasis and thrombosis. *Brit. J. Haemat.* 13:1, 1967.

Marcus, A. J.   Platelet functions. *New Eng. J. Med.* 280:1213, 1278, 1330, 1969.

Owen, C. A., Jr., Bowie, E. J. W., Didisheim, P., and Thompson, J. H., Jr. *The Diagnosis of Bleeding Disorders.* Boston: Little, Brown, 1969. Chap. 10, The Bleeding Patient.

Ratnoff, O. D. (Ed.).   *Treatment of Hemorrhagic Disorders.* New York: Hoeber Med. Div., Harper & Row, 1968. Chap. 1, An Approach to the Diagnosis of Disorders of Hemostasis.

Ratnoff, O. D.   Disordered Hemostasis in Hepatic Disease. In L. Schiff (Ed.), *Diseases of the Liver* (3d ed.). Philadelphia: Lippincott, 1969.

Troup, S. B., and Schwartz, S. I.   Hemostasis, Surgical Bleeding and Transfusion. In S. I. Schwartz (Ed.), *Principles of Surgery.* New York: Blakiston Div., McGraw-Hill, 1969.

Wasserman, L. R., and Gilbert, H. S.   Polycythemia vera and Myeloid Meta-plasia. In A. W. Ulin and S. S. Gollob (Eds.), *Surgical Bleeding: Handbook for Medicine, Surgery and Specialties.* New York: Blakiston Div., McGraw-Hill, 1966.

Williams, W. J.   Recent concepts of the clotting mechanism. *Seminars Hemat.* 5:32, 1968.

14. THE THROMBOCYTOPENIC PURPURAS

Robert T. Breckenridge

BLEEDING DUE TO decrease in the number of circulating blood platelets, the most common bleeding disorder, probably also is the most frequently unrecognized. Examination of the peripheral blood smear for the presence of platelets in any patient with hemorrhagic symptoms, and in every patient prior to surgery, would significantly reduce the number of patients encountered with serious and otherwise unexplained bleeding. If 8 to 12 platelets per oil-immersion microscopic field can be demonstrated in the blood smear of the bleeding patient, then the cause of the bleeding is not thrombocytopenia. If platelets are decreased on blood smear, the diagnosis of thrombocytopenia should be verified by a direct platelet count. Phase-contrast microscopy methods usually result in a normal range of 175,000 to 350,000 platelets per cubic millimeter. Normal values should be defined for each laboratory, since the range may vary.

Clear correlation between the platelet count and clinical bleeding sometimes is difficult to make. Accordingly, the precise number of platelets necessary for hemostasis is not firmly established. In general, platelet counts of greater than 50,000 per cubic millimeter are not associated with spontaneous bleeding. Platelet counts below 20,000 per cubic millimeter frequently are associated with petechiae and other hemorrhagic phenomena. Occasional patients with platelet counts in the 50,000 to 100,000 per cubic millimeter range, however, may bleed excessively during surgical procedures. In this setting the platelet count may decrease to a significantly lower range because of utilization of platelets during hemostasis at the site of surgical trauma and inability of the bone marrow to generate the necessary platelet replacement.

This work was supported in part by an operative grant from the Regional Medical Program and by U.S. Public Health Service Grant HE-04167-11.

HISTORICAL BACKGROUND OF THROMBOCYTOPENIA

Early medical writing contains references to purpuric rashes in association with a variety of illnesses. Lazare Rivière, writing in the seventeenth century, described patients with purpura during the course of "fevers." This may represent the earliest description of thrombocytopenia related to infection. Idiopathic thrombocytopenic purpura (ITP) was described first by Werlhof in 1735. These patients apparently had no underlying illness, and ITP occasionally is still referred to as Werlhof's disease.

By the late nineteenth century Krauss and Denys had noted that platelets were decreased in the peripheral blood smear in the presence of purpura and that platelets appeared again as the purpura disappeared. Since this description and the advent of the platelet count, thrombocytopenia has been reported in association with many illnesses. Examples are Osler's description of thrombocytopenia in patients with what we now know as systemic lupus erythematosus (SLE), the description of thrombocytopenia complicating infectious mononucleosis, and, more recently, the demonstration of thrombocytopenia following rubella vaccination.

A major development in the understanding of thrombocytopenia was the demonstration that certain medications may cause thrombocytopenia by an immune process. The pathogenesis of the thrombocytopenia appears to be damage of the platelet membrane by an antigen-antibody complex. The drug serves as a haptene and, together with plasma protein, behaves as antigen which induces the antibody response to the complex. The adsorption of this complex to the platelet surface apparently results in damage to the platelet with subsequent removal by the reticuloendothelial system.

The history of treatment for thrombocytopenia is marked by the suggestion in 1916 by Kaznelson that splenectomy be tried. The first patient so treated experienced an increase in platelets after splenectomy, but much later the thrombocytopenia recurred. One wonders if the surgical procedure would have continued in clinical popularity if the subsequent course of that patient had been appreciated. Steroid hormone therapy for thrombocytopenia was introduced by Robeson in 1948 and remains a useful adjunct to splenectomy in certain patients.

THE PLATELET IN HEMOSTASIS

Following vascular injury, constriction of blood vessels normally occurs and within seconds platelets begin to adhere at the site of injury. This initial platelet response occurs by interaction between the platelets and subendothelial collagen fibrils. The platelets adhere to the latter rather than to the endothelial surface. Seconds later platelet-to-platelet adherence occurs. This platelet interaction is thought to be mediated by the release of adenosine diphosphate (ADP) from the platelet. Interestingly, this "release reaction" is blunted in platelets from patients taking aspirin and certain other antiinflammatory agents.

At the time of vascular injury, tissue procoagulant activity (tissue thromboplastin) is thought to lead to trace amounts of thrombin formation in the platelets' plasma environment. The platelets loosely aggregated by the ADP-platelet interaction then begin to fuse and compact, forming the hemostatic platelet plug. This irreversible platelet reaction is known as viscous metamorphosis. The triggering of this complex morphologic and biochemical reaction results in some fashion from the action of thrombin on the platelet membrane.

The formation of the hemostatic platelet plug corresponds in time to the cessation of bleeding and determines the bleeding times as clinically measured. Of interest is the observation that patients who have taken aspirin may have prolongation of the bleeding time. This observation supports the idea that the early platelet-collagen-ADP interactions have significance in normal hemostasis. Patients already handicapped by thrombocytopenia should be cautioned to avoid taking aspirin since the remaining platelets might suffer a qualitative defect in addition to the quantitative defect represented by the thrombocytopenia. By inference, one might imagine that other agents interacting with the platelet might lead to defective hemostasis by interfering with normal platelet physiology.

DIFFERENTIAL DIAGNOSIS OF THROMBOCYTOPENIA

In all clinical settings, establishment of an etiologic basis for a diagnosis permits the most specific therapy. This also is true for thrombocytopenia. As in other clinical situations the history frequently is the most helpful portion of the evaluation of the thrombocytopenic patient. A variety of causes of thrombocytopenia exists, and these include drugs; exanthematous diseases, especially in the younger-age groups; and other viral illnesses. Virtually any exposure of the patient to such agents should be considered a possible cause of the thrombocytopenia. Since thrombocytopenia occurs in some 15% of patients with systemic lupus erythematosus, symptoms of serositis assume considerable significance in the clinical history.

The physical examination does not often supply an etiologic basis for the thrombocytopenia. Physical signs suggesting cirrhosis and portal hypertension, frank SLE, or exanthematous eruption may suggest that the thrombocytopenia is secondary to such illnesses. Prominent splenic enlargement is the exception in the adult with idiopathic thrombocytopenia. Accordingly, a large spleen in such a patient suggests that thrombocytopenia may be secondary to whatever process is producing the splenomegaly. A minority of adult patients with ITP have palpable splenomegaly, and when enlarged, the organ usually is only one or two fingerbreadths below the costal margin. Splenomegaly obviously does not exclude ITP. Splenic enlargement seems rather more common in the child with ITP than it is in the adult.

Many times the clinical history and the physical examination together do not offer an explanation for the thrombocytopenia. In this situation the laboratory assumes a more prominent role in establishing a basis for the thrombocytopenia.

Proper evaluation of the thrombocytopenic patient requires bone marrow examination. Significant diminution in the number of megakaryocytes or absence of megakaryocytes from the marrow suggests decreased platelet production as a mechanism for the thrombocytopenia. The presence of a normal number of megakaryocytes suggests that increased peripheral destruction of platelets may be responsible for the thrombocytopenia.

In the patient whose marrow is devoid of megakaryocytes (aplastic anemia or marrow replacement by nonmarrow tissue) the thrombocytopenia usually fails to respond to steroids or to splenectomy. If, on the other hand, megakaryocytes are present, the thrombocytopenia probably is caused at least in part by increased peripheral platelet removal. In many such patients a clinical response follows the use of steroid hormones or splenectomy, or both.

Evaluation in terms of systemic lupus erythematosus should be considered in each patient thought to have idiopathic thrombocytopenia. Approximately one-third of females with ITP subsequently develop systemic lupus erythematosus. In addition to the clinical observations and serologic data examination of serum proteins by electrophoresis may be of value. One study of patients with SLE and thrombocytopenia demonstrated that the gamma globulin fraction of the serum proteins represented about 20% of the total proteins. None of the patients with ITP in this study had such an elevation of gamma globulin.

Other than careful examination of the stained blood smear and equally careful evaluation of the bone marrow, we do not feel that many laboratory procedures are mandatory in the evaluation of the thrombocytopenic patient. Other laboratory procedures depend upon the clinical setting. Thus the patient suspected of having liver disease may require careful evaluation of the function of that organ, while the patient suspected of having a "consumption coagulopathy" requires measurement of various plasma clotting factors as well as a search for fibrin split products. As always, each patient requires individual evaluation.

MANAGEMENT OF THE THROMBOCYTOPENIC PATIENT

Ideal therapy for the thrombocytopenic patient requires the establishment of a precise cause for the thrombocytopenia. Thrombocytopenia secondary to viral infection is virtually always self-limited, as is the drug-related immune type of thrombocytopenia, so that splenectomy rarely is necessary in such patients.

An etiologic basis for the thrombocytopenia is not always possible to establish. Accordingly, therapy then represents a compromise. In this circumstance most patients are best treated as though the illness is of a self-limited type. Steroid hormones are administered if the platelet count is sufficiently low to present bleeding symptoms or signs, and splenectomy usually is considered only after a period of observation. In this clinic a period of at least 6 to 8 weeks is the rule.

The question of whether or not to hospitalize the patient newly diagnosed as having thrombocytopenia sometimes is difficult to answer. Hospitalization may remove the patient from a potentially harmful setting and places him where there is easier access to diagnostic procedures and supportive therapy. The hospital may represent a rather hostile environment, however, to certain patients. One must remember to avoid intramuscular injections, for example, in the thrombocytopenic patient and to use discretion in the obtaining of blood for study, since finger punctures and venipunctures may result in excessive bruising and bleeding. It is of some interest that the major threat of serious bleeding seems to occur during the first month of illness. If one gets a history of more prolonged thrombocytopenia without significant bleeding, one may be somewhat more comfortable about not hospitalizing the patient.

Platelet Transfusions

The availability of platelet concentrates has improved the care of the thrombocytopenic patient. The patient now may be carried through a bleeding crisis and the splenectomy done on an elective basis. Prior to the use of platelet concentrate transfusions, intracerebral hemorrhage usually went on to a fatal outcome. We now have seen patients with intracerebral hemorrhage who have stabilized with vigorous platelet transfusions and then undergone successful splenectomy days later. When used, platelet transfusions should be generous, for the in vivo yield of surviving platelets may be rather modest. In our experience it is not often that more than 60% of the transfused platelets, and often less, circulate hours following administration.

The patient with ITP usually removes transfused platelets from the circulation rapidly while the spleen is still present. For this reason we do not usually transfuse platelets until immediately prior to surgery unless some catastrophic bleeding is threatening or has occurred.

The in vivo survival of transfused platelets appears to dimish progressively after repeated transfusions. Although exceptions to this rule have occurred, particularly among children under treatment for acute leukemia whose platelet donors often are a parent, most hematologists withhold transfusions until life-threatening bleeding necessitates their use.

Steroid Therapy

When the diagnosis of ITP is made in a patient who has petechial or purpuric bleeding, we recommend hospitalization. The patient is treated with at least the equivalent of 300 mg of hydrocortisone daily. When evidence of bleeding has ceased or if platelets have returned, the patient can be discharged to be followed on an outpatient basis. Should platelets fail to return, the steroid therapy is continued for at least 3 or 4 weeks. At that time the dosage may be doubled for another 3 or 4 weeks. Occasionally at the higher dosage platelets may return. It is not clear to us whether this is related to the higher dosage or simply the greater passage of time. More often than not, the patient who failed to have platelets return at the lower dosage also fails with the higher dosage, but we feel the practice has merit. Should the platelet count fail to rise during steroid therapy, steroids are reduced gradually and the patient is considered a candidate for splenectomy. A maintenance dose equivalent to 100 to 150 mg of hydrocortisone is continued, usually as prednisone, 20 to 30 mg daily.

In our experience perhaps one-fourth of patients with ITP have return of platelets during steroid therapy. Perhaps one-half of this latter group relapse when steroids are discontinued.

Splenectomy

The patient who has a favorable response during steroid administration has the drug gradually reduced over a period of weeks in the hope of maintaining the remission. If the platelet count falls, the patient is considered a candidate for splenectomy. We feel that the return of platelets in response to steroids is of little predictive value for the response to splenectomy. Some 60% of the steroid-responsive patients respond favorably to splenectomy in a manner similar to the steroid-resistant group. The patient who has been shown to be steroid responsive, however, can be started again on prednisone prior to surgery in the attempt to increase the circulating platelets by the time of operation.

Pediatric patients usually are managed somewhat more conservatively in regard to splenectomy. Splenectomy only rarely proves necessary in the preadolescent patient. Probably this reflects the fact that many, if not most, of the thrombocytopenic episodes in children are postinfectious—usually a self-limited form of thrombocytopenia.

Although the majority of patients in all age groups respond with a lasting remission following splenectomy, on the average, patients in the older-age group respond somewhat less favorably. It is our feeling that most adult patients who appear to have ITP should be considered candidates for splenectomy. Surgery offers a more favorable outlook and if considered less hazardous than long-term steroid management.

Although some concern has been expressed about precipitating or worsening the course of systemic lupus erythematosus by splenectomy, this has not proved the experience in most centers. In fact if the lupus patient with thrombocytopenia has a successful response to splenectomy, the overall prognosis actually may be improved.

When splenectomy is performed, the surgeon should be a person experienced in this procedure. Technical competence obviously is a factor, and speed also is desirable. The surgeon should recognize that removal of the spleen is the primary concern and any other types of surgical observation or attention must be secondary to that prime goal. *After* the spleen has been removed the careful examination of the abdomen and search for accessory spleens can be undertaken. Although some patients have a relapse of thrombocytopenia following apparently successful surgery, it is not our practice to recommend reexploration with a search for accessory spleens. When the surgeon has been able to make a careful examination at the time of the original surgery, we have not found that reexploration has been of any value. Attention is called to the importance of examination of the peripheral smear in such patients. In those very rare patients in whom an accessory spleen is accounting for persistence of the thrombocytopenia, the peripheral blood smear may offer a clue. In such patients the usual postsplenectomy red cell changes are less apparent. Howell-Jolly bodies will not be found, nor will the poikilocytes characteristic of the postsplenectomy state.

Immunosuppressive Drugs

Within the past few years some patients with persistent idiopathic thrombocytopenia have been treated successfully with immunosuppressive drugs. This form of therapy deserves consideration as an alternative to long-term steroid therapy in the ITP patient with significant bleeding symptoms. The encouraging results reported initially have not been a uniform experience, unfortunately. In our view immunosuppressive therapy of the resistant ITP patient merits consideration, but its routine use in ITP should await clear evidence of its effectiveness. It is prudent to remember that idiopathic thrombocytopenia probably should be considered a *syndrome* with an irregular and remitting course. The remissions ascribed to any form of therapy thus may be coincidental.

Special Problems

The thrombocytopenic premenopausal female poses special problems. While most of these patients do not have disabling hemorrhage at the time of their menstrual period, major hemorrhage from the uterus can occur. When this happens it has become our practice to administer medroxyprogesterone, 50 mg daily for 2 days. In the majority of patients the bleeding diminishes strikingly or ceases within 2 or 3 days. If the patient continues to suffer serious uterine bleeding, dilatation and curettage are performed with the protection of platelet transfusions.

The pregnant thrombocytopenic patient presents several problems. If the pregnancy is in the first trimester, we feel that the patient can be managed in the same way as other patients with thrombocytopenia. If the patient is in the second or third trimester, however, splenectomy is associated with a greater risk of abortion. Patients discovered to be thrombocytopenic during the third trimester usually are treated conservatively until the pregnancy terminates. The patient then can be evaluated regarding splenectomy.

The physician should appreciate, and the patient made aware, that the newborn infant born of a mother with idiopathic thrombocytopenia may be born thrombocytopenic. This may occur even if the mother has been splenectomized. Since the antibody responsible for the thrombocytopenia may still be present in the mother's circulation and is a γG antibody, it can cross the placental barrier. The infant's spleen then is able to remove the platelets injured by the antibody. Trauma to the infant induced by prolonged labor or difficult forceps delivery must be avoided. In this setting the recommendation usually is made that the infant be delivered by cesarean section.

The care of the patient with idiopathic thrombocytopenia who has undergone splenectomy and remains thrombocytopenic also constitutes a special problem. A very few such patients experience spontaneous remission some months or years following the surgery. A few patients have modest improvement in the platelet count and diminution of bleeding symptoms following the reintroduction of steroids. An occasional female patient achieves remission of the thrombocytopenia with the onset of menopause. The remainder of such patients, and they constitute the majority, remain thrombocytopenic.

Our practice has been to treat the patient, *not* the platelet count. Some of these patients with moderately reduced platelet counts have no hemorrhagic symptoms and need no therapy. These patients occasionally may need treatment during bleeding episodes or if they require other forms of surgery. During such events steroids and platelet transfusions may be required. The use of platelet transfusions appears to be somewhat more effective in those patients who have previously had their spleens removed.

REFERENCES

Baldini, M.   Idiopathic thrombocytopenic purpura. *New Eng. J. Med.* 274: 1245, 1301, 1360, 1966.

Best, W. R., and Darling, D. R.   A critical look at the splenectomy–S.L.E. controversy. *Med. Clin. N. Amer.* 46:19, 1962.

Bouroncle, B. A., and Doan, C. A.   Refractory idiopathic thrombocytopenic purpura treated with azathioprine. *New Eng. J. Med.* 275:628, 1966.

Breckenridge, R. T., and Ratnoff, O. D.   A study of thrombocytopenia. *Blood* 30:39, 1967.

Cohen, P., Gardner, F. H., and Barnett, G. O.   Reclassification of thrombocytopenias by Cr^{51} labeling method for measuring platelet life span. *New Eng. J. Med.* 264:1294, 1350, 1961.

Dameshek, W.   Controversy in idiopathic thrombocytopenic purpura. *J.A.M.A.* 173:1025, 1960.

Dubois, E. L.   The Clinical Picture of Systemic Lupus Erythematosus. In E. L. Dubois (Ed.), *Lupus Erythematosus.* New York: McGraw-Hill, 1966.

Hardisty, R. M., and Ingram, G. I. C.   *Bleeding Disorders: Investigation and Management.* Philadelphia: Davis, 1965.

Jackson, D. P.   Treatment of Disorders of Blood Platelets. In O. D. Ratnoff (Ed.), *Treatment of Hemorrhagic Disorders.* New York: Hoeber Med. Div., Harper & Row, 1968.

Lüscher, E. F.   Platelets in hemostasis and thrombosis. *Brit J. Haemat.* 13:1, 1967.

Lusher, J. M., and Zuelzer, W. W.   Idiopathic thrombocytopenic purpura in childhood. *Pediatrics* 68:971, 1961.

Marcus, A. J.   Platelet function. *New Eng. J. Med.* 280:1213, 1278, 1330, 1969.

Ratnoff, O. D.   *Bleeding Syndromes.* Springfield, Ill.: Thomas, 1960.

Wintrobe, M. M.   *Clinical Hematology* (6th ed.). Philadelphia: Lea & Febiger, 1967.

15. TREATMENT OF HEMORRHAGIC DISORDERS ASSOCIATED WITH PLASMA DEFECTS

Leon W. Hoyer
George E. Miller
Robert T. Breckenridge

THE TREATMENT OF bleeding disorders has changed rapidly during the past few years. Satisfactory therapy is now available for most of these conditions, and it is likely that progress will continue. There are few fields in which the clinician's ability to treat his patients satisfactorily is more directly correlated with his awareness of diagnostic and therapeutic developments.

The management of patients with inherited hemorrhagic disorders due to lack of plasma factors is discussed in this chapter. The availability of partially purified, highly concentrated coagulation factors has facilitated the care of such patients and of certain patients with acquired bleeding disorders. Specific replacement therapy for the three most frequently encountered heritable bleeding disorders—hemophilia A (AHF, factor VIII deficiency), Christmas disease (PTC, factor IX deficiency), and von Willebrand's disease—are considered, as are those laboratory studies helpful in their diagnosis. Included in the references are recent reviews which provide detailed descriptions of the treatment of the less common hemorrhagic disorders.

Some of the data reported herein were obtained during the tenure of an operational grant from the Regional Medical Program. The cooperation of Mrs. Mary Gooley and the staff of the Hemophilia Center of Rochester and Monroe County made these studies possible.

DIAGNOSIS

Rational therapy of the inherited hemorrhagic disorders requires a precise diagnosis. Previously, when the only treatment available was fresh plasma, definition of the defect was less important. The development of specific coagulation factor therapy has made exact diagnosis essential. This precision in diagnosis requires a laboratory experienced in blood coagulation studies, for the coagulation factor assay procedures may be tedious and are subject to artifacts.

Few areas of clinical medicine exist in which the patient's history is of greater value. A carefully obtained and critically evaluated history may provide the only hint that the patient has a hemostatic defect. Abnormal bleeding from the umbilicus, bleeding after circumcision, and difficulty with ordinary cuts and bruises can alert the physician to the disorder. History of the response to the stress of any surgical procedure provides further information. It is important, therefore, to question the patient, and the parents, regarding tonsillectomy, dental extractions, or other surgical procedures that might have occurred. Plasma levels of clotting factors in excess of 5% usually provide protection from spontaneous hemorrhage but may be associated with disastrous bleeding following trauma or surgery. Severe hemophilia is diagnosed readily, but the mildly affected patient may escape detection only to suffer a major hemorrhage after dental extraction or appendectomy.

If the history is suggestive and the physical examination normal, one must rely on laboratory investigation to establish the diagnosis. The whole-blood clotting time is of little value in the preliminary evaluation of patients since it is insensitive to all but the most extreme deficiencies. The activated partial thromboplastin time is a much better screening test, as it is sensitive to all the plasma factors in the intrinsic coagulation system. An abnormal activated partial thromboplastin time—in the presence of a normal prothrombin time—should be followed by specific factor assays to identify the deficiency now known to be in the first stage of the coagulation mechanism.

If the history is suggestive of bleeding, a normal activated partial thromboplastin time should not be accepted as convincing evidence for normal coagulation. Specific factor assays should be done. This is especially important in the diagnosis of von Willebrand's disease (vascular hemophilia, decreased factor VIII with a long bleeding time). The factor VIII level may be only moderately depressed and, therefore, the activated partial thromboplastin time normal or only slightly prolonged. A specific factor VIII assay, a carefully done bleeding time, and an investigation of family members may be necessary to establish the diagnosis. In occasional patients with von Willebrand's disease an infusion of fresh-frozen plasma is required to make the differential diagnosis between von Willebrand's disease and true hemophilia. In the patient with hemophilia A, the infused factor VIII appears immediately on assay as a peak activity proportional to the infusion, followed by a decline in activity, with a factor VIII half-life in the range of 6 to 16 hours. The patient with von Willebrand's disease also has an initial factor VIII level commensurate with the amount transfused, but he may synthesize factor VIII over the next 8 to 10 hours. The further increase in factor VIII and slower disappearance has therapeutic implication as well as diagnostic value.

THERAPY

Some general considerations apply to all individuals with hemorrhagic disorders. Aspirin and aspirin-containing compounds should be avoided in these patients because their use adds a platelet defect to the existing plasma deficiency. In addition it is prudent to avoid intramuscular injections, lumbar punctures, or minor surgical procedures until the patient has received specific replacement therapy. Some physicians recommend a rather protective environment for their patients with hemorrhagic disorders, but this has not been our practice. While the younger patient must be protected from physical hazards, especially when he is beginning to walk, the older patient needs freedom for normal emotional development. Most hemophiliacs seem to do better when allowed reasonable latitude.

Replacement therapy should be specific for each disorder because there are differences in the stability of the missing factors, and in their half-life in vivo. The data presented for specific preparations is that obtained at the Hemophilia Center of Rochester and Monroe County, Rochester, New York.

HEMOPHILIA A

A variety of concentrates is available for the treatment of patients with factor VIII deficiency. Although none of these preparations consists exclusively of factor VIII, marked enrichment of this factor has been achieved when the activity per unit volume is compared with plasma (Table 15-1). While the factor VIII content is many times concentrated, fibrinogen remains a significant contaminant of the final product—as does the hepatitis virus.

The first concentrates were prepared by ethanol fractionation, for factor VIII is present in Cohn fraction I. Various modifications of this fraction were used for therapy until the discovery by Pool and her associates that cryoprecipitated factor VIII could be recovered by slowly thawing frozen plasma. Factor VIII also is precipitated by certain amino acids. This

Table 15-1.   Therapy of Hemophilia A (AHF, Factor VIII Deficiency) and Christmas Disease (PTC, Factor IX Deficiency)

Product	Units[a]/Volume (ml)	Cost[b]/Unit (¢)
Hemophilia A		
Fresh-frozen plasma	50–125/200–250	7–18
Cryoprecipitate	50–125/8	7–18
Hemofil	300/7	12
	900/26	9
Courtland	250/25	12
Christmas disease		
Frozen plasma	100–400/200	2–9
Konȳne	500/25	9

[a] One unit of factor VIII or factor IX is defined as that activity present in 1 ml of average normal plasma.

[b] Based on cost to the patient of $9.00/bag of cryoprecipitate or plasma and the current prices of commercially available concentrate (Jan. 1, 1970).

method is used in the preparation of the other two currently used concentrated products, Hemofil (Hyland Laboratories, Los Angeles, Cal.) and Courtland (Courtland Laboratories, Los Angeles, Cal.). Cryoprecipitates and these two commercial preparations provide adequate factor VIII in a small volume so that hypervolemia is rarely a problem. Further purification attempts appear to be associated with a decrease in factor VIII stability. More purified products probably will be developed, but those currently available equip us to deal effectively with virtually all clinical situations.

The commercial concentrates cost approximately $0.12 per unit factor VIII (a unit of factor VIII is that activity present in 1 ml of average normal plasma) at the present time. The cost to the patient of cryoprecipitate depends on the practices of the blood center from which the product is obtained. The processing charge for a bag of cryoprecipitate obtained from the Rochester Regional Red Cross Blood Bank is $9.00, so that the cost per unit factor VIII also is approximately $0.12 if the average recovery of factor VIII is 75 units per bag. Apart from considerations of cost, there are apparent advantages to both the cryoprecipitates (small number of donors and control of donor population, allowing a potential reduction in the risk of hepatitis) and the commercial preparations (preassayed so that a known amount of factor VIII activity can be given, storage at ordinary refrigerator temperatures, and ease of administration).

Therapy with factor VIII concentrates requires consideration of the recovery of the injected factor in vivo and persistence of the procoagulant activity in the patient's plasma (Table 15-2). Determination of the amount of factor VIII to be administered must take into account the patient's

Table 15-2. Treatment of Hemophilia A with Concentrated Antihemophilic Factor (AHF, Factor VIII)

Preparation	No. of Patients	No. of Episodes	Plasma Factor VIII (units[a]/100 ml) Before	Plasma Factor VIII (units[a]/100 ml) After	Expected Rise (%) Range	Expected Rise (%) Average	T 1/2 in vivo[b] (hr) Range	T 1/2 in vivo[b] (hr) Average
Cryoprecipitate	15	36	1–36	4–75	13–100	79	8–12	—
Hemofil	15	27	1–50	10–100	34–100	72	2–7	5
Courtland	19	34	1–27	7–100	38–100	85	7–12	10

[a] One unit of factor VIII is defined as that activity present in 1 ml of average normal plasma.
[b] Factor VIII survival during the first half-life. These data combine data from a published study (Prentice et al., 1967) and from the Hemophilia Center of Rochester and Monroe County.

plasma volume. In most instances this can be approximated roughly as 4% of the body weight. Occasionally, as in patients with blood loss and subsequent plasma expansion, one must use the hematocrit reading in the calculation of the plasma volume. This can be accomplished by multiplying the patient's weight in kilograms $\times$ 77.7 $\times$ (1 − hematocrit). As an example, a 50-kg hemophiliac with a normal hematocrit level has a plasma volume of 2000 ml. If his hematocrit reading had fallen to 20%, the plasma volume would be approximately 3100 ml and more factor VIII would be needed to obtain the same factor VIII levels.

Control of most spontaneous hemorrhages is obtained if the initial plasma concentration of factor VIII achieved is 30 units per 100 ml of plasma. Approximately one-half of the calculated initial dose is then given every 5 to 12 hours, depending on the in vivo half-life of the material used (Table 15-2). Surgery and major bleeding episodes require initial posttransfusion levels in excess of 40 units per 100 ml. Factor VIII concentrations should be maintained above 20 units per milliliter at all times. One also must take into consideration the incomplete recovery in vivo (Table 15-2) in the calculation of factor VIII requirements.

CHRISTMAS DISEASE

The recent development of a concentrate rich in factor IX has significantly changed the therapy of Christmas disease within the past two years. Factor IX is relatively stable in vivo and in vitro but apparently has a compartment distribution much greater than that for factor VIII. Consequently its recovery is less efficient, and an excess must be given initially to assure adequate in vivo levels. This limited plasma therapy and infusions in the past were complicated on occasion by pulmonary edema. Levels greater than 30 units per 100 ml were almost impossible to achieve. The factor IX concentrate now available (Konȳne, Cutter Laboratories, Los Angeles, Cal.) (Table 15-1) contains all the vitamin K–dependent clotting factors (factor IX), Stuart-Prower factor (factor X), factor VII, and prothrombin (factor II). Its usefulness in factor IX deficiency and in patients bleeding from coumarin excess has been demonstrated in several centers.

The initial dosage calculations are similar to those mentioned for factor VIII deficiency with the recognition that the recovery of factor IX is only 60% of that predicted. The initial dose must be increased to accomplish the desired therapeutic level. As an example, a patient with a 3000 ml plasma volume should be given 2000 units of the concentrate to obtain a plasma factor IX level of 40 units per 100 ml ($3000 \times 40/100 \div 0.6$). The levels of factor IX activity necessary for hemostasis are analogous to the factor VIII levels needed in hemophilia A. Spontaneous hemorrhages and minor bleeding episodes are treated with sufficient concentrate to obtain an initial plasma level of 30 units per 100 ml. Surgery and major bleeding problems require higher levels, and the amount of factor IX administered is that calculated to give an initial level of at least 50 units per 100 ml of plasma. The half-life of this material, after equilibration, may be as long as 20 to 24 hours. It has been our practice to give one-half the initial dose at 12-hour intervals for the first 2 days and treat only once a day thereafter.

The presence of the other vitamin K–dependent clotting factors, in addition to factor IX, makes Konȳne a useful therapy for severe bleeding due to coumarin excess and for patients with hereditary disorders associated with a lack of one of the vitamin K–dependent clotting factors. Factor deficiencies in patients with anticoagulant excess can be corrected immediately with this material, whereas the action of vitamin K requires several hours. Konȳne also is useful in the treatment of patients with bleeding secondary to severe liver disease, although proaccelerin (factor V) deficiency—common in these patients—is not corrected by this concentrate.

Von Willebrand's Disease

Therapy of von Willebrand's disease is somewhat different from that of the other inherited coagulation disorders. These patients *may* synthesize factor VIII following plasma transfusion. It is wise to establish whether this ability exists in each patient prior to undertaking surgery, for only some of these patients are able to make factor VIII. If the factor VIII level continues to increase several hours after plasma infusion, the patient can be transfused the evening prior to surgery and his ability to produce factor VIII can be utilized for hemostasis. It is obvious that factor VIII levels must be determined at frequent intervals in these patients. In the absence of such data, the patient with von Willebrand's disease should be prepared for, and carried through, hemorrhagic crises or surgery in the same manner as the true hemophiliac.

There is little information about synthesis of factor VIII after infusion of factor VIII concentrates—other than cryoprecipitate—in patients with von Willebrand's disease. It seems appropriate, therefore, *not* to rely on highly purified concentrates (Hemofil or Courtland) as "expectant" therapy in this disorder until more studies are available.

REFERENCES

Barrow, E. M., and Graham, J. B. Von Willebrand's Disease. In E. B. Brown and C. V. Moore (Eds.), *Progress in Hematology,* Vol. 4. New York: Grune & Stratton, 1964.

Bennett, E., and Dormandy, K. Pool's cryoprecipitate and exhausted plasma in the treatment of von Willebrand's disease and factor IX deficiency. *Lancet* 2:731, 1966.

Biggs, R., and Macfarland, R. G.   *Treatment of Haemophilia and Other Coagulation Disorders*. Philadelphia: Davis, 1966.

Breen, F. A., and Tullis, J. L.   Prothrombin concentrates in the treatment of Christmas disease and allied disorders. *J.A.M.A.* 208:1848, 1969.

Hardisty, R. M., and Ingram, G. I. C.   *Bleeding Disorders: Investigation and Management*. Philadelphia: Davis, 1965.

Hoag, M. S., Johnson, F. F., Robinson, J. A., and Aggeler, P. M.   Treatment of hemophilia B with a new clotting factor concentrate. *New Eng. J. Med.* 280:581, 1969.

Pool, J. G., and Shannon, A. E.   Production of high-potency concentrates of antihemophilic globulin in closed-bag system: Assay in vitro and in vivo. *New Eng. J. Med.* 273:1443, 1965.

Prentice, C. R. M., Breckenridge, R. T., Forman, W. B., and Ratnoff, O. D.   Treatment of haemophilia (factor VIII deficiency) with human antihaemophilic factor prepared by the cryoprecipitate process. *Lancet* 1:457, 1967.

Ratnoff, O. D. (Ed.). *Treatment of Hemorrhage Disorders*. New York: Hoeber Med. Div., Harper & Row, 1968.

Shulman, N. R., Cowan, D. H., Libre, E. P., Watkins, S. P., Jr., and Marder, V. J.   The physiologic basis for therapy of classic hemophilia (factor VIII deficiency) and related disorders. *Ann. Intern. Med.* 67:856, 1967.

16. DISSEMINATED INTRAVASCULAR COAGULATION

Leon W. Hoyer

IT IS PARADOXICAL that both hemorrhage and thrombosis may be caused by intravascular activation of the coagulation system. Many recent reports have considered the role of disseminated intravascular coagulation as a component in the pathophysiology of diverse clinical problems, and this productive concept has stimulated renewed interest in clinical hemostasis. Several other terms have been used instead of *disseminated intravascular coagulation*—perhaps because of its lengthy, awkward character. Even more ungainly, albeit alliterative, is the term *consumption coagulopathy*. Some hematologists use this term as a synonym for disseminated intravascular coagulation, but we have reserved the term for those conditions in which a significant bleeding diathesis is caused by the disseminated coagulation. *Defibrination syndrome* is a less satisfactory term, for it refers to only one aspect of the process and omits (by implication) those instances in which fibrinogen levels may be normal. *Diffuse intravascular thrombosis* is also overly restrictive in that secondary fibrinolysis may erase any morphologic evidence of the coagulation. Thrombosis is demonstrated infrequently in this syndrome.

PATHOGENESIS

The complexity of the coagulation system allows a fine balance so that excessive activity (and thrombosis) or insufficient activity (with bleeding) are avoided. This balance may be upset in several clinical settings and the protective mechanisms overcome.

The most obvious cause of disseminated intravascular coagulation is introduction of thromboplastic material into the circulation. Because thromboplastic activity is found in most tissues, many disease processes may activate the coagulation system in this way. Thromboplastic material enters the circulation directly in amniotic-fluid embolism, in some instances of disseminated carcinoma, and may be released during hemolytic transfusion reactions. Damaged tissues also may release thromboplastic material into the circulation, and it is in this way that shock, surgery, retained dead fetus, and abruptio placentae activate the coagulation sequence. Activation of the hemostatic mechanism is a frequently recognized complication of gram-negative sepsis. This has been attributed to the effects of circulating endotoxin on platelets and the coagulation sequence. It has recently been recognized that septicemia due to gram-positive organisms may also be associated with disseminated intravascular coagulation.

The reticuloendothelial system normally removes activated coagulation factors as well as strands of fibrin formed within the circulation. If this clearing capacity is compromised, the effect of any thromboplastic activity is magnified. The liver is especially important in the inactivation of coagulation factors, so that stasis and other causes of reduced hepatic blood flow may be followed by significant changes in the coagulation balance.

Tissue thromboplastin and other causes of disseminated intravascular coagulation activate hemostasis so that thrombin is generated from prothrombin (in the presence of factors V, VII, and X). This reaction may be viewed as the key to disseminated intravascular coagulation. *Thrombin* is a potent proteolytic enzyme which activates factors V, VIII, and XIII, causes platelet aggregation, and splits fibrinopeptides A and B from fibrinogen. Thrombocytopenia is recognized as the aggregated platelets are removed from the circulation, presumably by reticuloendothelial system clearance. The activated factors V and VIII transiently accelerate the coagulation process so that even more thrombin is generated.

Intravascular interaction of dilute thrombin with fibrinogen is quite different from uncomplicated extravascular coagulation at a wound site or in a test tube. The most important difference is the increased tendency in the former setting for fibrin monomer to complex with intact fibrinogen rather than polymerizing. The fibrinogen-fibrin monomer complex is stable in vivo and may be identified by in vitro tests for paracoagulation (cryoprecipitation, ethanol gelation, or protamine sulfate precipitation).

Significant reduction in plasma fibrinogen by thrombin proteolysis alone is very unusual. *Defibrination* requires involvement of the fibrinolytic system through the activating effect of small amounts of fibrin cleared from the plasma and the direct effect of tissue activator converting plasminogen to plasmin. Plasmin, a potent and relatively nonspecific proteolytic enzyme, attacks fibrinogen as well as fibrin, and a series of digestion products—fibrin(ogen) split products—is formed and the plasma fibrinogen level is reduced. The larger digestion products retain fibrinogen antigens and have anticoagulant properties. Their interaction with thrombin limits the amount of thrombin available to cleave fibrinopeptides from fibrinogen, and they interfere with fibrin polymerization. Platelet function is also impaired in the presence of these fragments.

Fibrin may be deposited in small blood vessels if secondary (protective) fibrinolysis is insufficient, and the partial vascular occlusion may result in red cell fragmentation similar to that seen in thrombotic thrombocytopenic purpura, disseminated carcinoma, and microvascular disease. Intravascular coagulation is perpetuated by the release of membrane thromboplastic material by the hemolyzed erythrocyte. The precipitating event in these situations may be obscured by the progressive hemolysis, platelet depletion, and intravascular coagulation.

DIAGNOSIS

Differentiation of disseminated intravascular coagulation with secondary (protective) fibrinolysis from primary fibrinolytic states may prove difficult in some instances. Therapy is very different in the two conditions, however, and every effort must be made to clarify the diagnosis. The usual findings in the two syndromes are given in Table 16-1. Standard coagulation tests may indicate an abnormality but do not distinguish disseminated intravascular coagulation from primary fibrinolysis. The thrombin time is perhaps the most useful single test in establishing that significant disseminated intravas-

Table 16-1. Coagulation Tests in Disseminated Intravascular Coagulation and Primary Fibrinolysis

Test	Disseminated Intravascular Coagulation	Primary Fibrinolysis
Fibrinogen	Low or normal	Low or normal
Prothrombin time	Long or normal	Long or normal
Thrombin time	Long	Long
Platelet count	Low	Normal
Euglobulin lysis time	Normal or short	Short
Factor V	Low	Low or normal
AHF (factor VIII)	Variable	Low or normal
Plasminogen	Low	Low
√Fibrin split products	Present	Present
Cryofibrinogen	Present	Absent
Incidence	More common	Very rare

cular coagulation *or* fibrinolysis is present, for few other conditions affect this test. The fibrin split products prolong the thrombin time, and this effect is central to the pathogenesis of bleeding in both syndromes. The platelet count is usually normal in primary fibrinolysis, though it may be reduced. The clot lysis tests, either dilute whole-blood clot lysis or euglobulin clot lysis, usually are normal or only slightly shortened in disseminated intravascular coagulation. Identification of cryofibrinogen, the complexes of fibrinogen with fibrin monomer which are insoluble at 4°C, is a simple and reliable test which we find to be specific. The presence of cryofibrinogen indicates plasma thrombin activity with formation of fibrin monomer; this does not occur with plasmin proteolysis alone. Unfortunately, this determination requires that the plasma be left for several hours at 4°C and, therefore, one must decide between disseminated intravascular coagulation and fibrinolysis on the basis of the *pattern* of the specific tests and by the clinical setting in which the coagulation abnormality is found. It is important to recognize that primary fibrinolysis is very rare, while disseminated intravascular coagulation complicates many disease states.

Measurement of plasma fibrinogen metabolism may provide the only way to identify minimal disseminated intravascular coagulation. By itself, however, shortened survival of ^{131}I-labeled fibrinogen does not distinguish disseminated intravascular coagulation from primary fibrinolysis. The diagnosis of mild disseminated intravascular coagulation is supported if heparin therapy prolongs the survival of labeled fibrinogen.

TREATMENT

In most cases the major objective is to relieve the patient's primary medical or surgical problem. If this stimulus to disseminated coagulation cannot be treated adequately, interference with the coagulation sequence is reasonable. Heparin's antithrombin effect is the most direct form of interference, and it has been used to block ongoing coagulation in a number of clinical settings.

As with many newly characterized disorders, enthusiasm for diagnosis and therapy has anticipated evidence for benefit from aggressive intervention. One must distinguish at least three clinical settings in which disseminated intravascular coagulation may be recognized. Therapy should be considered in light of the different potentials for benefit or harm.

Laboratory evidence for disseminated intravascular coagulation may on occasion be demonstrated in the absence of bleeding or other clinical signs. This condition obtains in the postoperative period in many patients, in some infectious diseases, and in some patients with metastatic malignancy. There is no reason to believe that the diagnosis of disseminated intravascular coagulation per se requires treatment in these instances. Careful observation and standard therapies are usually sufficient.

More aggressive treatment has been suggested for those patients in whom disseminated intravascular coagulation is accompanied by hypotension and oliguria, e.g., gram-negative sepsis. The role of intravascular coagulation in the pathogenesis of renal failure remains uncertain, but a rational basis for heparin therapy exists in these conditions. Controlled clinical trials are required to demonstrate whether or not routine use of heparin is indicated if hypotension accompanies gram-negative sepsis. The data now available do not isolate the effects of heparin therapy in these conditions. They do suggest that this therapy has potential clinical usefulness.

Disseminated intravascular coagulation is associated on occasion with significant secondary bleeding. Surgical or traumatic wounds may contribute to the blood loss, and every possible therapeutic step needs to be taken to remove the stimulus for the disseminated intravascular coagulation. One of the most common causes of disseminated intravascular coagulation, abruptio placentae, is an example in which vigorous operative therapy is the best treatment. Should the stimulus be less easily removed, as for example in metastatic carcinoma or leukemia, anticoagulation with heparin has been advocated. Treating a bleeding patient with heparin is precarious; it is certainly the last resort for the cautious physician. It is more reasonable, however, than simple replacement therapy with fibrinogen or fresh-frozen plasma—"stoking the fires"—for these infusions provide more substrate for the disseminated coagulation. They may, in fact, increase the bleeding as more fibrin split products are generated. Therapy with epsilon aminocaproic acid (EACA—Amicar, Lederle) alone, to inhibit the secondary (protective) fibrinolysis, is an invitation to disaster in these situations. Uncontrolled disseminated coagulation may cause massive disseminated thrombosis in these patients.

Heparin therapy provides the safer way to block the pathogenesis of this syndrome. Heparin may be given as a continuous intravenous infusion or by intravenous injections at 4- or 6-hour intervals. Sufficient heparin is given to keep the clotting time twice normal; this may require 10,000 to 40,000 units of heparin over the first 24 hours and during each subsequent day. Heparin therapy in these patients is empiric at best, and careful attention is required.

With more experience, better guidelines for treatment of severe disseminated intravascular coagulation may become apparent, but at this time only very general recommendations can be made. The bleeding manifestations of severe disseminated intravascular coagulation treated with heparin will decrease as the fibrin split products are cleared by the liver. They have a half-survival time in the circulation of 4 to 6 hours, so immediate hemostasis will not be expected. If the fibrinogen, factor V, or factor VIII levels are very low, it is appropriate to replace them after heparinization has been accomplished. Concentrates rich in fibrinogen and factor VIII are available, and factor V is present in fresh-frozen plasma. The prognosis is less dependent on coagulation factor replacement, however, than on satisfactory treatment of the underlying disease which has initiated the intravascular coagulation.

REFERENCES

Abildgaard, C. F. Recognition and treatment of intravascular coagulation. *J. Pediat.* 74:163, 1969.

Deykin, D. Clinical challenge of disseminated intravascular coagulation. *New Eng. J. Med.* 283:636, 1970.

Horowitz, H. J. Treatment of Defibrination Syndromes and Fibrinolytic Disorders. In O. D. Ratnoff (Ed.), *Treatment of Hemorrhagic Disorders.* New York: Hoeber Med. Div., Harper & Row, 1968. P. 158.

McKay, D. G. *Disseminated Intravascular Coagulation.* New York: Hoeber Med. Div., Harper & Row, 1965.

Mersky, C., Johnson, A. J., Kleiner, G. J., and Wohl, H. The defibrination syndrome: Clinical features and laboratory diagnosis. *Brit. J. Haemat.* 13:528, 1967.

Mosesson, M. W., Colman, R. W., and Sherry, S. Chronic intravascular coagulation syndrome: Report of a case with special studies of an associated plasma cryoprecipitate ("cryofibrinogen"). *New Eng. J. Med.* 278:815, 1968.

Pritchard, J. A. Treatment of Defibrination Syndromes of Pregnancy. In O. D. Ratnoff (Ed.), *Treatment of Hemorrhagic Disorders.* New York: Hoeber Med. Div., Harper & Row, 1968. P. 175.

Rodriguez-Erdmann, F. Bleeding due to increased intravascular blood coagulation. *New Eng. J. Med.* 273:1370, 1965.

Verstraete, M., Vermylen, C., Vermylen, J., and Vandenbroucke, J. Excessive consumption of blood coagulation components as cause of hemorrhagic diathesis. *Amer. J. Med.* 38:899, 1965.

17. FIBRINOLYSIS

Stanley B. Troup

DEPOSITION OF FIBRIN is a mammalian defense mechanism of prime importance. Removal of fibrin by its dissolution, fibrinolysis, is an equally important repair process. Fibrin formation is a common event that occurs in response to a variety of stimuli. Formation of the fibrin clot as a final event of the hemostatic effort has been discussed earlier (Chap. 13). Fibrin deposition occurs in response to virtually every inflammatory event to which man is subject. These vary from the alveolar exudates of pneumonia to the codeposition with antigen-antibody complexes in a variety of immunologically determined diseases. Deposition of fibrin may be a part of the limitation of spread of tumors as well.

Fibrinolysis may be viewed normally as a reparative process. While hemostasis is responsible for maintaining the integrity of the vascular system, fibrinolysis is charged with maintaining the patency of this system. Particularly does this seem true for the microcirculation. Less obvious, but important, is the maintenance of patency of other structures carrying liquid products. The lymphatic network, ureters, tear ducts, and the ducts of other exocrine glands represent such examples.

The topic of fibrinolysis is considered in this chapter from three points of view. The first is that of physiologic fibrinolysis, the normal reparative role described above. The second aspect is that of pathologic fibrinolysis. This deals with the hemorrhagic disorder due to accumulation in the plasma of fibrinogen and fibrin split products as a result of excessive proteolysis. Finally, therapeutic or induced fibrinolysis is discussed.

NORMAL FIBRINOLYSIS

Removal of fibrin in man is accomplished by the activity of at least one, possibly more, proteolytic enzyme system. This well-characterized system is that of plasminogen-plasmin. Plasminogen is a plasma globulin which func-

This work was supported in part by U.S. Public Health Service Grant HE-04167-11.

tions as a proenzyme, and plasmin is the proteolytic enzyme which evolves from it. This may be viewed as a parallel to the prothrombin-thrombin system in the blood clotting sequence. Quite likely the fibrinolytic system is equally complex. Plasminogen has been identified in virtually all body fluids but achieves its highest concentration in plasma. Unlike the substances normally necessary for the conversion of prothrombin to thrombin, the activators of plasminogen necessary to convert this substance to plasmin are present in vascular endothelium and in many tissues of the body.

The transformation from plasminogen to plasmin probably involves the splitting of an arginyl-valine bond. Interestingly, the active center of the plasmin molecule probably is the same as the active center of thrombin.

While plasmin prefers fibrin as its proteolytic substrate, it has a broad specificity. Fibrinogen also can be split by plasmin, as can the clotting factors V, VIII, IX, and prothrombin (factor II). Plasmin activity, possibly quite importantly, transforms the first component of complement (C_1) into the C_1 esterase, initiating that important part of the immunologic sequence. Not only can plasmin reach into the immunologic system, but also it is capable of activating plasma kinins. These peptides play a potent role in altering capillary permeability and participating in inflammatory reactions.

While probably of less interest, plasmin also can use as substrate hormones such as ACTH, growth hormone, and glucagon. The ability of plasmin to split certain synthetic amino acid esters permits measurement of plasmin activity in vitro.

Teleologic reasoning suggests that nature would provide means to limit the activity of such a potentially vigorous enzyme in plasma. At least two discrete products in human plasma have been identified which can inhibit the action of plasmin. Data have also been presented suggesting that inhibitors may be present normally which block the activation of plasmin from its precursor, plasminogen.

Plasminogen can be converted to plasmin in vivo in a number of ways. Liberation of plasminogen activator from vascular endothelium and other tissues occurs with hypoxia, hypoglycemia, or simply physical exercise. Pharmacologic activation of plasminogen occurs in response to injections of bacterial pyrogen, epinephrine, nicotinic acid, or acetylcholine. Stimulation of the central nervous system can result in marked activation, as evidenced by the effects of electroshock and pneumoencephalography. The administration of streptokinase also activates plasminogen, apparently after the streptokinase combines with a proactivator in plasma. Paradoxically, the proactivator may be plasminogen. The administration of urokinase, an enzymatic activator found in normal urine, also converts plasminogen to plasmin. These latter two activators can evoke inhibitors. Antibodies to streptokinase may appear, a naturally occurring streptokinase inhibitor separate from antibody may be present, and an activator inhibitor to urokinase also has been identified. In vitro activation of plasminogen can be accomplished by chloroform, streptokinase, urokinase, and by tissue particles, possibly lysosomes.

Two questions must follow the observations described. If the inhibitors of either the activation of plasminogen or the inhibition of the plasmin itself truly are effective, how then can fibrinolytic activity develop? If somehow this activity does develop, acknowledging the broad variety of substrates for plasmin, how then is plasmin activity largely limited to fibrin?

The scientific escape from the horns of this dilemma was provided by an important observation. Plasminogen has an affinity of a very high order for fibrin. Whenever fibrin is deposited, plasminogen is present with the fibrin. A sensible hypothesis followed: Normally when circulating plasminogen might be activated, the plasminogen antiactivators and antiplasmins present are equal to the task and little effective plasmin circulates. On the other hand, when plasminogen is laid down with fibrin in an area of inflammation or in a clot, the plasminogen is sheltered from its natural activator inhibitors, as is the plasmin that can evolve. If activators of plasminogen seep into the area of fibrin, resulting in plasmin formation from the plasminogen deposited there, the plasmin activity is in close proximity to its preferred fibrin substrate. The plasmin then can act even with small concentrations of its antiplasmins present. According to this ingenious hypothesis, every clot has incorporated in it the mechanism of its own dissolution.

PATHOLOGIC AND INDUCED FIBRINOLYSIS

Clinical interest in fibrinolysis centers in two areas. The treatment of pathologic fibrinolysis that arises most often secondary to intravascular coagulation, and much less frequently in response to a primary stimulus, is one focus of interest. The importance of successfully distinguishing these two is crucial. Potent agents are available to interrupt the fibrinolytic process. The danger of interrupting it while permitting intravascular coagulation to proceed is self-evident.

The other hope for potential clinical benefit is the induction of fibrinolysis in an attempt to diminish morbidity and mortality from thromboembolic disease. Effective activators of the fibrinolytic mechanism are available. The most promising are the activators of plasminogen. The two principal agents presently offering the greatest promise are urokinase and streptokinase. Controlled clinical trials are underway, and the next several years should provide us data that will permit sound judgments to be made.

PATHOLOGIC FIBRINOLYSIS

Primary pathologic fibrinolysis, as noted in the preceding chapter, is a very uncommon event. When pathologic fibrinolysis occurs, it almost always is secondary to intravascular coagulation. In those rare patients in whom increased fibrinolysis is a primary phenomenon, the principal plasma substrate is fibrinogen. Other plasma proteins of wide biologic activity also may be attacked; clinically important among them are factors V and VIII.

In the more common occurrence of fibrinolysis secondary to intravascular coagulation, the preferred substrate is fibrin, usually deposited in the microcirculation. Since no laboratory distinction presently can be made between the fibrin split products of the latter state and the fibrinogen split products of primary fibrinolysis, both clinical and laboratory distinction is difficult. Further, in the uncommon primary state, factors V and VIII may be diminished because of serving as substrate for the plasmin activity. In the process of intravascular coagulation these same products may be diminished because of their participation in the coagulation process.

The pathogenesis of the hemorrhagic disorder occurring in pathologic fibrinolysis has been dealt with in the preceding chapter. To recapitulate briefly, the products of fibrinogen or fibrin proteolysis (split products of fibrinogen or fibrin) accumulate in the plasma when proteolysis is excessive. These split products of various sizes are capable of interfering with hemostasis at virtually every point. They may interfere with platelet aggregation, complex with coagulation factors and interfere with formation of the prothrombin converting activity, inhibit thrombin activity, inhibit fibrin polymerization, and react with normal fibrin polymers to form abnormal polymers with diminished tensile strength.

The hemostatic defect that accompanies pathologic fibrinolysis in the last analysis is related to the fibrinolytic activity, but more directly to the presence of increased amounts of the fibrin (or fibrinogen) split products that appear because of the proteolysis.

While appearing rarely, *primary* fibrinolytic problems do occur. They may present as a consequence of a profound physiologic insult such as shock or anoxia, or following extensive surgical procedures. Not quite so uncommonly, but usually more modest in severity, the primary fibrinolytic state may be present in patients with hepatic cirrhosis. In this setting the liver fails to clear plasminogen activator from the circulation as it normally should. Now that activators of plasminogen are being administered with therapeutic intent, it is also possible to induce fibrinolysis, and a hemorrhagic state, without intravascular coagulation.

A striking inhibitor of plasminogen activation, epsilon aminocaproic acid, is available for treatment of primary fibrinolysis. This synthetic amino acid, an analog of lysine, can be administered by mouth or intravenously. Plasminogen activation promptly is diminished or halted, and the accompanying hemorrhagic problem disappears within hours since the half-life of the split products is about 9 hours. EACA has achieved worthwhile control of postprostatectomy bleeding as well. The product appears rapidly in the urine following its administration and here interferes with the activating ability of urokinase. The latter, in some patients, constantly may promote local lysis of clots on the surface of the prostatic bed.

As noted in the previous chapter, the use of epsilon aminocaproic acid should be limited because of the difficulty in distinguishing between primary and secondary fibrinolysis. Only when the former diagnosis can be established with certainty should this agent be used alone.

Induced Fibrinolysis

During the past decade or more, many attempts have been made to induce controlled fibrinolysis in man. Success in this effort would be of considerable value in the treatment of thromboembolic disease in man. Increased understanding of the physiology of fibrinolysis has put this goal within reach. An important point that has emerged is the realization that the level of plasminogen activator is the key to plasma fibrinolytic activity. The rapid lysis of a clot formed in the systemic circulation requires that substantial levels of plasminogen activator be present around the clot so that activator can penetrate the clot. This requirement is difficult to accomplish through normal physiologic mechanisms. In the microcirculation this is more easily achieved because of the potentially high level of activator adjacent to relatively small amounts of fibrin. In large vessels, however, the opposite is true.

Recognition of this requirement led to the experimental use of agents designed to increase the native fibrinolytic activity. The idea largely has been to facilitate the release of plasminogen activator from endothelium into the circulation. Nicotinic acid is an example of a substance that accomplishes this promptly. Plasminogen activator appears in the circulation within seconds following the intravenous use of this agent, but the activity usually is gone within an hour. Bacterial pyrogens accomplish similar results.

This approach has not been fruitful for several reasons. A limited endogenous store of activator is available, so that repeated injection soon exhausts the supply and later injections fail to be effective. Chills and fever further limit the use of pyrogen.

The next logical step appeared to be the circumvention of the endogenous release of activator by the use of a substance that could serve directly as a plasminogen activator. For many years streptokinase was the principal agent available. When carefully purified, this streptococcal product may be used for such a purpose.

Experimental studies in man have demonstrated clearly that induced venous thrombi can be lysed with the use of streptokinase. In these experimental circumstances relatively fresh thrombi have been lysed. Dissolution of an older thrombus or embolus constitutes a larger problem, but even in this situation streptokinase treatment has been successful in a generous number of patients. Pyrogenicity has been reduced, which has permitted a broader use of this agent, particularly in Europe. The use of streptokinase, since it is an antigenic protein, is limited for retreatment purposes; but it is clear that this product, when its use is carefully monitored, can effect clot dissolution without serious hazard to the patient.

Among the technical problems in its use is the initial determination of the patient's antibody titer to streptococcal products. A variable amount of the agent thus is necessary. When careful control is not achieved, a coagulation disorder due to excessive plasminogen activation can occur and result in severe bleeding. If care is used (and this requires good laboratory supervision), a controlled state of fibrinolysis can be maintained.

Because of the problems with streptokinase, attention turned to the possible use of a naturally occurring and, accordingly, nonantigenic product. This is urokinase, the activator normally present in human urine.

Urokinase probably is a product of the kidneys rather than of a plasma substrate that is cleared by the kidneys. Laboratory control has proved simpler with this agent than with streptokinase because patient response has proved more predictable. Treatment with urokinase is well tolerated by the patient and results, because of better control, in more modest disruption of the hemostatic mechanism.

Urokinase now has been evaluated under carefully controlled clinical circumstances, and the results establish that this product will dissolve thrombi and emboli without undue hazard. Studies now include patients with pulmonary emboli and central retinal artery occlusion, and early results are available in patients with coronary artery occlusion.

The largest experience with urokinase is in the treatment of pulmonary thromboembolic disease. About one-half of the treated clots have lysed. The reasons for failure in nearly half are not completely understood. The age of the clot probably is an important consideration. The ability to perfuse the involved area with urokinase probably is a significant factor when one remembers that the activator must diffuse into the clot to initiate the lytic process. Also, an optimal dosage schedule has not yet been decided.

The treatment has not been without complication. Excessive bleeding has been noted in approximately 50% of patients. This includes patients treated with heparin in addition to urokinase, so that bleeding cannot be attributed solely to the use of the activator. Anemia has appeared in some patients beyond that anticipated from the amount of bleeding. The cause of this is not immediately apparent. The anemia does not appear directly related to the induced fibrinolysis. The clotting defect induced by urokinase usually is relatively mild, and anemia has been noted to progress in some instances despite cessation of the treatment.

Establishing proof of the value of urokinase treatment has been difficult. Results thus far are encouraging but are not conclusive. Among the problems encountered in evaluation is the extent of spontaneous lysis of clots. It is clear that the pulmonary arterial system is capable of lysing thrombi actively, and possibly half the clots that travel to the lung are lysed in 24 hours without specific therapy. While thrombosis of the central artery of the retina appeared an attractive model, increasing study reveals that both the etiology and the natural history are so variable that large numbers of patients will be required to demonstrate possible worth of fibrinolytic treatment.

An area of intensive study, particularly in Europe, centers around the treatment of acute myocardial infarction. Since it is held that thrombosis of a coronary artery usually is the basis for myocardial infarction, it follows that reestablishing blood flow through the affected vessel, if accomplished rapidly enough, could diminish morbidity and mortality.

Results with urokinase are not available at this time. Purified streptokinase has been used in the treatment of early myocardial infarction. In a limited study the therapy has not been shown to achieve statistically significant improvement in the patients treated but has demonstrated that the therapy in itself is not harmful. A larger European study suggests that streptokinase-treated patients tolerate the treatment well, and these workers claimed significant improvement in the treated patients as opposed to controls. Larger trials employing urokinase presently are underway.

While an initial study of the treatment of cerebral thrombosis with fibrinolysis has suggested that this treatment is not of value, further evaluation is required. More careful study of diseases which are easier to evaluate and potentially less hazardous is necessary before a major study of cerebral occlusion is undertaken.

REFERENCES

Johnson, A. J., and Newman, J. The fibrinolytic system in health and disease. *Seminars Hemat.* 1:401, 1964.

Merskey, C., Johnson, A. J., Kleiner, G. J., and Wohl, H. The defibrination syndrome: Clinical features and laboratory diagnosis. *Brit. J. Haemat.* 13:4, 1967.

Ratnoff, O. D. Some relationships among hemostasis, fibrinolytic phenomena, immunity and the inflammatory response. *Advances Immun.* 10:145, 1969.

Sherry, S. Fibrinolysis. *Ann. Rev. Med.* 19:247, 1968.

Sherry, S. Fibrinolysis in health and disease. *Resident Phys.,* p. 79, February 1968.

Sherry, S. Urokinase. *Ann. Intern. Med.* 69:415, 1968.

Sherry, S. Fibrinolytic agents. *D.M.,* May 1969.

Von Kaulla, K. N. *American Lecture Series.* Springfield, Ill.: Thomas, 1963. Chapter on Chemistry of Thrombolysis: Human Fibrinolytic Enzymes.

18. DRUG EFFECTS ON ORAL ANTICOAGULANTS

Paul F. Griner

ADVERSE DRUG REACTIONS are responsible for up to 5% of hospital admissions to medical services, complicate the hospital course of an additional 10%, and are potent contributors to patient morbidity, mortality, and health care costs. A rapidly expanding body of knowledge relating to drug metabolism and toxicity has led to a more complete understanding of the mechanisms responsible for drug reactions. Many so-called idiosyncratic reactions can now be defined in more precise terms. Specific environmental and genetic factors have been elucidated in the pathogenesis of some untoward reactions to drugs. One such environmental influence is the phenomenon of drug interaction. That one drug may alter the effect of another has been known for many years. Although this phenomenon has been used to good advantage with certain drugs (probenecid and penicillin), there is increasing recognition of the harmful effects of some such interactions.

The intent of this chapter is to review interactions between oral anticoagulants and other drugs. Research in this field has been particularly fruitful. It is now known that drugs may modify the response to oral anticoagulants by (1) altering the absorption, distribution, or fate of the anticoagulant, (2) reducing the availability of vitamin K, or (3) affecting the synthesis of the vitamin K–dependent clotting factors. Conversely, the anticoagulant may alter the effect of other drugs.

Familiarity with the mechanisms involved in these interactions is essential for their recognition and for the promotion of rational anticoagulant therapy. In the following pages the action and metabolism of oral anticoagulants are briefly reviewed, the mechanisms of anticoagulant-drug interactions are presented, and the clinical significance of these interactions is discussed.

225

PHARMACOLOGY OF ORAL ANTICOAGULANTS

The mechanism of action of coumarin and indanedione anticoagulants has not been fully clarified. Hypotheses include (1) inhibition of the transport of vitamin K to its receptor protein in the liver cell and (2) competition between the anticoagulant and vitamin K for this receptor. There is tentative support for both concepts. The end result is an inhibition of hepatic synthesis or release of a number of proteins necessary for the formation of a fibrin clot (factors II, VII, IX, X). The 36- to 48-hour delay in the peak response to oral anticoagulants reflects the disappearance rate of the vitamin K–dependent clotting proteins. Synthesis of these proteins is dependent upon the endogenous production of vitamin K by gut bacteria or the ingestion of adequate amounts of the vitamin in the diet.

The gastrointestinal absorption of the oral anticoagulants is rapid and complete except for bishydroxycoumarin, whose absorption is erratic. The transport and distribution of these agents are accomplished through binding to plasma albumin. Approximately 97% of warfarin and 99% of bishydroxycoumarin are bound under normal conditions. The oral anticoagulants are almost completely metabolized by the liver with only minute quantities appearing unchanged in the urine. Recent studies suggest that some of the metabolites of warfarin possess anticoagulant activity in addition to that of the parent compound. The biologic half-life of warfarin and bishydroxycoumarin averages about 40 hours. The rate of metabolism of these drugs varies, however, by as much as sixfold among normal subjects. This phenomenon in part explains the differences among patients in daily doses required for effective anticoagulation. Hereditary resistance to oral anticoagulants has been described but is rare. Illness may influence the response to oral anticoagulants. Decreased requirements for these agents may be noted in patients with liver disease, hyperthyroidism, or fever. Increased requirements have been reported in the nephrotic state.

MECHANISMS OF DRUG EFFECTS ON ORAL ANTICOAGULANTS

The studies described in this section apply to coumarin anticoagulants unless otherwise noted. The pharmacologic properties of indanediones are similar to the coumarin derivatives. Whether any qualitative or quantitative differences exist between these two classes of anticoagulants in terms of interactions is not known for most drugs.

EFFECTS ON VITAMIN K SYNTHESIS OR ABSORPTION.   The administration of neomycin, sulfonamides, and broad-spectrum antibiotics may change the gut flora sufficiently to reduce vitamin K synthesis. Drastic cathartics and mineral oil are said to reduce the absorption of the vitamin. Under one or more of these conditions, an exaggerated response to oral anticoagulants may occur if dietary vitamin K is inadequate.

EFFECTS ON COUMARIN ABSORPTION.   Coumarins are weak acids, and their absorption may be reduced by the concomitant administration of antacids. Similarly, the administration of cholestyramine may result in decreased absorption of the anticoagulant through it chelating effect.

EFFECTS ON COUMARIN DISTRIBUTION.   As previously noted, coumarins are extensively bound to plasma albumin. Other drugs sharing the same binding site may displace the anticoagulant. Whether displacement occurs is dependent upon the concentration and relative binding affinity of the two drugs. The displaced (unbound) fraction of the anticoagulant is then free to exert its pharmacologic effect. For drugs such as warfarin, a small increase in the free fraction may be followed by a markedly enhanced anticoagulant effect. This mechanism has been shown to be responsible for the potentiating effect of phenylbutazone and its congeners upon warfarin.

Displacement of warfarin from its protein-binding site not only increases its pharmacologic effect but also facilitates its metabolism. Thus the biologic half-life of the anticoagulant is reduced (Fig. 18-1). This may not

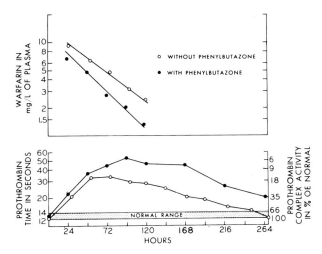

Figure 18-1.   Effect of administration of phenylbutazone on the prothrombin response and on the plasma level and disappearance rate of warfarin in a normal subject. Phenylbutazone, 600 mg/day, was given by mouth for 14 days before and 11 days after administration of a standard dose of warfarin, 1.5 mg/kg of body weight, given orally. (Reproduced in part from P. M. Aggeler et al., *New Eng. J. Med.* 276:496, 1967.)

be the case for all such drug interactions. For example, the hypocholesterolemic agent clofibrate appears to enhance the response to warfarin through noncompetitive displacement of the anticoagulant from its protein-binding site. Since this agent is less efficient in displacing warfarin than is phenylbutazone, no reduction in plasma levels of the anticoagulant can be demonstrated.

EFFECTS ON RECEPTOR SITE. It has been mentioned that wide variations exist in the rate at which anticoagulants are metabolized. It is also recognized that coumarin requirements vary within groups of patients who metabolize the anticoagulant at the same rate. To explain the latter phenomenon, genetic or acquired differences in the affinity of the hepatic receptor site for the anticoagulant have been proposed. For drugs such as D-thyroxine or norethandrolone, both of which enhance the response to oral anticoagulants, this mechanism may apply. These drugs do not appear to affect the absorption, distribution, or fate of bishydroxycoumarin or independently alter the hepatic synthesis of vitamin K–dependent clotting factors. Studies of the rates of synthesis and degradation of these clotting factors in anticoagulated subjects before and after administration of such drugs are necessary to confirm the hypothesis of altered receptor site affinity.

ALTERED METABOLISM OF COUMARINS. Oral anticoagulants undergo oxidative metabolism in the liver. The metabolism is mediated by enzymes located in the microsomal fraction of the liver cell. Oxidation is effected through an electron transport system. This system appears to be a common pathway for the metabolism of many drugs. One drug may decrease the rate of metabolism of another either by competing for this enzyme system or by inhibiting enzyme production. Phenyramidol (an analgesic–muscle relaxant) has been shown to enhance the effect of coumarin anticoagulants through such a mechanism. As a consequence of this interaction, the biologic half-life of the anticoagulant is prolonged and its effect enhanced (Fig. 18-2; Table 18-1). Conversely, one drug may *increase* the rate of metabolism of another by "stimulating" the synthesis of enzymes in the oxidizing system (enzyme induction). Such an interaction has been clearly documented between phenobarbital and coumarin anticoagulants (Fig. 18-3). As a consequence of this interaction, larger coumarin doses are required for effective anticoagulation. The implication of continuing the larger daily dose of the anticoagulant after stopping phenobarbital is clear: The gradual return of coumarin metabolism to normal may result in excessive anticoagulation and hemorrhage.

EFFECT ON SYNTHESIS OF VITAMIN K–DEPENDENT CLOTTING FACTORS. Some drugs enhance the action of oral anticoagulants by interfering with the

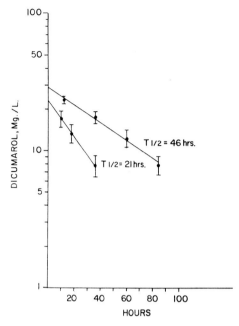

Figure 18-2. Metabolism of oral bishydroxycoumarin (150 mg) in 4 human subjects before and after oral phenyramidol (400 mg three times a day for 4 days). Each point represents the mean ± S.D. of four determinations. (From H. M. Solomon and J. J. Schrogie, *Biochem. Pharmacol.* 16:1219, 1966. © 1966, The Williams & Wilkins Co., Baltimore, Md. 21202, U.S.A.)

Table 18-1. *Effect of Phenyramidol on the Anticoagulant Response to Bishydroxycoumarin*

	Coagulation Activity[a] at 60 Hours (%)	
Subject	Before Phenyramidol	After Phenyramidol
E. H.	85	54
R. W.	100	32
M. R.	100	50
R. M.	100	45
Mean	96	45

[a] Coagulation activity was measured in human subjects given 150 mg of bishydroxycoumarin before and after treatment with phenyramidol.

SOURCE: J. M. Solomon and J. J. Schrogie, *J. Pharmacol. Exp. Ther.* 154:660, 1966 (© 1966, The Williams & Wilkins Co., Baltimore, Md. 21202, U.S.A.).

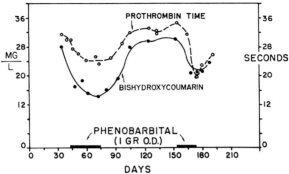

Figure 18-3. Effect of phenobarbital on plasma levels of bishydroxycoumarin and on prothrombin time in a human subject treated chronically with 75 mg/day of bishydroxycoumarin. (From J. J. Burns and A. H. Conney, *Proc. Roy. Soc. Med.* 58:955, 1965.)

hepatic synthesis of the vitamin K–dependent clotting factors. For example, quinidine, quinine, and salicylates may prolong the prothrombin time in normal patients in the absence of other changes in hepatic function. This effect is reversed by the administration of vitamin K. When one of these drugs is administered together with an oral anticoagulant, the prothrombin time may lengthen.

Recently it has been shown that oral contraceptives reduce the effect of oral anticoagulants, apparently without altering their metabolism. This interaction is accompanied by an *increase* in the activity of at least one of the vitamin K–dependent clotting factors (X). Further studies are necessary to define the mechanism of this interaction more clearly.

SIGNIFICANCE OF ANTICOAGULANT-DRUG INTERACTIONS

More than 30 drugs have been shown to alter the response to oral anticoagulants in man (Table 18-2). Some of these interactions are predictable, result in profound changes in the prothrombin time, and are commonly followed by hemorrhagic complications. Others are unpredictable or of minor consequence. The clinical significance of interactions between coumarins and each of these drugs, insofar as they are defined, is discussed in the following pages.

DRUGS KNOWN TO DECREASE THE EFFECT OF ORAL ANTICOAGULANTS

BARBITURATES. The anticoagulant effect of coumarin drugs is consistently reduced in patients receiving barbiturates. This effect can be demon-

Table 18-2. Drugs That May Alter the Response to Oral Anticoagulants

Clinical Significance	Anticoagulant Effect Enhanced	Anticoagulant Effect Reduced
Clear-cut; predictable	Phenylbutazone (Butazolidin) Oxyphenbutazone (Tandearil) Phenyramidol (Analexin) Norethandrolone (Nilevar) Methandrostenolone (Dianabol) D-Thyroxine (Choloxin) Glucagon Clofibrate (Atromid-S)	Barbiturates Glutethimide (Doriden)
Intermediate	Disulfiram (Antabuse) Methylphenidate (Ritalin) Acetylsalicylic acid Para-aminosalicylic acid Methyl salicylate Quinidine Quinine Acetaminophen (Tylenol) Antibiotics	Ethchlorvynol (Placidyl) Haloperidol (Haldol)[a] Oral contraceptives, estrogens Corticosteroids, ACTH Griseofulvin (Fulvicin) Meprobamate (Miltown)
Questionable	L-Thyroxine Thiouracils Diphenylhydantoin (Dilantin) Indomethacin (Indocin) Tolbutamide (Orinase) Chloral hydrate Monoamine-oxidase inhibitors Diazoxide Mefenamic, ethacrynic, and nalidixic acids	Antacids Cholestyramine

[a] Indanedione anticoagulants.

strated with as little as 60 mg of phenobarbital per day. Increased doses of anticoagulant are usually required to maintain prothrombin times within the therapeutic range. The interaction of bishydroxycoumarin and barbiturates is reduced but not abolished entirely if the anticoagulant is administered intravenously. (This phenomenon can be explained by the recent observation that the reduced response to bishydroxycoumarin in patients receiving some barbiturates may be a function not only of enzyme induction but of impaired gastrointestinal absorption as well.) The effects of this interaction may persist for many weeks following discontinuation of the barbiturate. Hypoprothrombinemia following continued administration of increased coumarin doses may thus be delayed. Bleeding complications following this interaction have been documented in man. The frequency of such complications has not been established. A recent report by MacDonald and Robinson, however, suggests that barbiturates and other drugs capable of enzyme induction were a factor in 14 of 67 bleeding reactions occurring during anticoagulant therapy.

These data permit the following recommendations: Close attention to the prothrombin time is necessary for patients receiving barbiturates and coumarin drugs concurrently. A reduction in anticoagulant dose should be anticipated following discontinuation of the barbiturate. The need for such a dose reduction may be delayed for some weeks. Alternative sedation should be sought for patients receiving oral anticoagulants when it is not possible to obtain frequent prothrombin times.

NONBARBITURATE SEDATIVES AND HYPNOTICS. Glutethimide (Doriden), ethchlorvynol (Placidyl), haloperidol (Haldol), and meprobamate (Miltown) may also reduce the effect of oral anticoagulants. The mechanism is presumed to be identical to that of barbiturates, namely, enzyme induction. This has been confirmed for glutethimide. The significance of the interaction appears to be at least as great for glutethimide as for barbiturates. The significance of anticoagulant interaction with ethchlorvynol and meprobamate remains to be determined. Haloperidol appears to interact only with indanedione anticoagulants.

Chloral hydrate has been widely cited as a hypnotic capable of reducing the response to oral anticoagulants through enzyme induction. Recent studies have shown this not to be the case; in fact, an enhanced anticoagulant effect theoretically may occur through displacement of the anticoagulant from its protein-binding site by trichloroacetic acid, a metabolite of chloral hydrate. However, in a controlled study chloral hydrate failed to influence the prothrombin time in 16 patients receiving long-term warfarin therapy at the University of Rochester, and it is concluded that this hypnotic can be employed safely in subjects treated with warfarin.

GRISEOFULVIN. Griseofulvin may antagonize the effect of oral anticoagulants. Enzyme induction has been shown to be responsible for this interaction. Although only a few examples of this interaction have been reported, pronounced reductions in prothrombin time were noted.

ANTACIDS, CHOLESTYRAMINE. More data are necessary to determine the influence of antacids and cholestyramine on the absorption of oral anticoagulants. Until their significance is more clearly defined, these drugs should be administered at a different hour than the anticoagulant.

ORAL CONTRACEPTIVES. Increased coumarin requirements have been documented in patients receiving diethylstilbestrol, oral contraceptives, and other compounds containing estrogen. Physicians prescribing oral anticoagulants should be aware of this phenomenon since anovulatory drugs are in such widespread use. The indications for anticoagulant therapy in patients receiving these drugs should be sufficient reason for their discontinuation.

CORTICOSTEROIDS, ACTH. Corticosteroids and ACTH may antagonize the effect of coumarin drugs. Further studies are necessary to define the mechanism and more clearly document the significance of this interaction.

OTHER DRUGS. Mercurial and thiazide diuretics are known to increase the requirement for oral anticoagulants. This may simply reflect improved liver function following relief of hepatic congestion. Antihistamines have been said to reduce the effect of oral anticoagulants, but there are no data to substantiate such an interaction.

DRUGS KNOWN TO INCREASE THE EFFECT OF ORAL ANTICOAGULANTS

PHENYLBUTAZONE, OXYPHENBUTAZONE. The pyrazolone derivatives are the most widely known drugs capable of enhancing the response to coumarin anticoagulation. This effect can be consistently produced in experimental subjects. The interaction may be a function of reduced metabolism of the anticoagulant in addition to its displacement from albumin. Lengthening of the prothrombin time may occur promptly upon administration of phenylbutazone and tends to persist for some days after discontinuation of the drug. Serious hemorrhage following the combined use of these drugs has been repeatedly documented. The use of phenylbutazone and oxyphenbutazone should be avoided in patients treated with oral anticoagulants.

CLOFIBRATE. The cholesterol-lowering agent clofibrate consistently enhances the response to coumarin anticoagulants. The magnitude of the response may be less than with phenylbutazone; no hemorrhagic complications due to this interaction have been reported. Clofibrate must be employed cautiously in patients receiving oral anticoagulants. Reduced anticoagulant requirements should be anticipated.

PHENYRAMIDOL (ANALEXIN). An enhanced response to both coumarin and indanedione derivatives is uniformly seen after treatment with phenyramidal, a muscle relaxant–analgesic agent. Increase in the prothrombin time may be demonstrated within 72 hours and is usually maximal by 7 days. The effect is pronounced. Since hemorrhagic complications have been described, this drug should not be administered to patients receiving coumarin anticoagulants.

METHYLPHENIDATE (RITALIN). It has recently been demonstrated that methylphenidate inhibits the metabolism of ethyl biscoumacetate. Its effect on the prothrombin time should thus be similar to that of phenyramidol. Further studies are necessary to confirm this effect.

NORETHANDROLONE (NILEVAR), METHANDROSTENOLONE (DIANABOL). Anabolic steroids have been shown to augment the response to coumarin anticoagulants. Marked prolongation of the prothrombin time may occur within a few days of their administration. The need to reduce the anticoagulant dosage should be anticipated in patients receiving norethandrolone and methandrostenolone. To what extent other androgenic steroids may share this effect is not yet known.

D-THYROXINE (CHOLOXIN), L-THYROXINE. D-Thyroxine potentiates the action of coumarin anticoagulants, possibly by the same mechanism as that proposed for anabolic steroids; that is, the drug may increase the affinity between the anticoagulant and its receptor site. The same precautions should be observed as for the anabolic agents when D-thyroxine is administered to patients receiving coumarin drugs. It remains to be seen whether L-thyroxine produces a quantitatively similar effect.

GLUCAGON. The protein glucagon has recently received attention as an inotropic agent in the treatment of severe heart failure. In large doses (exceeding 25 mg per day) it has been shown to potentiate markedly the action of warfarin. Bleeding complications have been described. The mechanism of this interaction has not as yet been clarified.

QUINIDINE, QUININE. The frequency with which quinidine and quinine exaggerate the response to oral anticoagulants is not known. It is probably low. Since these alkaloids are commonly administered to anticoagulated patients, it is important to recognize this effect. It is not necessary to reduce the anticoagulant dose when these agents are added. Close supervision of the prothrombin time is required, however.

ACETYLSALICYLIC ACID, METHYL SALICYLATE, PARA-AMINOSALICYLIC ACID (PASA). Large doses of salicylates (e.g., at least 2 gm of aspirin daily) are required to enhance the response to oral anticoagulants. However, since a single aspirin tablet daily is sufficient to impair platelet function, the use of acetylsalicylates is inadvisable in patients receiving anticoagulants.

ANTIBIOTICS. The effect of oral anticoagulants may be enhanced by antibiotics in a number of ways. A reduction in the synthesis of vitamin K by gut flora has been mentioned. Some antibiotics (e.g., chloramphenicol) appear to inhibit anticoagulant metabolism as well. Intravenous tetracycline may impair the hepatic synthesis of vitamin K–dependent clotting factors.

The extent to which antibiotics increase the response to oral anticoagulants has not been clarified. Physicians should bear these possible effects in mind when prescribing drugs from both groups.

ACETAMINOPHEN (TYLENOL). When patients receiving coumarin drugs are given acetaminophen, the anticoagulant response is slightly enhanced. A modest reduction in anticoagulant dose can be anticipated. The mechanism of this interaction is not known. No hemorrhagic complications have been reported. Since acetaminophen is present in a number of proprietary medications, it is important to be aware of this interaction.

DISULFIRAM (ANTABUSE). A single case of disulfiram-enhanced response to warfarin has been reported. Two hemorrhagic episodes complicating the interaction were documented. The mechanism of this interaction remains to be clarified. Disulfiram has recently been shown to impair the metabolism of ethylmorphine. A similar effect upon warfarin metabolism can be postulated. Frequent tests of prothrombin time are in order when disulfiram is administered to patients receiving oral anticoagulants.

DIPHENYLHYDANTOIN (DILANTIN). The metabolism of diphenylhydantoin is inhibited by coumarin but not by indanedione drugs. Diphenylhydantoin toxicity has been documented as a consequence of this interaction. Further studies are required to determine whether the converse of this interaction may occur, namely, coumarin response enhanced by the anticonvulsant.

TOLBUTAMIDE (ORINASE). The metabolism of tolbutamide may be inhibited by coumarins. Hypoglycemic episodes have been attributed to this interaction. The evidence for a similar effect of tolbutamide upon the metabolism of coumarins in man is conflicting. A reduction in the dose of either drug may be required when both are administered concurrently.

HEPARIN. The one-stage prothrombin time is prolonged by heparin. This effect must be recognized when patients are receiving oral anticoagulants and heparin concomitantly. Failure to do so may lead to inappropriately low doses of the oral anticoagulant. This artifact can be minimized by drawing blood for prothrombin time determinations 4 or more hours after the last heparin administration.

OTHER AGENTS. Diazoxide and ethacrynic, mefenamic, and nalidixic acids have recently been shown to displace warfarin from human albumin. These drugs should thus enhance the response to oral anticoagulants. Monoamine-oxidase inhibitors, indomethacin, phenothiazines, proteolytic enzymes, cathartics, mineral oil, narcotics, thiouracils, and hepatotoxins have all been suggested as additional agents that may enhance the response to coumarin drugs. At present, the data are not sufficient to permit evaluation of the clinical significance of these agents in patients receiving oral anticoagulants. Studies of the effects of alcohol upon anticoagulated subjects are conflicting. It is doubtful that alcohol, in moderation, significantly alters the response to coumarin drugs.

GENERAL RECOMMENDATIONS

The list of drugs capable of interacting with oral anticoagulants has increased rapidly in recent years. It will undoubtedly continue to grow. Further studies are necessary to establish the frequency and significance of interactions for many of these drugs. It is unrealistic to expect physicians to remember all agents with the potential to interact with oral anticoagulants. Practical methods of reinforcing physician awareness of these interactions must be developed. Possible methods include (1) anticoagulation sheets containing a list of potentially interacting drugs for use in the hospital or office, and (2) the use of pharmacy-based drug profile cards for hospitalized patients to permit the identification of potential interactions prior to drug administration.

Physicians prescribing oral anticoagulants *must* be made aware of *all* drugs received by their anticoagulated patients. They must critically examine the need for potentially interacting drugs in these patients and then employ them with caution. A drug interaction should be suspected when anticoagulation control is erratic or when unexpected changes in anticoagulant doses are required to maintain a stable prothrombin time. Suspected interactions should be confirmed. This can usually be accomplished by demonstrating a consistent change in prothrombin times or anticoagulant dose, or both, during administration of the suspect drug compared to control observations. Newly identified interactions should be reported, their frequency and significance established, and the mechanism of interaction defined.

REFERENCES

Aggeler, P. M., O'Reilly, R. A., Leong, L., and Kowitz, P. E. Potentiation of anticoagulant effect of warfarin by phenylbutazone. *New Eng. J. Med.* 276: 496, 1967.

Burns, J. J., and Conney, A. H. Enzyme stimulation and inhibition in the metabolism of drugs. *Proc. Roy. Soc. Med.* 58:955, 1965.

Goldstein, A., Aronow, L., and Kalman, S. M. *Principles of Drug Action:*

The Basis of Pharmacology. New York: Hoeber Med. Div., Harper & Row, 1968. Pp. 220–222, 259–266.

Griner, P., Rickles, F., Weisner, P., Raisez, L., and Odoroff, C.   Efficacy of chloral hydrate in subjects receiving warfarin. *Am. Intern. Med.* 74:540, 1971.

Koch-Weser, J.   Potentiation by glucagon of the hypoprothrombinemic action of warfarin. *Ann. Intern. Med.* 72:331, 1970.

MacDonald, M. G., and Robinson, D. S.   Clinical observations of possible barbiturate interference with anticoagulation. *J.A.M.A.* 204:97, 1968.

Morelli, H. F., and Melmon, K. L.   The clinician's approach to drug interactions. *Calif. Med.* 109:380, 1968.

O'Reilly, R. A.   Interaction of the anticoagulant drug warfarin and its metabolites with human plasma albumin. *J. Clin. Invest.* 48:193, 1969.

O'Reilly, R. A., and Aggeler, P. M.   Determinants of the response to oral anticoagulant drugs in man. *Pharmacol. Rev.* 22:35, 1970.

Schrogie, J. J., and Solomon, H. M.   The anticoagulant response to bishydroxycoumarin: II. The effect of D-thyroxine, clofibrate, and norethandrolone. *Clin. Pharmacol. Ther.* 8:70, 1966.

Solomon, J. M., and Schrogie, J. J.   The effect of phenyramidol on the metabolism of bishydroxycoumarin. *J. Pharmacol. Exp. Ther.* 154:660, 1966.

Solomon, H. M., and Schrogie, J. J.   The effect of various drugs on the binding of warfarin–^{14}C to human albumin. *Biochem. Pharmacol.* 16:1219, 1967.

Suttie, J. W.   Control of clotting factor biosynthesis by vitamin K. *Fed. Proc.* 28:1696, 1969.

Weiner, M., Shapiro, S., Axelrod, J., Cooper, J., and Brodie, B.   The physiological disposition of Dicumarol in man. *J. Pharmacol. Exp. Ther.* 99:409, 1950.

III
MYELOPROLIFERATIVE DISORDERS

19. THE KINETICS OF CELL PROLIFERATION IN ACUTE LEUKEMIA: FUTURE THERAPEUTIC IMPLICATIONS

Marshall A. Lichtman

THE LAST DECADE has seen rapid advances in the acquisition of knowledge regarding the mitotic cycle and the developmental and functional stages of the normal and leukemic granulocyte and lymphocyte. In addition, the mechanism of action and the cellular specificity of a variety of cytolytic and cytostatic drugs used in the treatment of neoplastic diseases of leukopoiesis have been under intensive study. Detailed consideration of these areas would involve mathematic and biologic considerations that are beyond the scope of this chapter. Nevertheless, an understanding of the leukemias as a group of diverse neoplastic diseases with different cell population dynamics, deserving different therapeutic approaches, requires some appreciation of the proliferative, maturational, and senescent phases in the life of the human lymphocyte and granulocyte. In addition, an understanding of the mechanism of action of chemotherapeutic drugs and their effects on normal as well as abnormal leukopoiesis has become fundamental to modern chemotherapy and will allow optimal benefits to accrue from such treatment.

The following discussion presents an overview of selected areas of knowledge regarding cell proliferation in acute leukemia as it may relate to the use of therapeutic agents.

The author is a Scholar of the Leukemia Society of America.

This work was supported by a General Research Support Grant; the Monroe County Cancer and Leukemia Society; and the U.S. Atomic Energy Project at the University of Rochester. It has been assigned publication no. UR-49-1300.

NORMAL CELL MITOTIC CYCLE

The cytologic changes that occur during mitosis are well known. With the availability of radioactive nucleic acid precursors, especially tritiated thymidine, and techniques for studying synchronized cultures of dividing cells, it has become apparent that only a small proportion of the time expended during the process of active cell replication is spent in recognizable mitosis. The cell mitotic cycle is divisible into four major stages, as shown in Figure 19-1: G_1, a period which precedes the onset of active deoxyribonucleic acid (DNA) synthesis and at which time the cell has an interphase amount of DNA (2n or diploid number of chromosomes); S, the period of active DNA synthesis when DNA is increasing toward twice the diploid amount; G_2, a short period which separates the end of DNA synthesis from the beginning of mitosis and during which time the nucleus has twice the interphase amount of DNA (4n); and M, the period of time of morphologically identifiable mitosis from prophase to telophase, at which time DNA is divided between two daughter cells, each resulting in a diploid cell (2n). The duration of the cell cycle differs with different cell types and with different conditions of growth. For a cell which replicates every 24 hours the act of mitosis may take only 90 minutes, whereas antecedent DNA synthesis may take 9 hours.

Although specific biochemical details of cell metabolism in the various

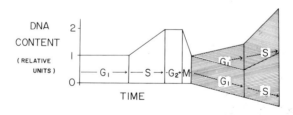

Figure 19-1. The cell mitotic cycle. Four periods are currently accepted as discrete cytochemical and cytomorphologic stages during cell reproduction. In G_1, no DNA synthesis or change in DNA content can be discerned. In S, DNA content lies between diploid (2n) and tetraploid (4n) quantity, and DNA synthesis is identifiable. In G_2, tetraploidy is present (4n) but DNA synthesis is nil. M represents the period of prophase, metaphase, anaphase, and telophase. In a logarithmically growing population, each daughter cell would proceed into the mitotic cycle as depicted. A great deal is yet to be learned about specific biochemical and biophysical events during the cell cycle and those intracellular and extracellular factors that control the movement or cessation of movement of cells through the cycle.

phases of the cell cycle await the results of current investigation, it has been suggested that G_1 is devoted to preparation for replication. Such preparations might include increases in intracellular organelles, ribosomes, and specific enzymes required for DNA synthesis during the subsequent S period. These preparations may so alter cytoplasmic mass as to be a trigger for the initiation of DNA synthesis. The period following DNA synthesis, G_2, may actually be a part of early mitosis during which time spatial changes in chromosomes occur. During this period preparation of the mitotic apparatus may be initiated. These details of the cell cycle may at first seem distant from current medical therapy. However, they provide different critical periods in cellular proliferation for the design and application of new cytolytic agents. Furthermore, the manipulation of populations of abnormal cells in vivo so as to coax them into various phases of the cell cycle could markedly enhance the therapeutic-to-toxic relationship of chemotherapeutic agents, as will be discussed subsequently. In addition, antimetabolites and antimitotic drugs affect the cell in specific phases of the mitotic cycle. An understanding of the success or failure of these drugs is dependent, in part, on knowing the growth pattern of the cells under treatment. Additionally, abnormalities of proliferation in leukemic blast cells can be assessed only in terms of how they deviate from normal during cell reproduction. Such differences could be exploited for therapeutic purposes.

NORMAL GRANULOCYTOPOIESIS

In the human being the mature granulocyte is a very short lived cell, having a brief sojourn in circulation and tissues, and the number available under steady-state conditions may be suboptimal in time of need. A storage compartment of ten times the blood granulocyte pool provides further access to mature or nearly mature granulocytes during periods of acute need. A system of stem cells maintains the capacity to sustain the granulocyte progenitor pool, thereby providing a continual supply of granulocytes for the lifetime of the organism. Several multiplicative divisions expand the mature cells available from one stem cell. This sequence of events is shown diagrammatically in Figure 19-2.

Stem Cells

A *stem cell compartment* is one in which numbers of cells are maintained indefinitely without inflow of cells from another compartment. Therefore the replication of stem cells serves the dual purpose of (1) providing cells which, under the influence of appropriate stimuli, are delivered into the maturational pathway to provide fully differentiated functional granulocytes, and (2) maintaining a pool of undifferentiated cells.

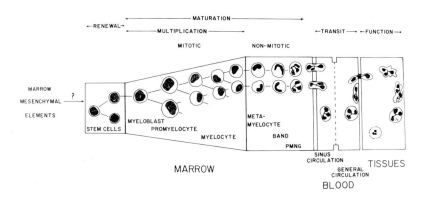

Figure 19-2. The several known compartments in normal granulocytopoiesis. Recent studies have begun to elucidate the stem cell and marrow mesenchymal cell compartments more fully. The egress of marrow mature granulocytes is in part related to their ability to traverse the small-diameter pores between hematopoietic cords and marrow sinuses. The factors governing delivery of cells in marrow sinuses to the circulation require further elucidation. They are presumably vasomotor and are represented by the broken line separating the marrow sinus blood from the general circulation. In marrows of leukemic patients the barrier retaining immature granulocytes is probably deficient, allowing the egress of immature cells whose biophysical characteristics would normally prevent their escape. Little is known regarding the exact life-span of either normal or leukemic cells in the tissue compartment. Inferences can be drawn from indirect observations to suggest that the polymorphonuclear granulocyte (PMNG) has a very short stay in the tissues, presumably ending in cell death with a negligible number returning to the circulation.

The stem cell compartment may be a complex system of cell pools operating in parallel and in series with each other, as will be discussed later. Uncertainty exists regarding the morphologic appearance of stem cells in human marrow. It has been suggested that a marrow cell similar morphologically to a small lymphocyte, although containing a different program of genetic information, may be the hematopoietic stem cell. A small cell with a high nuclear-cytoplasmic ratio may be an efficient way to package dormant genetic capacity in circulating cells. The active genetic content of the cell would determine its capacity to respond to specific stimuli. Hence the *hematopoietic stem cell,* a marrow "small lymphocyte," may be a phenocopy of an immunocompetent cell, a reticuloendothelial system "small lymphocyte." These are cells that look alike by light microscopy but respond, in the former case, to hematopoietic needs probably regulated by humoral stimuli, and in the latter case to antigenic stimulation.

Under unusual provocation mesenchymal elements of marrow, perhaps cells lining the haversian canals of bone, may replenish hematopoietic capacity. It is unknown whether this occurs on a day-to-day basis. The anatomic as well as the physiologic organization of the stem cell compartment remains an active area of hematologic investigation that awaits further clarification.

Multiplication and Maturation

The process of differentiation of stem cells leads to the development of readily discernible morphologic and biochemical cellular entities. Under normal circumstances, the stem cell compartment is capable of maintaining numbers of granulocytic, erythrocytic, and megakaryocytic cells in the absence of input from another compartment. The *myeloblast* (granuloblast)* is the currently accepted earliest recognizable precursor of the mature granulocyte. It is probable that the myeloblast is not a stem cell; rather it is an early member of the multiplicative pool of cells as outlined in Figure 19-2. Such cells are capable of cell division and maturation but are limited in the number of divisions they can undergo. Their daughter cells proceed into the maturation sequence. Hence these cells are not capable of continued self-renewal and cannot maintain hematopoiesis indefinitely. The granuloblast pool must, therefore, be maintained by the differentiation of an antecedent cell system. The term *uncommitted stem cell* has been used for this antecedent pool capable of furnishing granuloblasts, erythroblasts, and megakaryoblasts. The latter three blast cell types have been referred to as *committed stem cells;* however, they do not satisfy the definition of stem cells previously noted since they cannot sustain their own number without influx from a prior cell pool.

In the case of granulocytopoiesis, as noted in Figure 19-2, the multiplicative-maturational compartment describes the myeloblast, promyelocyte, and large myelocyte. During this sequence, specific granule synthesis occurs in parallel with limited multiplication of cell number. Even the limited multiplication allows a substantial expansion of cell number, making granulocytopoiesis more efficient, particularly in times of increased need. This is followed by a nonproliferative phase which includes the late (small) myelocyte, metamyelocyte, band, and segmented granulocyte. Although multiplicative (mitotic) potential is lost, it is during this sequence of further differentiation that cytoplasmic reorganization takes place which enhances the cell's ability to deform in order to negotiate restricted passageways, to adhere to vessel walls, to migrate, and to ingest microorganisms. These capabilities are poorly developed prior to the metamyelocyte stage but they are essential for normal functional capacity. The mature polymorphonuclear granulocyte enters the storage compartment of the marrow, to escape in a random fashion shortly thereafter. Although the accumulation of tenfold more bands and polymorphonuclear granulocytes in marrow than in blood has been made an active process by the use of the term *storage com-*

---

* Electron microscopic and histochemical studies suggest that most myeloblasts in human marrow are already committed to granulocyte differentiation.

partment, it may simply be the result of random factors related to the rate of mature granulocyte production and the rate at which the granulocytes can search out and pass through pores in the barrier separating hematopoietic cords from sinuses, and the subsequent entry of sinus granulocytes into the general circulation (Fig. 19-2).

ACUTE LEUKEMIA

Acute leukemia is characterized by the failure of production of differentiated, functionally useful granulocytes. Unlike normal blast cells which mature, lose their mitotic capacity, and die in a finite period of time, leukemic blast cells accumulate in excessive numbers in marrow and, later, tissues. However, the morbidity and mortality in leukemia are related primarily to the concomitant reduction in quantity of normal blood cells, resulting in varying degrees of granulocytopenia, anemia, and thrombocytopenia. The resultant predisposition to bleeding and infection remains the major cause of death in patients with leukemia.

LEUKEMIC CELL MITOTIC CYCLE

Studies of leukemic blast cells have demonstrated quantitative deviations from normal in cell proliferation. Although in the past production of leukemic cells has traditionally been thought of as a *hyperproliferative state,* studies of individual cells in established acute leukemia indicate that leukemic blast cells generally take longer to go through the mitotic cycle than do normal myeloblasts. Hence the time spent in DNA synthesis and in other phases of the cell mitotic cycle are longer in the leukemic blast cell. Furthermore, the fraction of cells which can be identified as dividing in acute leukemia at the time of diagnosis is significantly less than the fraction of granuloblasts in mitosis in normal marrow. Nevertheless, in absolute terms, because of the far greater size of the population under study, the number of cells being produced is greater in leukemic marrow than in normal marrow. Moreover, the birth of new cells usually exceeds the death rate of cells, leading to a progressive accumulation of leukemic blast cells in marrow and tissues. Evidence also suggests that the density of the cell population in the marrow of leukemic patients is inversely related to the fraction of cells in the mitotic cycle. If one studies patients after chemotherapy, during early relapse when the marrow population is less dense, the fraction of cells dividing is greater than it is in patients prior to therapy. Comparisons must be defined in relation to the total cell population density, and it is currently impossible to study normal blast cells under similar circumstances in vivo.

In addition, occasional cases of established acute leukemia may show cell production rates equal to or greater than those of normal myeloblasts.

Also it is increasingly evident that leukemic blast cells as identified morphologically represent a heterogeneous population of cells, the normal counterparts for which are unclear. Indeed it is uncertain whether the predominant leukemic blast cells seen morphologically on examination of the marrow are the cells which sustain the leukemic process. It is conceivable that a counterpart of the morphologically unidentifiable stem cell may be predominantly responsible for the renewal of leukemic cells (leukemic stem cells). The predominant cell seen morphologically in acute leukemia may be analogous to the multiplicative compartment of normal marrow and would be better compared to the promyelocyte and myelocyte in terms of the time required to complete the mitotic cycle and of the fraction of cells dividing. Such comparisons of new cell production might result in entirely different interpretations of the relative mitotic capacity of leukemic cells. Therefore the current emphasis on the relative hypoproliferation of the individual leukemic blast cell may be no more accurate than the former emphasis on the hyperproliferation of this cell.

In so-called hypoproliferative leukemias, in which the disease may smolder for long periods without treatment, the relationship between birth of new blast cells and death of blast cells is such that little change in the patient's clinical status occurs over protracted periods of time. It is assumed that the body burden of leukemic cells is also relatively constant since blood and marrow examinations do not indicate progressive accumulation of cells, at least for a period of time. Since little is known regarding the death rate of medullary or extramedullary leukemic blast cells, one might better call this variant *hypoaccumulative leukemia* since proliferation or mitotic activity may not be greatly reduced; rather, cell death may be accelerated. This condition is characterized by disorderly and suboptimal hematopoiesis, but often enough functional cells are present to sustain useful life for months or years without specific drug treatment. Controlled clinical trials are needed to better characterize the blast cell kinetics and the usefulness of specific chemotherapy in this not uncommon situation.

LEUKEMIC HEMATOPOIESIS

Hematopoiesis in the patient with acute leukemia could be considered in terms of the total absence of normal stem cells with only leukemic stem cells remaining, or cohabitation of the marrow by normal and leukemic stem cells, the normal stem cells being reduced in numbers and prevented from differentiating in significant quantity. Although support can be mustered for either hypothesis, presently the weight of evidence favors the presence of dual stem cells, normal and leukemic, in cases of acute leukemia that develop de novo. There may not be normal stem cells in acute leukemia developing from chronic granulocytic leukemia and myeloid metaplasia, however, and this may account for the poor remission rate in these diseases, since it is held that normal stem cells remaining in the marrow of leukemic patients are responsible for the remissions that occur with chemotherapy.

The presence of an enlarging leukemic blast cell population in the marrow suppresses the multiplication ability of normal stem cells and impairs their entry into the maturational compartments. How the leukemic cells gain hegemony and the precise nature of the interactions between leukemic and normal cells remain unclear. The fact that the fraction of leukemic blast cell dividing is inversely related to cell density in the marrow indicates that at least a degree of control over cell production rate remains, even in the leukemic population. Whether this density-related, relative inhibition of leukemic cell division is due to cell-cell interaction, microenvironmental limitations, or a feedback loop mechanism is not known. Obviously this effect is inadequate to prevent extensive replacement of the marrow by leukemic cells.

The deficiency of red cell and platelet production, which is an almost invariable concomitant of acute leukemia, has been thought to be a secondary phenomenon due totally to the deleterious effects of the accumulation of leukemic blast cells in the marrow on normal hematopoietic stem cells. Under such circumstances, normal erythropoietin- and thrombopoietin-sensitive cells are prevented from responding by cell division and maturation into erythrocytes and megakaryocytes. The primordial abnormal cell in acute leukemia (leukemic stem cell) may, however, represent an alteration in a precursor cell which under normal circumstances is capable of differentiation into mature red cells, granulocytes, and megakaryocytes (i.e., an uncommitted stem cell). Hence the anemia and thrombocytopenia associated with acute leukemia in many cases may represent a primary abnormality. The presence of intrinsic physical, chemical, and antigenic abnormalities of the red cell and chromosomal aberrations in erythroblasts in leukemia are compatible with primary involvement of erythroid precursors in the leukemic process.

The various morphologic manifestations of acute leukemia may also be explained on this basis. For example, erythroleukemia, which initially shows pathologic erythroid proliferation as well as abnormal granulocytic proliferation, may represent a more prominent expression of the disordered erythropoiesis of the leukemic stem cell in this particular situation. The morphologic characteristic of the disease may be variable, depending on the level of the stem cell compartment or clone of stem cells involved and their predisposition to manifest leukemic erythroid, granulocytic, monocytic, and megakaryocytic partial differentiation.

Although the central defect in acute leukemia is the failure of efficient and regulated maturation of immature cells, evidence suggests that varying degrees of differentiation may be present in leukemic cells. In chronic granulocytic leukemia mature cells are, in morphologic and in several functional respects, very similar, often indistinguishable from normal despite the presence of histochemical and karyotypic differences. In the typical situation the degree of maturation of acute leukemic cells into functionally useful cells is of such a limited magnitude that the patient's life is in jeopardy. It is, however, of theoretical and practical interest that the leukemic lesion of stem cells may have a quantitative distribution, with some cells being affected so mildly that they may undergo nearly full maturation.

In some situations, particularly with forms of myelomonocytic leukemia, partial maturation of the leukemic cell may be identifiable and closely correlated with morphologic appearance. It is common in myelomonocytic leukemia to have cells which are qualitatively abnormal develop with an appearance recognizable as that of a monocytoid cell. This may also be true in acute granulocytic leukemia, in which the appearance of qualitatively abnormal (leukemic) promyelocytes, myelocytes, polymorphonuclear granulocytes, erythrocytes, and megakaryocytes may be observed. There seems to be a quantitative spectrum of derangements in leukemic cells which on the one extreme is manifested by virtually no evidence of differentiation, as in rapidly progressive acute granulocytic leukemia, to the other extreme in which there is relatively normal differentiation, as in chronic granulocytic leukemia. Between these two extremes, varying degrees of disordered maturation and blast cell accumulation may occur and may be represented clinically as preleukemic states, refractory anemias, hypoaccumulative leukemias, subacute leukemias, and several morphologic variants (myelomonocytic, basophilic, eosinophilic, erythroid, and megakaryocytic leukemias).

In addition to degrees of maturation identifiable by standard morphologic criteria, cells with the morphologic appearance of blasts may represent cells whose mitotic capacity has been reduced. This is shown diagrammatically in Figure 19-3. Studies of tritiated thymidine incorporation using autoradiography have shown that blast cells incorporating tritiated thymidine (i.e., actively synthesizing DNA presumably in preparation for division) tend to be large blast cells, whereas the small blast cell has a lower thymidine-labeling index and is more often not actively mitotic. Hence reduced blast cell size and decreased mitotic activity have been correlated. In addition, fewer blast cells in the circulation are actively dividing as compared to blast cells in the marrow. It has been suggested that the cells released from the marrow tend to have undergone a form of maturation

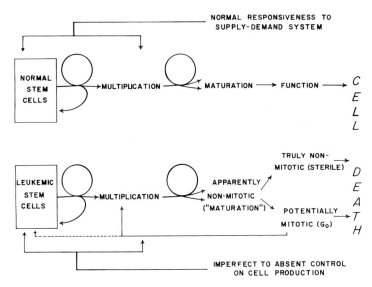

Figure 19-3. Comparison of normal and leukemic granulocytopoiesis. Little is known regarding cell death rates in the various compartments during either normal or leukemic granulocytopoiesis. In the normal marrow granulocyte death is probably infrequent. In some leukemias intramedullary death of cells may be an important factor in the rate of accumulation of leukemic blast cells.

which has lowered their mitotic capacity and perhaps favored their release from marrow, drawing an analogy to normal granulocytopoiesis.

Although leukemic blast cells may undergo a sequential reduction in size, mitotic capacity, and perhaps other characteristics which are not accompanied by morphologic evidence of maturation, leukemic blast cells do not conform to a normal, orderly growth pattern. They usually have only a limited ability to mimic normal differentiation, and they cannot perform the function of the mature granulocyte since they fail to undergo the cytoplasmic reorganization necessary to allow for efficient migration into tissues, phagocytosis, and intracellular killing of microorganisms. Furthermore, they continue to divide at a population density at which normal stem cells would be expected to be completely inhibited. In addition, their absolute birth rate is inevitably greater than their death rate so that a steady state is not maintained and accumulation of leukemic cells occurs.

This accumulation of cells in acute leukemia is also due to the longer survival of immature granulocytes in the circulation and possibly in tissue. The leukemic blast cell disappears from the circulation at only one-fifth the rate of the normal mature granulocyte. This difference is probably related to the biophysical properties of the cytoplasm of all immature granulocytes, which limit their ability to adhere to vessels, deform, and migrate into tissues. They may, however, be transiently sequestered in the splenic circulation and later reenter the circulation, explaining the biphasic kinetic patterns of labeled immature granulocytic cells.

The mitotic capacity of individual leukemic blast cells is relatively heterogeneous. How deviant this heterogeneity is from normal is difficult to assess, for reasons previously noted regarding the difficulties in studying normal counterparts at similar population densities. Within the leukemic blast cell population, the mitotic cycle time is variable. Important technical considerations arise when estimating such variables as thymidine incorporation by cells, since the length of exposure to radioactive thymidine may be too short to label cells which are slowly moving through the cell cycle and not in S phase while label is present. Indeed a fraction of cells spend prolonged periods of time in apparent dormancy, without dividing, and are not labeled with thymidine even with prolonged exposure. The term G_0 has been applied to such cells. Although such leukemic cells are apparently dormant, it has been shown that under given circumstances they may reenter the mitotic cycle and divide. The rate at which G_0 cells enter mitosis and their inherent susceptibility or resistance to chemotherapy are important considerations in the treatment of leukemia.

KINETIC CONSIDERATIONS IN CHEMOTHERAPY

Acute lymphocytic and granulocytic leukemia have not been considered separately because the pattern of mitosis of the leukemic blast cell population is similar in the two diseases. However, responsiveness to specific drugs, frequency of remission induction, and length of remission are considerably different for these two cell types, indicating that apparent cell production rates are not sole indicators of responsiveness to drugs. The normal counterpart of the granulocytic leukemic blast cell has been discussed. The normal counterpart of the lymphocytic leukemic blast is even more problematic and makes estimates of the normality or abnormality of single cell and population growth patterns extremely difficult. To some extent the acceptance of the lymphoblast as a neoplastic transformation of a lymphoid cell is based on inference; and although immunologic and cytochemical data support the lymphoid nature of such a leukemic process, this cannot be considered conclusive. Since the stem cell compartment may be complex, it is conceivable that the differences in acute leukemias may be related to the compartmental level of the mutant stem cell, or that a difference in the nature of the inducing leukemogenic agent may determine in part the difference in the biology of the leukemia that develops.

The ideal chemotherapeutic agent has been described as having, among other characteristics, the ability to destroy leukemic cells selectively. The goal of discovering agents with selective action against tumor cells seems somewhat less illusory with the discovery that L-asparaginase can inhibit neoplastic cells that require L-asparagine for growth, having little deleterious effect on normal hematopoietic tissues because of their ability to synthesize L-asparagine de novo. The drug is not without other forms of toxicity, however. The recent discovery that serine is a requirement for cells cultured from patients with chronic granulocytic leukemia, whereas it is not required by normal cells, also offers hope for further enhancement in the specificity of leukemic treatment. Unfortunately, as demonstrated by the clinical experience with L-asparaginase, relative selectivity for neoplastic cells does not ensure the degree of sensitivity of such cells that would lead to eradication.

TIMING, DOSE, AND COMBINATIONS OF CHEMOTHERAPEUTIC AGENTS

Although a burgeoning body of knowledge portends further advances in the treatment of leukemia, until recently, rather than cell kinetic patterns leading to artful chemotherapy, the studied use of drugs in patients with leukemia and in experimental animal leukemias has provided insight into cell population dynamics. Chemotherapy of leukemia remains basically empirical, with clinical trials determining the effectiveness of different drugs, dosages, and administration schedules. However, recent understanding gained from observations in animal and human leukemia has led to improvements in the therapeutic approach with resultant increased frequency and duration of remissions in acute leukemia. Chemotherapists are beginning to apply results of kinetic studies to new approaches to drug therapy schedules.

Animal models of leukemic disease studied by Skipper and co-workers have indicated that increased survival is related to the size of the population of leukemic cells destroyed, not to a fundamental difference in the nature of residual cells, such as a reduction in growth rate of tumor. Their studies have also shown that the relationship of cell kill to a given drug dosage is a proportional one. Therefore a given dosage of an antileukemic agent kills the same percentage of cells, not the same number of cells, over a wide range of cell population size. This principle had been known in studies of bacterial cells. *First-order kinetics* is the mathematic term applied to the constant percentage reduction in a population regardless of size. The dose-response curve for chemotherapeutic agents is a very steep one, indicating that a large increase in cell kill occurs for a proportionately smaller increase in drug dose. These studies suggested that intensive short-term therapy (to the limit of host tolerance with supportive care) should be more efficacious than low-dose, long-term therapy. This is particularly true in circumstances in which logarithmic growth and short mitotic cycle time are present. An example of the effects of different drug schedules is shown in Figure 19-4.

Furthermore, in animal models, unless all leukemic cells are destroyed, the disease recurs. Similarly the injection of one or a very few leukemic cells can transmit the disease and kill the animal. The duration of remission (the duration of subclinical disease) is also related to the residual number of leukemic cells. These observations may be applicable in certain respects to man, since it is assumed that the disease in man may start as the altera- tion of a single cell, that the disease manifestations are related, in part, to the accumulated number of leukemic cells, and that cell production rate— by determining the number of leukemic cells—will be an important deter-

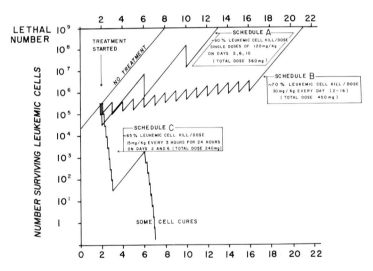

Figure 19-4. Results of cytosine arabinoside treatment of L1210 mouse leukemic cells in vivo from the work of Skipper and colleagues. With an inocu- lum of about 4×10^4 cells and logarithmic growth, a lethal number of cells is reached in 8 days. The effect of giving 8 spaced doses per day (Schedule C) totaling 120 mg/kg/day on each of 2 days can result in elimination of the cell population, whereas the same dose given as a single injection on each of 3 days for a larger total dose (360 mg/kg as opposed to 240 mg/kg) results in "a smaller effect in cell burden and a rapid restitution of the leukemic cell popula- tion," demonstrating the importance of utilizing the kinetic characteristics of a cell population to advantage. It also highlights the erroneous conclusions which could be reached about potential drug efficacy if the influence of dose–time relationships of drug administration to cell population kinetics cannot be defined. (From H. E. Skipper in Dameshek and Dutcher (Eds.), *Perspectives in Leu- kemia,* 1968. By permission of the author and Grune & Stratton.)

minant of duration of remission. Animal models having logarithmic growth rate of leukemic cells must be credited with taking thinking regarding chemotherapy of leukemia out of a state of total empiricism and with stimulating logical approaches to the study of the interaction of chemotherapy, cell population kinetics, and clinical disease. Unfortunately these tractable animal models are considerably simpler biologically and more predictable than is the human disease. It is not surprising and should not be discouraging that precise interpositions cannot be made.

The child with acute lymphatic leukemia has been estimated to have one trillion leukemic cells at the time of diagnosis, and the adult with acute granulocytic leukemia considerably more, making gargantuan the difficulty in eradicating all cells. For example, if 99.999% of cells are destroyed in the induction of a complete remission in acute lymphocytic leukemia (estimates indicate a remission will occur with less reduction in cell number), this would reduce the body load of leukemic cells to a still substantial ten million cells. It is likely also that many of these residual cells are in cloistered sites, poorly accessible to antimetabolites, such as behind the blood-brain barrier or in gonads and thymus.

The primary goal of therapy is to reduce the leukemic cell burden to the lowest possible number within the tolerance of the host. The maximum amount of drug compatible with host survival appears to be optimal with respect to maximum reduction of leukemic cells. The advances in supportive care described in Chapter 22 have made it possible to improve host tolerance and have allowed chemotherapists to induce a period of severe marrow hypofunction due to therapy. This intentional induction of hematopoietic aplasia in an effort to reduce the marrow and tissue leukemic blast population to the lowest levels possible requires the supervision of experienced personnel, since the immediate risks to the patient are heightened. This approach must aim for the reduction in the marrow blast population rather than just the blood population. Such treatment has increased the remission rate in patients with acute granulocytic and lymphocytic leukemia.

It is unclear what competitive factors are involved in releasing inhibition of normal or near-normal hematopoietic stem cells under these conditions. It is unlikely that differences in cell production rates, determined solely by relative population densities, are totally responsible. It can be argued that increased effectiveness of therapy is related in part to the ability to induce a greater reduction in leukemic cell load. This is in keeping with animal studies indicating an inverse relationship between residual leukemic cell burden after therapy or the number of leukemic cells transplanted into experimental animals and duration of life. Moreover, in children with acute lymphocytic leukemia, studies of the proportions of marrow blasts during relapse support the important relationship of reduction in marrow blast numbers to duration of remission. Remissions can be prolonged by maintenance therapy, which can be shown to slow the accumulation of marrow blast populations, often referred to in terms of the doubling time or the time required to increase the blast population twofold. The mechanism of the rare occurrence of extremely long disease-free periods after induction therapy and discontinuation of maintenance therapy is unexplained. It must be due either to the extermination of all actively mitotic leukemic stem cells or, more likely, to a change in the growth potential of residual leukemic stem cells—again indicating the (in this case fortunate) difference from animal models with their predictable reproliferation, even from a single or very few residual cells.

In the treatment of acute leukemia, the use of multiple drugs has developed as a means of intensifying therapy. This approach is the result of the availability of drugs with both different modes of action and different toxicities. This allows greater antineoplastic effect without a proportional increase in a specific toxic effect. In addition it enables one to use drugs with different modalities of action on cells, resulting in an additive or sometimes synergistic cytocidal effect. Quantitative studies of subjects with acute leukemia indicate that with combined therapy the body burden of leukemic cells is further reduced and remission rates are increased; and in patients in whom remission has been induced, the duration of remission in the absence of maintenance therapy is significantly longer after multiple-drug treatment. Strict analogies to animal models are hazardous; however, it is likely that the reduced number of residual cells is one important factor in the lengthened duration of remission. In contrast to animal models, other factors relating to changes in the intrinsic mitotic capacity of residual cells, a lag in mitotic capacity after chemotherapy, or the ability of environmental homeostatic mechanisms to act temporarily on the reduced leukemic cell mass must also be involved.

Unfortunately, for unknown reasons as yet not correlated with growth patterns of leukemic blast cells, remissions occur in only 40% of patients with acute granulocytic leukemia even after intensive multidrug therapy. Furthermore the remissions are of relatively short duration. The characteristics of the disease which correlate with the ability to enter remission are not entirely clear. The height of the peripheral white blood count is roughly correlated with remission rate. The lower the count, the greater is the likelihood of remission, generally. This may be a reflection of the body burden of leukemic cells. Hence, the lower the count, the lower the total number of leukemic cells, the more likely chemotherapy will be successful. Such simplistic inferences are weak, however, and even in patients in whom significant reduction in blast population occurs with resultant marrow aplasia, remission is not assured. What other factors determine remission induction and remission duration? Why do rare patients have prolonged remissions, in some cases without maintenance chemotherapy?

Killmann has articulated an intricate model of the stem cell compartment which addresses itself to these and other questions. He conceives the stem cell compartment as being composed of clones of cells (groups with identical genetic expression) which are *sleepers* or *feeders*. Sleeper stem cells are in a dormant state blocked from entering hematopoietic production lines. The feeder stem cells are more advanced, self-renewing, and provide cells for hematopoietic cell differentiation. Should a feeder pool be injured or spent, it could be replaced from a sleeper pool. Killmann further suggests that in acute granulocytic leukemia the pattern of remission and relapses may relate to a sleeper-feeder stem cell hypothesis, the detailed support for which can be found in his writings. Hence if the feeder clone is leukemic and is heavily populated, normal sleeper clones if they exist, or clones of a lower degree of abnormality than frankly leukemic cells, are prevented from proliferating. After therapy, if the leukemic feeder clones can be severely depressed and sleepers are recruited, the possibility of a clone change exists.

The nature of the sleeper clone which will be recruited depends on several conditions. If recruitment is from a normal sleeper clone, remission will ensue. The presence of normal chromosomal karyotype in patients with acute granulocytic leukemia in remission with previously abnormal karyotype supports the concept of a clone change. The absence of gross chromosomal abnormality in nearly half of patients with acute leukemia indicates that the change to a normal diploid number of chromosomes does not ensure the normalcy of the new clone. Although Killmann suggests that remission duration will be dependent on the length of life of the normal (or near-normal) clone, it is possible that the life of this clone may be abnormally foreshortened by the as yet poorly understood interaction or competition of the reproliferating leukemic clone. A very important factor in the duration of remission may relate to the partial responsiveness of the leukemic sleeper clone to feeder inhibition. This may also be an important consideration in the propensity of abnormal and ultimately leukemic clones to develop in the marrows of chronically hypoplastic bone marrows. Since marrow leukemic blast cell production rate may be partially responsive to cell density, leukemic sleeper clones may also retain some control features which may govern remission duration. Such mechanisms may make more intelligible rare sustained remissions, the latent period after radiation exposure before leukemia becomes clinically apparent, and other clinical observations. Interacting factors such as virological, immunologic, cell reparative systems, and others may also be involved.

In addition, if the fraction of residual normal stem cells is greater and their time of cell reproduction shorter, normal hematopoiesis may be favored temporarily. Such normal hematopoiesis may retard the reproliferation of leukemic cells for a time. Since leukemic stem cells are not fully responsive to negative feedback controls, they will eventually restart to proliferate, increase in population, and again suppress normal hematopoietic stem cells, resulting in leukemic blast cell replacement.

Currently, descriptive hypotheses are being expounded by various investigators which encompass many of the observed patterns of clinical disease expression. Some experimental data are available to provide a framework for such theses. These exercises are important since they attempt to distill and integrate accumulated observations and provide logical hypotheses to be tested experimentally. However, it must be emphasized that they are not yet founded on a substantial body of experimental data and hence should not restrict one inordinately in considering alternative suggestions.

CHEMOTHERAPY AND THE CELL MITOTIC CYCLE

The mitotic activity of leukemic cell populations is important in responsiveness to drugs. This is shown diagrammatically in Figure 19-5. Antimetabolites which are used in the therapy of leukemia are referred to as mitotic cycle–dependent agents. Drugs such as methotrexate, 6-mercaptopurine, and cytosine arabinoside interfere with DNA synthesis and are effective only at the time cells are actively synthesizing DNA. This means that the cell must be in the mitotic cycle, and more specifically in the DNA

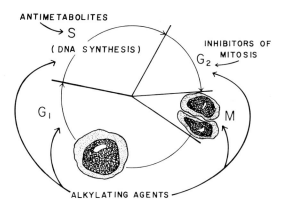

Figure 19-5.   The time in the mitotic cycle during which dividing cells are susceptible to various categories of chemotherapeutic agents.

synthesis phase of the cell cycle, for drug effect to be applied. Since thymidine incorporation studies indicate that only a fraction of leukemic blast cells are in DNA synthesis when a pulse of drug is given, attempts to prolong infusions of antimetabolites have been used to increase the duration of effective blood concentration of drugs and thereby the number of cells exposed during DNA synthesis. Administration of cytosine arabinoside by prolonged infusion has provided better results than shorter administration periods. In the case of some cycle-dependent antimetabolites, a pulse dose has proved maximally effective. This depends on the duration of therapeutic blood levels and the duration of a significant intracellular pool of the drug after cessation of therapy.

Knowledge of such characteristics of specific drugs is as important as cycle time in determining drug schedule. The interactions on the cell of antimetabolites, antimitotic agents, antibiotics, and yet-to-be-discovered agents involves more than cycle phase. Drug metabolism, alternative metabolic pathways, transmembrane transport capacity, and other factors are involved. Studies have already shown that antimetabolic action appears to be enhanced during the S phase if cells are increasing in number rather than maintaining steady-state numbers.

ENHANCEMENT AND RECRUITMENT

Evidence has suggested that reduction in marrow leukemic blast cell population density may increase the proportion of leukemic cells dividing. In addition, certain antimetabolites may result in a partial synchronization of the transit of leukemic cells through the mitotic cycle. Therapeutic schedules to take advantage of these possible manipulations of cell populations in vivo are being studied in several laboratories. Recent partial synchronization of acute lymphatic lymphoblasts in the DNA synthesis period in vivo has been accomplished with the use of cytosine arabinoside administered for 1 to 2 minutes. This technique provides an enhancement in the number of cells "trapped" in DNA synthesis. This accumulation of cells in S phase provides a large population susceptible to a second mitotic cycle–dependent agent such as the periwinkle alkaloid, vincristine, which may act in the G_2 period. Vincristine therapy after synchronization in the S phase would greet a large number of cells entering G_2 and susceptible to the drug. If, as has been suggested, random growth of normal cells occurs more rapidly after cytosine arabinoside S-phase trapping, a therapeutic advantage might result, since the proportion of normal cells susceptible to an antimetabolite acting during a specific phase of the mitotic cycle would be less than the proportion of synchronized leukemic cells susceptible to such a second challenge.

DORMANT BLAST CELLS

A further important problem in current leukemia therapy is the nonproliferative blast cell. Although some of these cells may have entered an irreversible nonmitotic state destined to undergo cell death, evidence suggests that some dormant blast cells are capable of reentering a proliferative phase after a prolonged period of dormancy, as noted in Figure 19-3. Such cells could escape the effects of therapy to divide and accumulate at a later time, especially when the inhibiting effect of a large cell population is removed by chemotherapy. These cells have been likened to normal G_0 cells such as the hepatocyte. The hepatocyte, although usually dormant, will be induced to mitosis after partial hepatectomy until liver mass is restored.

The volume of individual leukemic blast cells is often broadly distributed. The large blast cell is more likely to be in the cell mitotic cycle; its daughter cell may remain smaller and be nonmitotic. Some blast cells are sequestered in a variety of extramedullary tissues inaccessible to systemic chemotherapy, and they may play an important role in recrudescence of the disease. When searched for by techniques not ordinarily used, leukemic blast cells can be found in tissues during apparently complete remissions. It is possible that after successful chemotherapy and remission induction, there may be recruitment of such cells. These formerly dormant leukemic blast cells are induced to divide in part by the reduction in leukemic cell mass. They might then be susceptible to further therapy with antimetabolites.

Clinical studies are already in progress using techniques to induce recruitment. Extracorporeal irradiation, one such technique, is of particular interest because of its unexcelled cytolytic effect. The ability to irradiate blood extracorporeally allows reduction in the cell population without infringing on normal marrow stem cells. Increased marrow mitotic activity has been demonstrated in leukemic patients after extracorporeal irradiation. At this time, antimetabolites could be given with the intention of heightened efficacy due to a reduction in total leukemic cell numbers and a larger fraction of remaining cells dividing, including cells which would have initially been dormant. Further studies are needed to determine the clinical usefulness of such techniques.

The ability to initiate therapy with agents like L-asparaginase, which have little hematopoietic toxicity, may also allow recruitment with little initial marrow toxicity. In addition, the use of agents which are not cycle dependent should be studied more intensively as adjuvant therapy with antimetabolites and antimitotic agents. Formerly, alkylating agents were felt not to be useful in the treatment of leukemia. However, drugs like cyclophosphamide and bis-chloroethyl-nitrosourea (BCNU) have been of considerable usefulness in recent years. Since some alkylating agents are not primarily dependent on mitotic cycling for their action, they could affect nonmitotic (G_0) cells as well as cells not in the S phase of the cell cycle. Since recruitment may not involve all cells with mitotic potential, alkylation may be another avenue of attack against these cells. Some alkylating drugs appear to be most effective on cells in the mitotic cycle; however, they act in all phases of the cycle and thereby provide cytocidal effects against a broader population of cells.

If the time required to double a leukemic cell population is about 5 days as estimated from serial marrow examinations, a single leukemic cell could produce clinical relapse in 6 months. Although earlier clinical studies were consistent with exponential growth, the recent results of studies of duration of unmaintained remission after intensive therapy are not consistent with such an assumption. Since it is unlikely that residual cell numbers are reduced to very small quantities, it is most likely that residual leukemic cells are not continually doubling in number and that many may be nonmitotic (temporarily). Whether this is due to the shock of therapy, requiring cellular reparative processes to allow later proliferation, a selective residue of less mitotic cells, or a change in the effect of controlling influences on the leukemic blast cell is unknown.

Clinical studies indicate that certain drugs are superior for remission induction in acute leukemia (e.g., vincristine, L-asparaginase in acute lymphoblastic leukemia), while others may be more effective in remission maintenance. This does not appear to be due to development of drug resistance since the inducing drug can be used repeatedly. Although this is not a hard and fast distinction, it is of interest, since it supports the difference in growth pattern of residual leukemic cells and highlights the need to avoid strict extrapolations from animal models to human disease.

Further prolongation of remission duration may rest with the ability to learn more regarding the nature of residual cells and the drugs which might destroy them. Also the ability to reduce the actively dividing population by techniques which are not damaging to those hematopoietic elements responsible for remission, such as extracorporeal irradiation, corticosteroids, and selective agents like L-asparaginase, will allow greater tolerance for later use of alkylation and other more hematotoxic agents for residual nonproliferative cells.

DIURNAL VARIATION

The presence of a diurnal variation in marrow mitotic activity is of considerable interest. The variation is, however, too slight to make the time of day at which a drug is administered a significant therapeutic advantage. Nevertheless, with the acquisition of further knowledge regarding control of the rate of cell mitosis, the ability to manipulate mitotic activity by physiologic means may provide a useful adjunct in chemotherapy.

MARROW TRANSPLANTATION

The eradication of all or most proliferative hematopoietic cells with irradiation or chemotherapy and their replacement with normal marrow elements from a histocompatible donor have been attempted as a means of curing leukemia. Thus far such attempts have not resulted in permanent cure and only very rarely in documented amelioration of the disease. Marrow transplantation, unlike solid organ homotransplantation, requires not only the surmounting of immunologic barriers but the organization of the single cells of donor marrow into a viable, regulated, functioning arrangement in the recipient's marrow stroma. Furthermore, the transplantation of immunocompetent donor cells has led to graft-versus-host reactions (referred to as "secondary disease"). Moreover, the required elimination of most if not all leukemic stem cells adds further to the difficulties involved in this form of treatment. The role of marrow transplantation in the treatment of leukemia awaits the outcome of current studies of the cytologic, immunologic, and pharmacologic variables involved.

IMMUNE FACTORS

A future role of immunotherapy in primary or secondary treatment of acute leukemia is under study in several centers around the world. In the *surveillance hypothesis,* a challenge by neoplastic clones of cells in healthy subjects is continual and is usually repulsed by immunologic defenses. This theory has been revitalized by several observations. Tumor-specific antigens on the surface of cancer cells from experimental animals and man have been observed on careful analysis. Furthermore, an increased frequency of neoplastic diseases, including lymphoma and leukemia, have been observed in patients with immune deficiencies. The occurrence of neoplasia in host or transplanted tissues in subjects given long-term immunosuppression therapy and the regression of tumors after the cessation of immunosuppressive drugs have further strengthened the important relationship between immune mechanisms and oncogenesis in man. Indeed, tissue transplantation is an iatrogenic provocation to a system which may have evolved to prevent the proliferation of mutant autologous neoplastic cellular transformations. In addition, recent studies have identified antibodies in human cancer patients which are capable of preventing the inhibitory effect of the patient's own lymphocytes on the patient's tumor cells in vitro. Other provocative observations can be cited to support the current investigative interest in the role of immune factors in oncogenesis.

Presumably the proliferation of leukemic cells is not related to an immunologic deficiency of the host as a general phenomenon; however, this does not negate the possible importance of immunologic factors in terms of either contributing to etiology or acting as an adjuvant in control of the disease. An important interrelationship may exist between the ability of the immunocyte population to inhibit or reject a neoplastic clone. The kinetics of proliferation of both competing populations, immunocytic and neoplastic, may determine the hegemony of one or the other. This may relate to the ability to maintain extended remissions without therapy in some patients with acute leukemia in whom a marked reduction in leukemic cells is induced with chemotherapy. Since it is highly improbable that current therapy can reduce the population of leukemic stem or blast cells to near zero, the contribution of other factors must be considered. Immune surveillance clearly merits further study in this regard, as does the antigenic character of leukemic cells. It is unlikely that immune manipulations alone can deal with a large neoplastic cell body burden; however, the adjuvant role of immunity remains an important possibility. Not inconsequential is the possible deleterious effect of chemotherapy on the proliferative response of immunocytes. This may be particularly true during certain periods when inhibition of immune responsiveness may be most detrimental to the host's ability to participate in controlling residual neoplastic cells. Currently, both active and passive immunotherapy is being evaluated as to its role in cytocidal therapy.

ANTIVIRAL THERAPY

If, as is currently hypothesized, the essential alteration in acute leukemia involves the incorporation or activation of viral nucleic acid in the hematopoietic stem cell, chemotherapeutic or immunologic therapy directed against viral particles may be envisaged. The kinetics of viral replication and the control of such factors may be an entirely new horizon in the future of therapy of acute leukemia.

Disease prevention is a goal preferable to cure and may be more readily attainable, as it has been in other viral diseases for which preventive therapy by vaccination is highly effective whereas treatment of established disease remains unsuccessful (e.g., poliomyelitis, measles). It should be emphasized that leukemia does not appear to behave like other infectious viral diseases in terms of person-to-person (horizontal) spread. However, the addition of bovine and feline leukemia to that of avian and murine, as having a viral causation, has rekindled interest in animal-to-human transmission. The ability to grow feline leukemia virus in human cells in culture is very provocative in this regard. Interacting factors are probably involved to complete the neoplastic transformation. Hence, viral infestation may be an "initiating" event which is inadequate to produce disease unless a "promoting" factor is superimposed, such as exposure to radiation. Identification of promoting agents, particularly if they are potentially controllable environmental factors, may also allow preventive measures to be taken. These concepts are discussed more fully in Chapter 20.

In summary, the kinetic pattern of normal and leukemic immature and mature granulocytes and the cell mitotic cycle and self-renewing, multiplicative and maturational compartments in granulocytopoiesis have been described. Comparisons of normal and leukemic granulocytopoiesis have been drawn and recent conceptualizations of leukemic hematopoiesis have been reviewed.

The importance of animal models in understanding the relationship of cell kinetic patterns to chemotherapy has been noted. The deviation from animal models of human leukemic cell production rates and the response of human leukemic cell populations to chemotherapy have been noted. The more recent studies of human leukemic blast cell kinetics and the potential importance of these kinetic patterns to chemotherapy have been reviewed. The cell mitotic cycle, cell production rate, fraction of population dividing, and cell death rate were reviewed, as they may relate to a better understanding of current therapy and to approaches to future therapy. Because of the theoretical as well as practical difficulties in dealing with the complex behavior of cell populations in human leukemia, the success of new approaches cannot be predicted and must be tested by clinical trials in a controlled manner to be certain of their usefulness. The definite recent gains in chemotherapy of acute leukemia as a result of new drugs and regimens support the importance of further studies for improved chemotherapy while searches for preventive or curative modalities are being made.

ACKNOWLEDGMENT

The illustrations for this chapter were prepared by Linda Billingham, to whom the author expresses his appreciation.

REFERENCES

Athens, J. W.   Granulocyte kinetics in health and disease. *Nat. Cancer Inst. Monogr.* 30:135, 1969.

Boggs, D. R.   The kinetics of neutrophilic leukocytes in health and disease. *Seminars Hemat.* 4:359, 1967.

Clarkson, B. D.   Review of recent studies of cellular proliferation in acute leukemia. *Nat. Cancer Inst. Monogr.* 30:81, 1969.

Cronkite, E. P.   Kinetics of granulocytopoiesis. *Nat. Cancer Inst. Monogr.* 30:51, 1969.

Frei, E., III, and Freireich, E. J.   Progress and perspectives in the chemotherapy of acute leukemia. *Advances Chemother.* 2:269, 1965.

Gavosto, F., Pileri, A., Gabutte, V., and Masera, P.   Non-self-maintaining kinetics of proliferating blasts in human acute leukaemia. *Nature* (London) 216:188, 1967.

Henderson, E. S.   Treatment of acute leukemia. *Seminars Hemat.* 6:271, 1969.

Killmann, S. A.   Acute leukemia: The kinetics of leukemic blast cells in man. *Series Haemat.* 1:38, 1968.

Killmann, S. A.   A Hypothesis Concerning the Relationship Between Normal and Leukemic Hematopoiesis in Acute Myeloid Leukemia. In F. Stohlman, Jr. (Ed.), *Hematopoietic Cellular Proliferation.* New York: Grune & Stratton, 1970.

Lichtman, M. A.   Cellular deformability during maturation of the myloblast: Possible role in marrow egress. *New Eng. J. Med.* 283:943, 1970.

Lichtman, M. A., and Weed, R. I.   Surface characteristics of human immature and mature granulocytes: Relationship to granulocyte function. *Blood* 34:825, 1969.

Mauer, A. M., Lampkin, B. C., and Nagao, T.   Prospects for New Direction in Therapy of Acute Lymphoblastic Leukemia. In F. Stohlman, Jr. (Ed.), *Hematopoietic Cellular Proliferation.* New York: Grune & Stratton, 1970.

Skipper, H. E.   Cellular Kinetics Associated with "Curability" of Experimental Leukemias. In W. Dameshek and R. M. Dutcher (Eds.), *Perspectives in Leukemia.* New York: Grune & Stratton, 1968.

Southam, C. M.   Immunotherapy of Leukemia: Theoretical and Experimental. In W. Dameshek and R. M. Dutcher (Eds.), *Perspectives in Leukemia.* New York: Grune & Stratton, 1968.

20. THE ETIOLOGY OF LEUKEMIA

Arnold I. Meisler

THE CAUSE of leukemia is unknown and a review of the subject must, therefore, be highly speculative. On the other hand, sufficient laboratory, clinical, and epidemiologic evidence has accumulated to permit a plausible, unifying theory. Such a formulation can be useful not only as a summary of what is known about leukemogenesis, but also in indicating directions for future investigation. This review is not meant to be exhaustive, in part due to the exigency of space, but also because material was excluded that seemed unclear, ambiguous, or poorly documented. A further qualification is that chronic lymphocytic leukemia is not considered, since it is thought by some that this disorder does not represent a leukemic state.

I hope in this brief survey to develop the concept that human leukemia has a multifactorial basis. There may, however, be a final common path which involves the interplay of a virus and an abnormal host genome. The latter renders the cell susceptible to leukemic transformation by a virus which, under most circumstances, is a harmless, ubiquitous passenger. This hypothesis is developed in the light of recent information defining individuals who appear to be highly susceptible to the development of leukemia and of observation on the prevalence of viral particles in tumor tissue.

CYTOGENETIC ABNORMALITIES

On epidemiologic grounds, Miller has identified five classes of individuals whose probability of developing leukemia is greater than 1 in 100. Common to all but one of these groups is the presence of cytogenetic abnormali-

The author is a scholar of the Leukemia Society of America.
Supported by Grant P-496 from the American Cancer Society.

ties of an inherited or acquired nature. These groups are summarized in Table 20-1.

Groups 2 and 4 in the table include individuals with acquired karyotypic abnormalities in whom chromosomal breakage and rearrangements have occurred secondary to radiation. It should be noted that chemical agents such as benzene are known to be leukemogenic and to produce chromosomal alterations. The magnitude of risk is unknown at present because of the lack of access to a large enough group of individuals heavily exposed to the solvent. More recently, chromosomal rearrangement and breakage with subsequent leukemia have been described in chloramphenicol toxicity. Among other acquired disorders showing these chromosomal aberrations and leukemia, cases of pernicious anemia and sideroblastic anemia have been documented. The pertinent references are included in a recent review by Fraumeni.

Bloom's syndrome, the third entity in Table 20-1, has recently been reviewed in detail by German. It is characterized by photosensitive telangiectasia of the face, stunted growth, and an unusual propensity to develop acute leukemia; it is transmitted by an autosomal recessive gene. Culture of the patient's skin in vitro reveals chromosomal breakage and rearrangement. Similar karyotypic abnormalities have been noted in cases of Fanconi's anemia and ataxia telangiectasia, heritable conditions which appear to predispose to leukemia.

Down's syndrome in which G trisomy occurs, the fifth group in Table 20-1, is the prototype for congenital aneuploidy predisposing to leukemia. There have also been a significant number of case reports suggesting that Klinefelter's syndrome, in which there is an XXY sex chromosome complement, also may predispose to leukemia. Evidence for the latter relationship is still not conclusive. The rare D trisomy has been described with leukemia in two instances despite the short life-span of infants with the syndrome.

According to Miller's data, the child whose identical twin has previously developed leukemia faces the greatest risk of developing the disease. It is still not clear whether this risk extends beyond 7 years of age. Miller is attempting to clarify this point by classifying the 15,500 male twins who served in the U.S. Army during World War II in terms of probable zygosity and coincidence rates for leukemia.

One may reasonably ask whether the karyotypic abnormality is indeed necessary for the development of leukemia. Surely the affected twins, and for that matter all other previously normal individuals who develop leukemia, do not all belong to one of the categories in the table. This is certainly not the inference intended. On the other hand, no information is available concerning the karyotype of these individuals immediately prior to the time that they became ill. It is possible that some sort of noxious environmental exposure could produce chromosomal abnormalities which are necessary to

Table 20-1. Groups Having Exceptionally High Risk of Leukemia

Group	Approximate Risk	Time Interval	References
1. Identical twins whose co-twins are leukemic	1 in 5 [a]	Weeks or months	MacMahon & Levy (1964)
2. Radiation-treated patients with polycythemia vera	1 in 6	10–15 years	Modan & Lilienfeld (1965)
3. Bloom's syndrome patients	1 in 8 [b]	Within 30 years	Sawitsky et al. (1966)
4. Hiroshima survivors who were within 1000 meters of the hypocenter	1 in 60	Within 12 years	Brill et al. (1962)
5. Down's syndrome patients	1 in 95	Within 10 years	Barber & Spiers (1964)
6. Radiation-treated patients with ankylosing spondylitis	1 in 270	Within 15 years	Court-Brown & Doll (1965)
7. Sibs of leukemic children	1 in 720	Within 10 years	Miller (1963) Stewart (1961)
8. U.S. Caucasian children < 15 years of age	1 in 2880	Within 15 years	U.S. Vital Statistics (1964)

[a] Of 11 identical twin pairs with leukemia, the co-twin was affected in 5 instances.
[b] Three leukemics among 23 persons with Bloom's syndrome.
SOURCE: Modified from R. W. Miller, *Cancer Res.* 27:2420, 1967.

initiate the events that culminate in clinical leukemia. Since the unaffected twin whose sibling developed leukemia is so highly at risk, he would be a likely individual to follow with serial karyotyping to determine whether an abnormality develops prior to the onset of the leukemic state.

A discussion of chromosomal abnormalities preceding or predisposing to leukemia would not be complete without mentioning chronic myelogenous leukemia (CML). This problem is discussed in Chapter 27, but a position can be stated. It is now well established that roughly 85% of cases of CML have an abnormal small chromosome 21, designated the Philadelphia chromosome, Ph[1]. The chromosome is present in erythroid precursors and megakaryocytes, but not in lymphocytes stimulated to divide by phytohemagglutinin. In a recent review Zuelzer and Cox proposed, I believe correctly, that since this chromosome has been identified in the blood of individuals prior to the development of CML, it cannot be regarded as a "secondary stigma of neoplastic cells." They feel that it must somehow be causally related to chronic granulocytic leukemia. With this I cannot entirely agree.

For example, though we know that there is a high incidence of leukemia in Down's syndrome, not all patients with Down's syndrome develop leukemia. In a like manner it is known that ionizing radiation and viruses can produce entirely similar chromosomal defects, yet there is no evidence that all these individuals develop leukemia. It may be, then, that although a chromosomal abnormality is a necessary precursor to the disease, it is not sufficient. Furthermore, it is not entirely clear that CML can truly be called leukemia. There is obviously an abnormality in cell proliferation, but this is not adequate to make a diagnosis of leukemia unless we define it as such. Herein lies the great conundrum of malignant disease. What is it? How can it be defined? There is no real reason, perforce, that CML must be classified as a malignant disease. It kills the patient by virtue of its becoming acute leukemia, and thus it could actually be placed at the head of Miller's classification of predisposing causes, i.e., the risk of developing leukemia is 100% in those who show the Philadelphia chromosome. By the objective criteria of malignancy, once these have been discovered it may be that the conversion to a truly leukemic cell occurs before morphologic evidence is apparent.

With regard to radiation-induced leukemia, it is apparent that the type of myeloproliferative or lymphoproliferative lesion induced by radiation varies, depending on the age of the populations exposed and the condition of irradiation with respect to the total dosage, the dose rate, and the distribution of radiation within the tissues of the body. The types of neoplasm associated with irradiation before birth and during infancy are acute leukemias indistinguishable from those prevalent in the general population during childhood and, as might be expected, acute lymphocytic leukemia predominates. Similarly, irradiation of adults is predominantly associated with myeloid leukemia, acute as well as chronic. This has been reviewed by Upton. He has also shown that the incidence of leukemia induced by irradiation at any given age "approximates a constant multiple of the natural incidence at the particular age in question, rather than a constant number of additional cases." It appears that the developing fetus is uniquely susceptible to radiation exposure. Upton estimates that the incidence of leukemia in childhood is increased roughly 40% by a dose of less than 5 rads received in utero.

Thus far I believe that an association between increased susceptibility to leukemia and chromosomal anomalies has been shown. Furthermore, it seems clear that radiation, which characteristically produces chromosome breakage and rearrangement, may induce leukemia which conforms in every way to spontaneously occurring leukemia with regard to age distribution, type, and course. Of great relevance are the experiments by Todaro et al. They have shown that skin fibroblasts grown in tissue culture from patients predisposed to the development of leukemia, as in Down's syndrome, have a five- to fiftyfold increased susceptibility to transformation by the oncogenic virus SV_{40}. In the parlance of workers in the field of tumor viruses, transformation means that the cell has acquired certain properties such that, when injected into the host of origin, it will form a tumor. Of interest is the fact that cells from infants showing the rare E trisomy, a condition which results in death shortly after birth, are also highly susceptible to transformation by SV_{40}. We take this to mean that if the infants were to live long enough, a relatively large proportion would develop leukemia. As expected, cells irradiated in vitro also show an increased susceptibility to transformation.

VIRUS AS A CAUSAL AGENT

The possibility of leukemia's being an infectious disease must be considered. I mean this in the sense that infection is tantamount to overt clinical disease as, for example, a nonimmune individual given an intravenous injection of poliovirus would almost always develop some manifestation of the disease. In general, there is no excess of leukemia in individuals having the closest contact with the disease—married partners, children born of women afflicted with the disease during pregnancy, and physicians treating the disease. In mice it is known that leukemia can be transmitted to their young by viruses present in breast milk. In data on breast-feeding collected from 541 leukemic children under 15 years of age, compared with those from 486 neighborhood control children, there was no significant difference in the frequency or duration of breast-feeding.

With regard to blood transfusion, a study was done on 500 leukemic children as compared to neighborhood controls to see if a greater proportion of the leukemic children had received exchange transfusions for blood type in compatibility in the newborn period. There was no significant difference. A study was conducted by Hempelmann and associates in which they traced the records of blood donors in 12 counties in upstate New York. They determined which of these donors subsequently developed leukemia and then located the recipients of this blood and found no increased incidence of leukemia in the recipients. We may conclude then that if a viral agent can be implicated in leukemogenesis, there must be a wide variation in susceptibility to the agent, and infection with the agent is not sufficient to produce the disease.

To this date a wide variety of malignant animal tumors have nevertheless been identified as being caused by viruses. The animals include horses, cattle, dogs, chickens, cats, ducks, guinea fowl, turkeys, rabbits, foxes, deer, gray squirrels, woodchucks, and pheasants. In material obtained from human tumors, examination under the electron microscope revealed particles that are indistinguishable from the C-type RNA viruses first demonstrated to be oncogenic in chickens by Ellerman and Bang, and by Rous about 60 years ago, and in mice by Gross in 1951. While the complete infectious form of the virus is rarely observed under natural conditions, in certain inbred mouse strains with high leukemia incidence, such as AKR and C58, and some lines of chickens, overt virus is commonly observed and is demonstrable even prior to birth. A summary of the pertinent literature is beyond the scope of this review, and so only a few of the most relevant observations can be cited. Whether or not these particles are of etiologic importance in the causation of leukemia or are merely harmless passengers in these cells, which are somehow more suitable hosts by virtue of their being tumor cells, is a moot question. A truly definitive proof would involve satisfying the requirements of Koch's postulates. In human tumor these rigid requirements may be impossible to fulfill because of ethical considerations. In tissue culture there are enormous technical problems having to do with host cell selection and induction of the virus genome from a state, presumably integrated into host cell DNA, to a vegetative or permissive state in which new particles are synthesized. Moreover, to compound the difficulty, there is no compelling reason to believe that the virus must persist once malignant transformation has occurred. In such a case retrospective study for viral recovery would be valueless. Suffice it to say, in these systems only positive results are meaningful. Koch's postulates have been fulfilled in tissue culture, however, in the cases of the Rous sarcoma virus and the papovavirus SV_{40}.

One of the most promising leads thus far implicating viruses in leukemogenesis is the by now well known Burkitt's lymphoma which occurs in certain regions of equatorial Africa, most commonly in children between the ages of 5 and 12. The distribution of the disease in areas where the climate favors the breeding of mosquitoes has led to the suggestion that the disease may be carried by an arthropod vector. Of great interest is the fact that the Epstein-Barr (EB) virus, a herpes-type agent, is apparently present in cells from the Burkitt's lymphoma patients, as well as from cells of patients with infectious mononucleosis. Furthermore, serum from patients with either disease will react in some cases with membrane antigen of cells from the other disease. Thus infectious mononucleosis cells will react with Burkitt's serum and vice versa. If the Burkitt's lymphoma story is substantiated, we will have an example in human beings of the phenomenon well known in animal cells in culture of a virus causing cytocidal infection in the cells of one individual and malignant transformation in the cells of another. What determines the outcome of an infection is at present unknown. The presence or absence of the membrane antigen is of no predictive value since in polyoma virus infection in vitro, membrane antigens appear on the surface of the cell whether malignant transformation or lytic infection is produced.

I believe the evidence is overwhelming that a virus is implicated as a cause of leukemia. The animal models so widespread in nature make it impossible to believe that man is somehow an exception. The important question now is not whether a virus causes leukemia, but rather what is the mechanism of malignant transformation, and what determines whether a cell will be transformed or lysed by a given virus? A recent discovery of enormous importance is Temin's finding that the RNA tumor viruses contain an enzyme which permits the transcription of the viral RNA genome into complementary DNA. This provides a mechanism by which the viral genetic information can be integrated into host cell DNA. In this latent form, the virus may cause cell transformation without the production of mature virus.

INTERACTIONS RESULTING IN CELL TRANSFORMATION

It is clear that chromosomal breakage and aneuploidy in some instances predispose to leukemia. On the basis of Todaro's experiments mentioned earlier, certain types of cells with an abnormal karyotype appear to be very much more susceptible than normal cells to transformation by oncogenic viruses. The activation of a latent leukemogenic virus and induction of lymphoma in C57BL mice by radiation is well documented. Leukemogenic activity of cell-free filtrates from lymphomas induced by radiation in C57BL mice (a strain that ordinarily shows a low incidence of leukemia) has been shown. In a similar manner, induction of lymphomas in C57BL mice by methylcholanthrene, urethan, or diethylnitrosamine was accompanied by the development of murine leukemia viral antigens in most of the tumors significantly before the lymphomas appeared. Inoculation of cell-free filtrates of these chemically induced lymphomas was able to produce tumors in newborn mice.

In the experiments mentioned, it seems clear that a leukemia-producing virus resided in the mouse cells and could be activated by radiation or chemical carcinogens, agents known to produce abnormalities of the karyotype. This suggests that in those areas with a high incidence of Burkitt's lymphoma, it might be useful to determine the incidence of karyotypic abnormalities among unselected children. A prospective study might reveal not only an increased incidence of chromosomal abnormalities, but also an increased incidence of the disease in children carrying chromosomal abnormalities. At the same time, an increased incidence of infectious mononucleosis may also be found.

It should be emphasized, however, that the karyotypic abnormalities we are concerned with are not the gross changes seen in the overtly cancerous cell, nor may they even be as distinct as some of those present in the diseases discussed earlier. It is, in fact, quite conceivable that the defects in the genome are beyond our present limits of detection. Karyotyping is, after all, even in the best hands a very gross procedure. Again we must concede therefore that only a positive finding, i.e., a microscopically visible abnormality in the chromosomes, can have meaning.

Recently Huebner and Todaro proposed a somewhat similar hypothesis. They believe that sufficient evidence is at hand to state that most or all vertebrate species have C-type RNA virus genomes incorporated into the cellular DNA which permits them to be passed in a vertical manner from parent to offspring.

Depending on the host genotype and various modifying environmental factors, either virus production or tumor formation or both may develop at some time in these animals or in their cells grown in culture. This hypothesis implies that the occurrence of most cancer is a natural biological event determined by spontaneous or induced derepression of the endogenous specific viral oncogne(s). Viewed in this way, ultimate control of cancer will, therefore, very likely depend on delineation of the factors responsible for derepression of virus expression and of the nature of the repression involved.

In addition, the inadequacy of present cancer chemotherapy attests to the fact that the cure of cancer cannot be achieved until the factors that distinguish the malignant cell from the normal are delineated.

REFERENCES

Dameshek, W. Chronic lymphocytic leukemia: An accumulative disease of immunologically incompetent lymphocytes. *Blood* 29:566, 1967.

Fraumeni, J. F.   Clinical epidemiology of leukemia. *Seminars Hemat.* 6:250, 1969.

German, J.   Bloom's syndrome: I. Genetic and clinical observations in the first twenty-seven patients. *Amer. J. Hum. Genet.* 21:196, 1969.

Huebner, R. J., and Todaro, G. J.   Oncogenes of RNA tumor viruses as determinants of cancer. *Proc. Nat. Acad. Sci. U.S.A.* 64:1087, 1969.

Igel, H. J., Huebner, R. J., Turner, H. C., Kotin, P., and Falk, H. L.   Mouse leukemia virus activation by chemical carcinogens. *Science* 166:1624, 1969.

Lieberman, M., and Kaplan, H.   Leukemogenic activity of filtrates from radiation induced lymphoid tumors of mice. *Science* 130:387, 1959.

Miller, R. W.   Persons with exceptionally high risk of leukemia. *Cancer Res.* 27:2420, 1967.

Moorehead, P. S., and Saksela, E.   The non-random chromosomal aberrations in SV_{40} transformed human cells. *J. Cell. Comp. Physiol.* 62:57, 1963.

Nowell, P. C., and Hungerford, D. A.   Chromosome changes in human leukemia and a tentative assessment of their significance. *Ann. N.Y. Acad. Sci.* 113:654, 1964.

Temin, H. M., and Mizutani, S.   RNA-dependent DNA polymerase in virions of Rous sarcoma virus. *Nature* (London) 226:1211, 1970.

Todaro, G. J., Green, H., and Swift, M. R.   Susceptibility of human diploid fibroblast strains to transformation by SV_{40} virus. *Science* 153:1252, 1966.

Upton, A. C.   The Role of Radiation in the Etiology of Leukemia. In C. J. D. Zarafonetis (Ed.), *Proceedings of the International Conference on Leukemia-Lymphoma.* Philadelphia: Lea & Febiger, 1968.

Zuelzer, W. W. and Cox, D. E.   Genetic aspects of leukemia. *Seminars Hemat.* 6:228, 1969.

21. CONTRIBUTIONS OF CYTOGENETICS TO HEMATOLOGY

Kong-oo Goh
Robert S. Heusinkveld

ADEQUATE VISUALIZATION of the human chromosome became possible during the late 1950s and gave rise to the science of human cytogenetics. This new science, consisting primarily of the study of human chromosome morphology and number, has contributed profoundly to our understanding of some human diseases, but early hopes that it would reveal the causes of neoplasia have thus far been frustrated. Nevertheless cytogenetics has provided intriguing and occasionally clinically useful insight into the biology of some hematologic diseases, and it is the purpose of this chapter to highlight some of the major contributions of cytogenetics to clinical hematology.

DEFINITIONS

chromosome   A discrete gene-carrying nuclear structure which appears during mitosis and transmits genetic information to daughter cells.
centromere   The small portion of a normal chromosome which does not take up stains used to identify chromosomes. The position of the centromere in relation to the whole chromosome is one of the characteristics used to identify individual chromosomes and to classify them into groups.
chromatid   One of the two identical parts of each metaphase chromo-

Part of this work was done by Dr. Goh while he was associated with Oak Ridge Associated Universities, Oak Ridge, Tenn., under direct contract with the U.S. Atomic Energy Commission. Dr. Heusinkveld's contribution was supported by U.S. Public Health Service Grant AM-01004.

some. During telophase the chromatids separate, one going to each daughter cell. Each chromatid has two arms which join at the centromere.

acrocentric chromosome A chromosome with a very short arm; sometimes called a *telocentric chromosome.*

diploid (2n) The number of chromosomes in a zygote or in a somatic cell. The normal human diploid chromosomal number is 46.

aneuploid An abnormal number of chromosomes—either more (hyperdiploid) or less (hypodiploid) than the diploid number.

pseudodiploid A metaphase cell containing a normal total number of chromosomes but having an abnormal number or distribution of chromosomes.

polyploid The number of chromosomes is equal to a multiple of the normal haploid chromosomal number.

karyotype A display of photographed chromosomes prepared by pairing and grouping chromosomes cut out from photographs of a cell at metaphase. In man the paired chromosomes are segregated into groups labeled alphabetically from A to G, plus the pair of sex chromosomes; or, using a different convention, are numbered according to size from 1 to 22 (largest to smallest) plus the pair of sex chromosomes.

ACUTE LEUKEMIAS

A great variety of abnormal karyotypes have been found among leukocytes obtained from patients with acute leukemias. No specific abnormality appears to be associated with acute leukemias, and neither the development of abnormality nor its degree is related to prognosis. Therefore cytogenetic analysis is not of great clinical value in the diagnosis and management of the acute leukemias.

CHRONIC MYELOCYTIC LEUKEMIA

In 1960 Nowell and Hungerford found a small abnormal chromosome in metaphases from the immature peripheral granulocytes of patients with chronic myelocytic leukemia (CML) (Fig. 21-1). This chromosome, characteristic of CML, was named the Philadelphia chromosome (Ph[1]) after the city where it was first described. CML is the only hematologic disorder characterized by the presence of a specific marker chromosome.

The Philadelphia chromosome is not an extra chromosome. It replaces a normal G chromosome and is thought to arise from a simple deletion, or

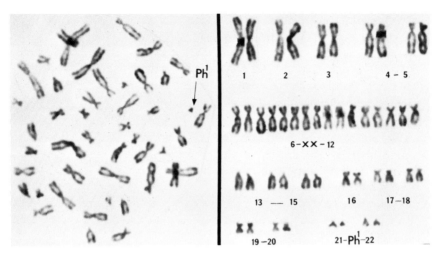

Figure 21-1. Metaphase and karyotype of a cell with a Philadelphia (Ph¹) chromosome from a woman with chronic myelocytic leukemia.

deletion with translocation of the deleted long arm, of a G chromosome. The Ph¹ is found in all typical cases of CML and is probably specific for this disease. The Ph¹ has occasionally been described in patients with myeloproliferative diseases other than CML, but even these few cases could be considered as part of the clinical spectrum of CML.

In several series the Ph¹ has not been found in about 10% of patients carrying the clinical diagnosis of CML. However, comparison of the Ph¹-positive and Ph¹-negative patients with CML revealed distinct differences between the two groups. The Ph¹-negative group was in either extreme end of the age group, responded less well to alkylating agents, and had a distinctly poorer prognosis. In particular, among the Ph¹-negative patients busulfan did not produce the complete remissions so characteristic of early uncomplicated Ph¹-positive CML. The clinical differences between the Ph¹-positive and Ph¹-negative CML are so clear-cut that they should be regarded as different diseases. We believe that Ph¹-negative CML is more accurately regarded as being a variant of acute myelogenous leukemia.

The greatest contribution of cytogenetic analysis to clinical hematology is its ability to distinguish CML from other myeloproliferative disorders such as myeloid metaplasia and, as discussed above, acute myelogenous leukemia. In addition, CML may be accompanied by such intense eosinophilia that confusion with an eosinophilia syndrome or acute eosinophilic leukemia may occur. Occasionally patients with CML may not be seen until after the onset of the "terminal transition" when the diagnosis may be obscured either by myelofibrosis or by large numbers of blasts, mimicking acute leukemia.

The practical consequences of separating Ph¹-positive CML from other hemopathies are not negligible. For example, splenectomy may benefit patients with myeloid metaplasia complicated by hypersplenism but is rarely indicated for patients with CML. Cytogenetic differentiation of acute leukemia from CML may help guide therapy, for patients with acute leukemia do not respond to busulfan. Instead, their anemia and thrombocytopenia may be aggravated by busulfan. Ph¹-positive CML with eosinophilia does not differ from CML without eosinophilia, and it may be expected to respond initially to busulfan. Acute eosinophilic leukemia behaves like acute myelogenous leukemia and is most resistant to therapy. The blastic phase of CML is usually refractory to chemotherapy, and careful consideration should be given before undertaking aggressive treatment in the hope of inducing a remission—a potential disservice which might occur should the blastic phase of CML be confused with acute myelogenous leukemia. In our opinion, the Ph¹ should be sought whenever a diagnosis of CML is equivocal and when CML enters the differential diagnosis of what appears to be some other myeloproliferative disorder. The specificity of the relation between CML and the Ph¹ has made cytogenetic analysis of considerable diagnostic value in differentiating CML from other myeloproliferative diseases.

Some insight concerning the etiology of CML has been gained as a result of the presence of its "marker chromosome." Twin studies indicate that the Ph¹ is usually an acquired postzygotic anomaly, for when one member of a set of monozygotic twins develops CML, the Ph¹ is found only in the cells of the affected twin. In only one instance has the Ph¹ been identified in both members of a set of identical twins. These facts suggest that the pathogenesis of CML does not usually involve a genetic predisposition and that environmental factors may be more important. Acute leukemia differs from CML in that if one twin develops leukemia, the risk of leukemia in the second twin is distinctly increased.

Chromosome analysis of direct bone marrow preparations from patients with CML shows that almost all metaphase cells are Ph¹-positive, even metaphases of polyploid cells (megakaryocytes) and hemoglobin-containing cells. These observations establish that all the myeloid elements of the marrow, erythroid and megakaryocytic as well as granulocytic, are abnormal in CML. Furthermore, the absence of normal metaphases suggests that in CML the entire normal myeloid apparatus is replaced (or possibly transformed) by abnormal cells. Most remarkable is the observation that even during complete peripheral and marrow remission, *virtually all bone marrow metaphases contain the Ph¹*. How these abnormal cells can be induced to behave normally for long periods of time is an intriguing mystery. The Ph¹ is uniformly present during the blastic phase of CML,

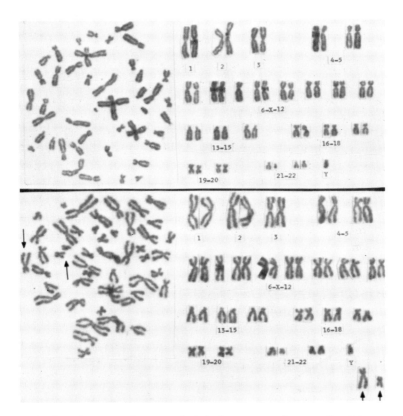

Figure 21-2. Two metaphases and their karyotypes from a direct bone marrow preparation of a man with acute blastic crisis of chronic myelocytic leukemia. A Ph[1] chromosome is seen in the upper karyotype. In addition to the Ph[1] chromosome, there are two additional chromosomes (*arrows*) in the bottom karyotype.

often accompanied by additional abnormalities (Fig. 21-2). Blastic crises may or may not be heralded by the appearance of aneuploid cells, but when aneuploidy does appear during the course of CML, the terminal transformation generally occurs shortly thereafter.

Before leaving the subject of CML, it is important to note several considerations essential to the correct interpretation of cytogenetic studies of CML. First of all, only immature granulocytes undergo mitosis; thus the blood of patients with CML in remission contains lymphocytes that do not have the Ph[1] chromosome. Furthermore, in many studies phytohemagglutinin (PHA) has been added to peripheral blood and marrow cultures. This substance stimulates lymphocytes to undergo mitosis after a lag period of 48 to 72 hours. Therefore cultures containing PHA and terminated at 72 hours may contain a large proportion of mitotic lymphocytes. Failure to appreciate these facts has led to erroneous interpretations of the data from some of the early cytogenetic investigations of CML.

POLYCYTHEMIA VERA

No consistent chromosomal abnormality has been found in polycythemia vera (PV). An increased incidence of cells with aneuploidy, polyploidy, and chromosomal breaks has been demonstrated in some patients; however, these may have been the result of therapy. The only practical application of cytogenetics to polycythemia vera is to assist in identifying the occasional patient with CML who presents with polycythemia, thrombocytosis, and only moderate granulocytosis.

AGNOGENIC MYELOID METAPLASIA

By conventional criteria, agnogenic myeloid metaplasia (AMM) and CML may resemble each other. When ambiguity exists, cytogenetic analysis will differentiate them. Only 1 well-documented case of Ph[1]-positive AMM has been reported, and the investigators who reported it believed that the patient had both AMM and CML simultaneously. Possibly the case represented typical AMM which evolved into CML. An alternate explanation is that the Ph[1]-like chromosome observed was not a true Ph[1].

EOSINOPHILIC LEUKEMIA

Cytogenetic studies have been reported from 14 patients with eosinophilia bearing a diagnosis of either eosinophilic leukemia or "hypereosinophilic syndrome." The Ph[1] was present in 5 of the 14. It is difficult to analyze these reports because either the clinical data or the chromosomal analyses are incomplete. As some degree of eosinophilia is almost always present in CML, it is possible that cases of "eosinophilic leukemia" with a Ph[1] are in fact CML.

We have studied 2 patients thought to have eosinophilic leukemia and did not find any Ph[1] chromosomes in any of the 73 metaphases analyzed. In 1 patient we found 10% abnormal metaphases in the cultured peripheral leukocytes, and in another patient, 20% abnormal metaphases from the direct bone marrow preparation. A very large acrocentric chromosome, a type of abnormal chromosome occasionally found in patients with various types of cancer or leukemia, was found in metaphases from both patients. It is our opinion that eosinophilic leukemia exists as a distinct entity and that "Ph¹-positive eosinophilic leukemia" is simply CML with prominent eosinophilic hyperplasia. Our opinion is based on the absence of the Ph¹ in many patients with an eosinophilic leukemia and the finding of a different abnormal chromosome in the 2 cases we have had an opportunity to study.

CHRONIC LYMPHOCYTIC LEUKEMIA

In 1962 Gunz and his associates reported finding an abnormal chromosome among the relatives of 2 patients who had chronic lymphocytic leukemia (CLL) and in a patient with CLL whose brother had died of the same disease. The abnormal chromosome appeared to belong to group G (21–22), and the authors called it a Ch¹ or Christchurch chromosome, after their native city. They suggested that individuals carrying this chromosome might be predisposed to CLL. This hypothesis has not been confirmed. No Ch¹ chromosomes have been reported in other cases of familial CLL, outside of Christchurch, and Ch¹ chromosomes have been found in patients who did not have CLL.

Several investigators have reported normal chromosomal patterns in CLL, based on the analysis of very few metaphases per patient. We have studied 6 patients with CLL in different clinical stages. Of 236 karyotyped metaphases, 40% were pseudodiploid. Pseudodiploid metaphases were found in all patients but in varying proportions (20 to 80%), depending on the clinical stage of the disease. The highest percentage was present before treatment when the white count was rising. The lowest percentage was present after treatment when the white count had been reduced to normal. Forty-three morphologically abnormal chromosomes were found among these pseudodiploid karyotypes.

The disparity between our experience and that of most others is not readily explicable. The total number of metaphases reported to be normal by others is impressive, but the number of metaphases analyzed per patient has been small. Hauschka has suggested that pseudodiploid metaphases may simulate normal chromosome patterns and that painstaking analysis of apparently normal diploid cell populations is required to distinguish pseudodiploid from normal metaphases. In other words, a threshold exists which determines the degree of variation necessary for a chromosome to be classified as "abnormal," and this threshold is not the same for all investigators. To check our threshold, we examine 104 karyotypes from 4 patients with diseases other than CLL and found that only 2.9% were pseudodiploid.

CONGENITAL DISEASES ASSOCIATED WITH LEUKEMIA

Bloom's syndrome, Fanconi's anemia, constitutional aplastic anemia, and xeroderma pigmentosum are all congenital diseases frequently complicated by the development of acute leukemia. Karyotypes from nonleukemia patients with each of these diseases are characterized by a high frequency of chromosome breaks. Although there is no proof that chromosome breakage causes malignant transformation, the finding of a tendency to such breakage and rearrangement years before the onset of leukemia suggests that these two phenomena are related. The mechanism of chromosome breakage in these diseases is unknown. It has been suggested that an equilibrium may exist between chromosome breakage and chromosome repair. In xeroderma pigmentosum there is good evidence that DNA repair is defective. Thus, cytogenetic analysis supports the impression that leukemias may somehow be associated with fundamental perturbations of chromosome structure and function but has failed to reveal the nature of this association.

REFERENCES

Baikie, A. G., Court-Brown, W. M., Buckton, K. E., Harnden, D. G., Jacobs, P. A., and Tough, I. M.   A possible specific chromosome abnormality in human chronic myeloid leukaemia. *Nature* (London) 188:1165, 1960.

Bauke, J.   Chronic myelocytic leukemia: Chromosome studies of a patient and his non-leukemic identical twin. *Cancer* 24:643, 1969.

Bentley, H. P., Reardon, A. E., Knoedler, J. P., and Krivit, W.   Eosinophilic leukemia: Report of a case, with review and classification. *Amer. J. Med.* 30:310, 1961.

Forrester, R. H., and Louro, J. M.   Philadelphia chromosome abnormality in agnogenic myeloid metaplasia. *Ann. Intern. Med.* 64:622, 1966.

Goh, K. O.   Cytogenetic studies in blastic crisis of chronic myelocytic leukemia. *Arch. Intern. Med.* (Chicago) 120:315, 1967.

Goh, K. O.   Large abnormal acrocentric chromosome associated with human malignancies: Possible mechanism of establishing clone of cells. *Arch. Intern. Med.* (Chicago) 122:241, 1968.

Goh, K. O., and Swisher, S. N.   Specificity of the Philadelphia chromosome: Cytogenic studies in cases of chronic myelocytic leukemia and myeloid metaplasia. *Ann. Intern. Med.* 61:609, 1964.

Goh, K. O., and Swisher, S. N.   Identical twins and chronic myelocytic leukemia: Chromosomal studies of a patient with chronic myelocytic leukemia and his normal identical twin. *Arch. Intern. Med.* (Chicago) 115:475, 1965.

Hardy, W. R., and Anderson, R. E.   The hypereosinophilic syndromes. *Ann. Intern. Med.* 68:1220, 1968.

Nowell, P. C., and Hungerford, D. A.   A minute chromosome in human chronic granulocytic leukemia. *Science* 132:1497, 1960.

Sandberg, A. A., Cartner, J., Takagi, N., Maghadam, M. A., and Crosswhite,

L. H.   Differences in chromosome constitution of twins with acute leukemia. *New Eng. J. Med.* 275:809, 1966.

Tough, I. M., Court-Brown, W. M., Baikie, A. G., Buckton, I. E., Harnden, D. G., Jacobs, P. A., King, M. J., and McBride, J. A.   Cytogenetic studies in chronic myeloid leukaemia and acute leukaemia associated with mongolism. *Lancet* 1:411, 1961.

Whang-Peng, J., Canellos, G. P., Carbone, P. P., and Tjio, J. H.   Clinical implications of cytogenetic variants in chronic myelocytic leukemia (CML). *Blood* 32:755, 1968.

APPENDIX

The following are names and addresses of some of the physicians and scientists in the United States who are doing cytogenetic studies. Inquiry about availability of clinical cytogenetic studies may be directed to them.

Alabama	Dr. W. H. Finley University of Alabama Medical Center Birmingham 35233
California	Dr. S. Ohno City of Hope Medical Center Duarte 91010
Colorado	Dr. H. A. Lubs University of Colorado Medical Center Denver 80220
District of Columbia	Dr. C. B. Jacobson Reproductive Genetic Unit George Washington University School of Medicine Washington 20005
Georgia	Dr. J. G. Hollowell Medical College of Georgia Augusta 30902
Illinois	Dr. J. D. Rowley Argonne Cancer Research Hospital Chicago 60637
Maryland	Dr. J. Whang-Peng National Cancer Institute Bethesda 20014
Massachusetts	Dr. W. J. Mitus Blood Research Laboratory Tufts University School of Medicine Boston 02111
Michigan	Dr. A. B. Bloom Department of Human Genetics University of Michigan Medical School Ann Arbor 48104

Dr. W. W. Zuelzer
Children's Hospital of Michigan
Detroit   48202

Mississippi

Dr. H. A. Thiede
Department of Obstetrics and Gynecology
University of Mississippi School of Medicine
Jackson   39216

New Hampshire

Dr. K. Benirschke
Department of Pathology
Dartmouth Medical School
Hanover   03755

New York

Dr. A. A. Sandberg
Roswell Park Memorial Hospital
Buffalo   14203

Dr. J. German
The New York Blood Center
New York   10021

Dr. K. Hirschhorn
Department of Pediatrics
Mount Sinai Hospital Medical School
New York   10029

Dr. O. J. Miller
Department of Obstetrics and Gynecology
Columbia University College of Physicians and Surgeons
New York   10032

Dr. K. O. Goh
Monroe Community Hospital
Rochester   14620

Ohio

Dr. M. MacIntyre
Case Western Reserve University School of Medicine
Cleveland   44106

Dr. J. Warkany
University of Cincinnati College of Medicine
Cincinnati   45219

Oregon

Dr. F. Hecht
Division of Medical Genetics
University of Oregon Medical School
Portland   97201

Pennsylvania

Dr. D. A. Hungerford
Institute for Cancer Research
7701 Burholme Avenue
Fox Chase, Philadelphia   19111

Dr. P. C. Nowell
Department of Pathology
University of Pennsylvania School of Medicine
Philadelphia   19104

Dr. N. Wald
Graduate School of Public Health
University of Pittsburgh School of Medicine
Pittsburgh   15213

Tennessee	Dr. G. Littlefield Medical Division Oak Ridge Associated Universities Oak Ridge 37830
	Dr. E. Engel Vanderbilt University School of Medicine Nashville 37203
Texas	Dr. M. W. Shaw Department of Biology M.D. Anderson Hospital Houston 77025
Utah	Dr. C. P. Miles Department of Pathology University of Utah College of Medicine Salt Lake City 84112

22. MANAGEMENT OF ADULTS WITH ACUTE LEUKEMIA

Robert I. Weed

EMOTIONAL NEEDS OF THE PATIENT

Acute leukemia in adults, perhaps more than any other illness, should strongly reinforce the credo of the good internist, i.e., to examine, consider, and treat the whole patient. In the frustration of dealing with a condition whose fatal prognosis is all too often regrettably clear, the physician who has been responsible for primary medical care of the patient may prefer to turn over total care of the patient to the hematologist. However, the role of the primary physician should be preserved, although modified, particularly in those cases in which there has been a long relationship between the patient and his own physician and the latter is in a position to continue to administer to the patient's general health needs. Obviously when the patient is hospitalized for complicated chemotherapy, sometimes it may be preferable for the consultant to assume primary responsibility. Even under these circumstances, though, if both primary physician and consultant take care of patients at the same hospital, it is usually possible for the primary physician to maintain charge of the case with daily advice from the consultant.

Emotional frustrations similar to those of all physicians dealing with incurable disease are felt by the hematologist who deals with leukemia on a day-to-day basis, as discussed in Chapter 23. The physician in this situation has a responsibility not only to gain familiarity with details of the use of newer chemotherapeutic agents, but also to view skillful administration of chemotherapy as one part of overall management which requires not only a knowledge of pharmacology but continuing thoughtful attention to all the patient's needs. Although a truism applicable to almost every situation, in the management of adult leukemia it is particularly important that the physician examine his own attitude toward the disease before dealing with the patient.

Until curative therapy for leukemia becomes available, the most important problem in its management is for the physician to understand and deal with the emotional reactions of his patient, as discussed in Chapter 23. At a time when friends, and often family, may find themselves unable to communicate openly with the patient for reasons of fear or guilt or both, there is a distinct satisfaction for the physician who establishes a positive and firm supportive relationship with his patient and senses the latter's appreciation.

ANEMIA

Apart from direct attack on the fundamental problem of disordered leukocyte differentiation and multiplication, a common practical problem is the management of anemia. Anemia is an invariable complication of leukemia but may occur for a variety of reasons. In classic, actively proliferating acute leukemia, marrow replacement by malignant blast cells may "crowd out" the erythroid precursors. Ideally, specific chemotherapy to empty the marrow of leukemic infiltration should permit return of red cell production. This is commonly the gratifying result in treatment of lymphoblastic leukemia, whether it occurs in children or adults, but the disappointing incidence of remissions in myeloblastic leukemia—ranging from 20% to the highest reported values of 50%—still leaves a large percentage of patients requiring continual transfusion; even those who go into remission may need several transfusions prior to the remission. Variables such as the ability of the cardiovascular system to compensate for anemia and the activity of the 2,3-DPG compensatory mechanism discussed in Chapter 10 make it difficult to set down precise levels at which the hematocrit or hemoglobin should be maintained. The rapidity with which the anemia develops, i.e., several days or weeks, or suddenly following a brisk hemorrhage or an acute episode of hemolysis, determines the relation of symptoms of hypoxia to anemia. Compensatory mechanisms are brought into maximum operation when the anemia develops slowly rather than acutely. Consequently, symptomatology is important. Many patients can readily identify the point at which they begin to feel weak, tired, short of breath, or somewhat dizzy, but the specific hematocrit levels at which these symptoms appear may vary from less than 18% to values between 26 and 30%. From a physiologic point of view, it is almost never indicated to maintain the hematocrit level above 30%, and often in younger patients with an intact cardiovascular system it is possible to permit the hematocrit to get down to levels of 20% before transfusion is necessary to restore hematocrit values to between 25 and 30%. All the considerations and precautions reviewed in Chapter 11 should be kept in mind.

In addition to marrow replacement, however, some adults have an indolent form of leukemia in which the marrow is either normocellular or hypocellular and there is leukopenia in the peripheral blood. In this case the erythroid precursors do not appear to be "crowded out" but rather unable to develop normally in the presence of the leukemic process. For such patients transfusion alone may be the only indicated form of therapy for a period of months or even 1 or 2 years.

Finally, hemolytic anemia may accompany acute adult leukemia. Although "autoimmune" hemolytic anemia is a significant complication of chronic lymphocytic leukemia, it is very rare in acute leukemias. More common, however, is the problem of isosensitization after multiple transfusions, as discussed in Chapter 11.

INFECTION

Infection is the most common fatal complication of acute leukemia in adults, accounting for approximately 40% of deaths. Unlike chronic lymphocytic leukemia, until debilitation becomes extreme, immunologic deficiencies in circulating antibody or delayed hypersensitivity generally do not constitute a predisposing defect in acute leukemia. The absence of mature granulocytes and monocytes, however, removes a major mechanism of host defense against infection.

Certain important points in the management of infection in adult leukemia require particular emphasis. First of all, it is clear that any unexplained fever in a leukemic patient must be considered related to an underlying infection. This is so not only because of the statistical importance of infection as a cause of death but also because occurrence of a febrile reaction to the leukemia process itself is rare. Proper search for and identification of an infectious agent may permit elimination of the complication and, in fact, in some cases spontaneous remission of the leukemia may even follow an episode of severe infection.

Bacteremia with or without pneumonia is the most common clinical type of infection, and gram-negative organisms (primarily *Escherichia coli, Pseudomonas,* and *Proteus*) are the most frequent offenders, followed by *Staphylococcus aureus.* The gastrointestinal tract—because of ulceration, infiltration, or the presence of gram-negative organisms as normal flora— appears to be the primary source in many cases.

In choosing antibiotic therapy for management of bacterial sepsis, it is most important to recognize that in acute leukemia characterized by absence from the blood of mature granulocytic and monocytic forms capable of phagocytosis and destruction of bacteria, the use of bacteriostatic agents may be ineffectual. Appropriate cultures are most important to aid in the selection of the proper bactericidal agents, since the latter offer the only hope for arrest of the infection in the absence of the normal ancillary contribution of phagocytic cells. Unfortunately, in many patients positive cultures are not always available and consequently treatment must be started using an empirical selection of bactericidal agents to cover both gram-positive and gram-negative infections. If the patient is thrombocytopenic, agents that must be given intramuscularly should be avoided; otherwise hematoma formation may ensue and be difficult to distinguish from a soft tissue abscess or may actually lead to abscess formation.

Patients who have mature granulocyte counts less than 500 per cubic millimeter, whether a consequence of the leukemic process itself or of chemotherapy directed against the leukemia, are clearly predisposed to the complication of bacterial infection. Because gram-negative sepsis is a frequent complication of acute leukemia and because the site of origin is so often the gastrointestinal tract, it would be highly desirable to sterilize the gut or to maintain a low count of potential pathogens within the intestine. For this reason programs of prophylactic treatment with nonabsorbable antibiotics have been recommended, with rotation of agents to minimize emergence and overgrowth of resistant strains. Such a program is outlined in Table 22-1. Oral antibiotic prophylaxis should be considered for the patients at highest risk, particularly to tide them over a period of induced marrow aplasia which may be a necessary first step toward the induction of a remission. The oral prophylactic regimen is very expensive, however, and can seldom be undertaken unless there is some third-party support avail-

Table 22-1. Nonabsorbable Oral Antibiotic Regimens for Gastrointestinal Prophylaxis

ANTIBACTERIAL AGENTS (Regimens A and B are interchangeable; choose one and add both antifungal agents)	
Regimen A	*Dosage*
Paromomycin sulfate	500 mg
Polymyxin B sulfate	70 mg
Vancomycin hydrochloride	250 mg
Regimen B	
Gentamycin sulfate[a]	200 mg
Vancomycin hydrochloride	250 mg
ANTIFUNGAL AGENTS	
Amphotericin B[b]	500 mg
Nystatin	3.6 million units

All antibiotics except nystatin are given in flavored solution every 4 hours. Nystatin is given as 6 tablets or 6 cc suspension every 4 hours.

[a] Supplied by Schering Corp. as Garamycin syrup.
[b] Supplied by E. R. Squibb & Sons as Preparation AJS.
SOURCE: From G. P. Bodey et al., *Cancer* 24:972, 1969.

able. Patients may find the regimen bothersome and some even find it impossible because of the great numbers of pills, the unpleasant taste of some of the preparations, and the induction of nausea.

Transfusion with sufficient numbers of mature granulocytes to enable patients to control infection would be ideal, but this approach is of limited practicability at present. The low number of granulocytes present in normal blood, the fragility of white cells when handled, and the dilution space within the body all constitute severe limitations. The leukocytes from 40 units of normal blood would be required to raise the peripheral white count by 1×10^3 per cubic millimeter in an average-sized adult male. Although cell-separating devices to recirculate a donor's blood in order to harvest the leukocytes hold promise for the future, such instruments are still in experimental and developmental stages.

At present the only way to provide granulocytes is by use of donors with chronic granulocytic leukemia (CGL) who have granulocyte counts greater than 100,000 per cubic millimeter. The risks include those associated with any transfusion, including isoimmunization interfering with future transfusions, reactions attributable to prior isoimmunization resulting from prior red cell or whole-blood transfusions, plus the long-term possibility of a graft-versus-host reaction.

If the potential life-saving benefit to a patient with sepsis appears to outweigh the long-term risks and an appropriate donor is available, leukocyte transfusion may be tried. Leukocytes are prepared by sedimentation of red cells, gentle centrifugation of the leukocyte-rich plasma, and resuspension of leukocytes in saline solution prior to infusion. Immunologic activity may be reduced by incubation for 2 hours at 37°C prior to administration of the cells. Best results in combating infection appear to follow infusion of 2×10^{11} or more leukocytes. Although it seems desirable to use leukocytes from an ABO-compatible donor, this is not essential. In fact, CGL-transfused blood has produced a successful graft in leukemic recipients in spite of high titer of AB isoantibody produced by the recipient against an incompatible donor graft.

FUNGAL INFECTION. Antecedent antimetabolites, alkylation chemotherapy, and corticosteroid administration appear to predispose to fungal infections as a complication of acute leukemia. *Histoplasma* and cryptococcosis infections may be acquired outside of the hospital while aspergillosis, mucormycosis, and candidiasis are common in-hospital fungal infections complicating the course of acute leukemia in adults. Oropharyngeal candidiasis is an annoying problem which accounts for approximately one-half of all fungal complications in this group of patients. Fortunately, this form of *Candida* seldom disseminates and can usually be well managed with nystatin mouthwashes. Disseminated *Candida, Histoplasma,* and *Cryptococcus* infections must be treated with intravenous amphotericin B.

VIRAL INFECTIONS. Viral infections are relatively less common in adults with acute leukemia. Herpes zoster, although common in chronic lymphocytic leukemia and certain lymphomas, is rarely encountered in adults with acute leukemia. Adults with leukemia are obviously at risk for viral hepatitis and cytomegalovirus infection in proportion to the number of blood transfusions required. Cytomegalic inclusion disease must be considered as a possible underlying cause for unexplained fever and interstitial pneumonia in occasional patients with acute leukemia. If available, diagnostic work-up should include culture of the urine for cytomegalovirus as well as study of changes in complement-fixing antibody titers. No specific therapy is available, but establishment of the diagnosis obviates the necessity for therapeutic trials of a variety of antibiotics and, if the patient survives the acute phase, recovery from the cytomegalic disease may ensue spontaneously.

PARASITIC INFECTIONS. Parasitic infections must be considered, and foremost among such infections is interstitial pneumonia produced by *Pneumocystis carinii*. The physician must be alert to the possibility of this complication, as it is often characterized by rapidly progressive pneumonia associated with an alveolar-capillary block syndrome. Diagnosis should be established by methenamine silver stains of sputum or, preferably, lung biopsy material, since sputum is often negative. However, biopsy may be contraindicated because of thrombocytopenia and, if the clinical picture suggests *Pneumocystis,* a 6- to 14-day trial of pentamidine isethionate (4 mg per kilogram of body weight per day) should be tried. Symptomatic response is often rapid and accompanied by improvement in pulmonary function tests. Finally, pneumonia produced by *Strongyloides* has been reported as a complication of acute leukemia.

Infectious complications provide a particular threat to the patient with acute leukemia and a diagnostic challenge to his physician. The combination of an obscure fever and an inability to manufacture granulocytes may impede diagnosis, since the patient's inability to make pus may be misleading. For example, the absence of exudate may readily obscure a diagnosis of streptococcal pharyngitis in acute leukemia. Yet if properly identified, infectious complications are often more amenable to specific therapy than the leukemic process itself. Therefore no stone should be left unturned in attempting to identify an offending organism.

HEMORRHAGE

After infection, bleeding problems are the next most common cause of death in acute leukemia. Thrombocytopenia secondary to faulty production because of leukemic involvement of the bone marrow is by far the most common predisposing basis for the hemorrhagic manifestations of leukemia. As in the case of anemia, symptomatology is influenced by the rapidity with which the thrombocytopenia develops. If the situation is chronic, a low platelet count may not be associated with symptomatic bleeding. While bleeding on the basis of thrombocytopenia seldom occurs at platelet counts above 50,000 per cubic millimeter, it is often surprising how well some patients can tolerate platelet counts below 20,000 per cubic millimeter without bleeding problems, providing that the thrombocytopenia developed slowly and that no major challenge is presented to the hemostatic mechanism.

Trauma or gastrointestinal lesions, including peptic ulcers, may precipitate spontaneous episodes of hemorrhage because of the markedly increased consumption of platelets, which aggravates the thrombocytopenia, thereby initiating a vicious circle. The presence of active bleeding may make it difficult to interpret the efficacy of platelet transfusions since, in the face of a major hemorrhage, many platelets may be consumed without any effect on the platelet count. The most important measure of therapeutic success, however, is cessation of bleeding.

The recent recognition that platelets can be effective after periods of storage up to 72 hours when kept at room temperature has made possible much more extensive use of platelet transfusions for the support of leukemic patients, particularly during periods of active bleeding or profound thrombocytopenia induced by chemotherapy. The availability of platelet packs in which the platelets are concentrated and the volume load reduced has made it possible to give leukemic patients the platelets from 20 units of blood without imposing a significant cardiovascular load. Continuing platelet transfusions, however, are commonly associated with the development of isoantibodies, thereby reducing the effectiveness of subsequent transfusions. For this reason platelet transfusions should be reserved for the situations in which active bleeding is occurring or obviously threatened as indicated by progressively falling platelets, or the development of minor evidences of bleeding predisposition, such as increasing numbers of cutaneous petechiae, or both. Although not generally available at present, testing for major histocompatibility antigens (HL-A) in the future appears to offer great promise in avoidance of isosensitization, thereby prolonging the period during which platelet transfusions are useful.

Female patients in the reproductive-age group pose a special hemorrhagic problem at the time of each menstrual period. Since this is a predictable problem as thrombocytopenia develops, it should be anticipated and prophylactic measures undertaken to prevent vaginal bleeding from becoming massive and platelets from falling so low that additional internal or cerebral bleeding may be superimposed. Nonsurgical sterilization by irradiating the ovaries is an excellent permanent solution and preventive measure which should be considered in all menstruating adult females. However, ovarian irradiation will not stop vaginal bleeding already underway, and even if given prior to a menstrual period, it may be followed by at least one final menstrual flow. In such cases, for those patients in whom vaginal bleeding is already a problem, and for those women in whom sterilization is unacceptable or undesirable, hormonal suppression of bleeding should be attempted. Patients who have been taking estrogen or estrogens and progesterone or oral contraceptives may do well by continuous maintenance of their hormone ingestion. In our hands, estrogen therapy has been ineffective in inducing cessation of bleeding already underway. Medroxyprogesterone, however, has proven useful in some patients both for cessation and for maintenance of suppression; 50 mg three times daily is given initially. If stopped, an abbreviated menstrual period may ensue in 48 to 72 hours. Alternatively, continued suppression with the aim of producing endometrial atrophy may be attempted by administering 10 mg of medroxyprogesterone daily.

A much less common hemorrhagic complication of leukemia is that seen in patients with promyelocytic leukemia. Granulocytic precursors and eosinophils are known to contain active profibrinolysins, and therefore in the past it has been suggested that activation of fibrinolysin in this disease predisposes such patients to their hemorrhagic problems. More recent evidence, however, has suggested that the primary problem is intravascular coagulation with secondary fibrinolysis. Cautious administration of heparin may be both diagnostic and therapeutic.

OTHER COMPLICATIONS

HYPERURICEMIA. In patients with leukemia or other neoplastic diseases, there is often a very significant increase in nucleic acid breakdown which may be greatly increased by chemotherapy. The enhanced purine catabolism results in hyperuricemia which may lead to gouty arthritis, renal calculi, and, most serious of all, progressive uric acid nephropathy.

Allopurinol, a xanthine oxidase inhibitor which was developed to suppress the oxidative degradation of mercaptopurine, has proved to be of great value in controlling the hyperuricemia associated with neoplasia and its treatment. The drug inhibits conversion of hypoxanthine and xanthine to uric acid by enzyme inhibition and can be used in the face of renal disease. To lower an elevated uric acid, or prior to institution of chemotherapy to prevent hyperuricemia, or both, 100 mg of allopurinol three or four times a day should be administered.

LOCAL INVOLVEMENT.   In addition to the most common complications already mentioned, occasionally symptomatology due to local infiltration of the skin, central nervous system, or other local vital areas may occur. Under these circumstances local irradiation may be of value. In the case of the central nervous system, if there is evidence of leukemic involvement of the brain in a localized area as manifested by cranial nerve involvement, treatment with 1000 R may produce substantial improvement in the central nervous system manifestations. Leukemic meningitis, on the other hand, should be treated by intrathecal methotrexate, 0.5 mg per kilogram of body weight (not to exceed 20 mg per dose) to be administered twice weekly until evidence of meningeal involvement has disappeared, as manifested by fall in the spinal fluid cell count and protein level to normal values. If the marrow is already depressed by chemotherapy, folinic acid, 3 mg every 4 hours, may be given to block the methotrexate effect outside the nervous system.

ANTILEUKEMIC CHEMOTHERAPY

Prior to the choice of any "specific" chemotherapeutic agent, it is essential to evaluate whether chemotherapy is indicated and whether it is likely to be useful. Treatment of acute lymphoblastic leukemia is indicated in both children and adults, and often treatment is rewarded by remission. The results of treatment of acute myeloblastic leukemia in adults, however, have been disappointing both in terms of an effect on survival and on remission rate, which at best may be 30 to 50%. The uncertain results and significant toxicity associated with many forms of treatment provide a major incentive for examining whether vigorous chemotherapy is justified in each individual patient.

Approximately 10 to 15% of patients with acute myeloid leukemia, diagnosed on the basis of morphology, have a disease characterized by slow clinical progression. Although distinctly pathologic, the bone marrow may be relatively hypocellular and the peripheral white count may be low, although characterized by the presence of a variable percentage of myeloblasts. Because the leukemic cell population does not appear to be expanding and invading normal tissue in such patients, their major problems are anemia or thrombocytopenia, or both. Initiation of specific chemotherapy, rather than being beneficial, may result only in suppression of an already hypoactive marrow. Actually such patients may do well for many months or occasionally for 1 to 2 years, managed only by supportive transfusions, and in these patients the decision should be made not to treat with chemotherapy.

Apart from this slowly progressive group, certain other groups of patients have forms of acute leukemia which are usually resistant to chemotherapy. These include patients with acute blastic transformation of chronic granulocytic leukemia, myeloid metaplasia, and erythremic myelosis (Di Guglielmo syndrome) whose disease has entered into a blastic crisis. Even though the results of treatment in this group are very poor, the prognosis—once blastic transformation has occurred—is so poor that one may be justified in trying chemotherapy, since rarely patients may show some significant improvement.

In patients having acute leukemia from the onset, chemotherapy should be instituted when there is clear evidence of active proliferation of leukemic cells manifested by a marrow replaced by blast forms, or a markedly elevated or rapidly increasing peripheral white blood cell (blast) count, or evidence of tissue or organ infiltration. Therapy is intended to destroy leukemic tissue in the hope that normal cell production can be resumed. The rationale for selection of specific agents, as well as a discussion of present efforts to increase the rational basis for choice of agents, is discussed in Chapter 24.

Once the decision has been made to institute chemotherapy, clearly the ideal immediate goal of treatment is to achieve a complete remission. Hematologic remission is defined as disappearance of blast forms from the peripheral blood, reduction of blast forms in the bone marrow to less than 5%, and restoration of granulocytes to greater than 3000 per cubic millimeter (sufficient to protect against infection). Although the future holds promise that we will be able to cure leukemia or control it indefinitely, the long-term goal of today is to prolong the *useful* survival of adult patients with acute leukemia.

Unfortunately, the potent chemotherapeutic agents presently available are all potentially toxic in one way or another. In fact, in order to achieve remission it is usually necessary to render the marrow essentially aplastic and then hope for a return of normal elements. This is a calculated risk, but it clearly means that the physician in charge must be prepared to cope with the problems of bleeding and infection that often ensue during periods of severe marrow depression. Each agent also has its own unique toxicities, and it is the responsibility of the physician to inform his patient about them so that the patient can recognize the earliest manifestations of toxicity. The toxicities of the individual agents are discussed in Chapter 24 on chemotherapy of leukemia in adults.

Evaluation of the results of a chemotherapeutic regimen in a given patient should not be based on the totally objective criteria of hematologic remission on the one hand or duration of survival on the other. Rather the benefits of inducing a remission should be considered in the light of the discomfort and disability associated with therapy. For example, a decision to choose an agent that may have a higher statistical record of remission induction may be tempered by knowledge that its administration requires hospitalization with intravenous infusions, accompanying gastrointestinal toxicity, anorexia, and loss of time away from friends and loved ones. Although difficult to define and include as a statistic, meaningful survival rather than simple duration of survival should be the objective. If vigorous therapy with a very toxic agent is undertaken with the hope of prolonging life for another month, it should be because the physician understands that his patient wishes everything to be done. Conversely, some patients who have had previous and often complicated courses of treatment may actually indicate that they prefer not to go through further therapy. Such a discussion and decision obviously will take place only when there is the type of close relationship between patient and physician discussed at the beginning of this chapter. Even if the patient wishes no further chemotherapy, treatment must continue in the form of understanding and concern for minor and major discomforts as the physician carries out his responsibility to help the patient to die with dignity.

REFERENCES

Bodey, G. P., Freireich, E. J., and Frei, E., III.   Studies of patients in a laminar air flow unit. *Cancer* 24:972, 1969.

Crosby, W. H.   Various views on chemotherapy: To treat or not to treat acute granulocytic leukemia. *Arch. Intern. Med.* (Chicago) 122:79, 1968.

Dameshek, W.   Treatment of Acute Granulocytic Leukemia. In W. Dameshek and F. Gunz (Eds.), *Leukemia* (2d ed.). New York: Grune & Stratton, 1964.

Dameshek, W.   Treatment of AGL. *Arch. Intern. Med.* (Chicago) 123:725, 1969.

Goodell, B., Jacobs, J. B., Powell, R. D., and DeVita, V. T.   *Pneumocystis carinii:* The spectrum of diffuse interstitial pneumonia in patients with neoplastic diseases. *Ann. Intern. Med.* 72:337, 1970.

Grumet, F. C., and Yankee, R. A.   Long-term platelet support of patients with aplastic anemia: Effect of splenectomy and steroid therapy. *Ann. Intern. Med.* 73:1, 1970.

Lee, S. L., and Rosner, F.   Treatment of AGL. *Arch. Intern. Med.* (Chicago) 123:205, 1969.

Moore, E. W., Thomas, L. B., Shaw, R. K., and Freireich, E. J.   The central nervous system in acute leukemia. *Arch. Intern. Med.* (Chicago) 105:451, 1960.

Maggie, F. M., Ball, T. J., Jr., and Ultmann, J. E.   Allopurinol in the treatment of neoplastic disease complicated by hyperuricemia. *Arch. Intern. Med.* (Chicago) 120:12, 1967.

Neimetz, J., and Nossel, H. L.   Activated coagulation factors: *In vivo* and *in vitro* studies. *Brit. J. Haemat.* 16:337, 1969.

Schwarzenberg, L., Mathé, G., Amiel, J. L., Cattan, A., Schneider, M., and Schlumberger, J. R.   Study of factors determining the usefulness and complications of leukocyte transfusions. *Amer. J. Med.* 43:206, 1967.

Sullivan, M. P., Vietti, T. J., Fernbach, D. J., Griffith, K. M., Haddy, T. B., and Watkins, W. L. Clinical investigations in the treatment of meningeal leukemia: Radiation therapy regimens vs. conventional intrathecal methotrexate. *Blood* 34:301, 1969.

Troup, S. B., Swisher, S. N., and Young, L. E. The anemia of leukemia. *Amer. J. Med.* 28:751, 1960.

Viola, M. V. Acute leukemia and infection. *J.A.M.A.* 201:923, 1967.

Zarafonetis, C. J. D. (Ed.). *Proceedings of the International Conference on Leukemia-Lymphoma.* Philadelphia: Lea & Febiger, 1968.

23. PSYCHOLOGICAL PROBLEMS IN LEUKEMIAS AND LYMPHOMAS

William A. Greene

THE PHYSICIAN faced with a patient with leukemia or lymphoma must deal with a number of psychological problems. First are those associated with his own attitude toward these diseases; second is his confidence in his ability to implement effectively diagnostic and therapeutic measures, and third are his understanding and capacity to attenuate emotional distress manifested by the individual patient threatened by such an illness.

What is said here pertains most directly to the care of adult patients with leukemia, has some relevance to the care of the patient with lymphoma, and may be considered as concerns the patient with neoplasia in general. Pertinent information on children and their parents is available in the reports of a colleague, S. B. Friedman, from his extensive pediatric experience. This is not a discussion of the fatally ill or the terminally ill patient. Rather it is presented with the impression that the prognosis of the adult patient with leukemia or lymphoma is often too ominously perceived. The frequent association, leukemia today—dead tomorrow, is unrealistic. The average life expectancy for all patients with all types of leukemia—acute, subacute, and chronic—is about 2 years, and much longer for those with lymphoma. It should be emphasized that the way the relationship between physician and patient is first established will determine and hopefully facilitate management during the course of the illness and the eventual terminal phase.

PRODROMAL PSYCHOLOGICAL DISTRESS

Mention should be made of studies suggesting that psychological distress may contribute to the manifest development of these diseases. Emotional

The work on which this paper is based was supported by U.S. Public Health Service Program Grant MH-11668.

reactions incident to the patient's frustrations with unachieved goals, the upheaval of moving to a distant location, or despair in the wake of loss of a significant person have been implicated in the onset and course by myself and others. Presumably such factors operate through neuroendocrine and neuroimmunologic processes. The clinician should be cognizant of these studies showing a high incidence of emotional distress engendered by social change antecedent to the clinical onset in most patient groups. These disrupting life circumstances frequently account more for the patient's anxiety or despair than the fact of his being sick or learning that he has leukemia or Hodgkin's disease.

WHAT DO YOU TELL THE PATIENT?

A paramount question in the mind of the physician and members of the family when the diagnosis is being considered or has been made is what to tell the patient. This is usually voiced in terms of what should he know or what does he know. Often the patient knows more than those around him think he knows. It is important to appreciate what these questions mean. They have a number of meanings: First, does the patient know that he has leukemia or Hodgkin's disease? Second, does he know that he will die with the disease? And third, does he know when he will die? It is crucial to consider these several meanings of the questions before deciding how to answer.

That He Has Leukemia?

That he has leukemia is best shared with the adult patient. The same applies to most adolescent patients when their parents can permit it. In spite of the difficulty of imparting this information, it is preferable in the long run to tell the patient with leukemia or lymphoma his diagnosis and that you, the physician, are concerned but can comfortably proceed with treatment. This is preferable for initiating and making possible the maintenance of a confident mutual relationship. There is no place for euphemistic terms such as anemia, inflammation, mononucleosis, or gland trouble.

There are ways of telling the patient his diagnosis which do attenuate the pessimism usually associated with the diagnosis of leukemia or lymphoma. To put matters in perspective it is well to tell the patient that the symptoms —lump, bleeding, cough, fatigue, anorexia, pain—that he has had for a number of weeks or months indicate that he has been sick with leukemia or Hodgkin's disease for that length of time. Saying "What you have had is leukemia," is different from, "You have leukemia." It is also reasonable to assume, and to tell him, that he has had the disease for some time even before he recognized the symptoms. In this way one conveys to the patient that he has had leukemia for a number of months or even a year or more.

This gives him the opportunity from his own experience in the past with the disease to project himself into the future with leukemia at least for another year or so.

To approach the problem even earlier, it is helpful when seeing a patient with suspected leukemia or lymphoma to ask the patient in the initial interview whether he has considered or wondered how he may be sick. A number of patients will readily bring up their concern about leukemia or Hodgkin's disease. Others will mention fatigue, infections, emotional distress, gland trouble, but indicate that they have other possibilities in mind too ominous to mention, usually by saying, "That's all, I guess." This should be the physician's cue to ask whether the patient has considered the possibility of leukemia. These exchanges afford the physician the opening to let the patient know that he too considers leukemia a possibility and that if this proves to be the problem he will decide with the patient how to proceed with treatment. Such early considerations of the possibility of a diagnosis of leukemia or lymphoma and the availability of therapeutic measures to cope with the disease may forestall an acute communicative dilemma for the physician and patient when a diagnosis is definitely established.

In many communities there are one or more physicians, internists, or hematologists who are known to be relatively expert in treatment of serious blood or lymph gland disorders. When referred to such a physician, patients infer that their ailment is suspected of being such a disorder—which in the minds of most patients, relatives, and neighbors means leukemia or Hodgkin's disease. Not to consider openly with patients the possibility of leukemia or lymphoma when it is suspected during the usual work-up is to beat around the bush and to lose the chance of making a difficult problem less acutely frantic when the diagnosis is established. If the diagnosis proves to be leukemia or lymphoma, physician and patient have already started working together in the light of the patient's preparing for the fact that he has the disease.

In the context of this relationship, it is preferable for the physician to be alone with the patient and to state that the diagnosis is leukemia, Hodgkin's disease, or lymphosarcoma, with the measures for treatment, the general outlook for prognosis, and the extent to which the patient will be able to carry on his daily activities immediately or following treatment. One or more members of the family, a spouse or parents or children, may be included at the time or afterward, depending on the wish of the patient. In this way one gives the patient a choice, respecting his autonomy on the one hand and his possible need for the support of family members on the other. Details are clarified as the patient asks questions. Hopefully, the physician can communicate the diagnosis and the prospects without feeling too ashamed that curative measures are not better and without feeling too guilty at telling the patient how he is sick.

On being told that they have leukemia or lymphoma, most patients become somewhat anxious, restless, perhaps depressed and tearful for 2 or 3 days. This is a normal, healthy reaction which soon subsides and lays the ground for a subsequent relationship between the physician and his patient. When treatment is begun around some equivocating type of diagnosis, such reactions may not subside. At times it may be important for the physician to proceed with direct communication to the patient even though members of the family may feel that this should not be done. Frequently their assumptions about the fragility of the patient are a function of their own distress.

That He Will Die?

Of course, the answer to the question of whether or not the patient is going to die is yes, and most patients with leukemia or lymphoma intermittently recognize that this is so. They can quite readily tolerate the realistic statement by the physician that their life will be foreshortened with the disease.

To discuss with the patient what may be the approximate duration of his attenuated life with the disease is different from focusing on the fact that he will die from the disease. Particularly this is so when such prognostications are coupled with consideration of the many activities in which he may continue to participate, what disabilities or degree of suffering he may encounter, and the several types of therapy available. Physicians and family members are prone initially to voice overoptimistic predictions of survival to these patients. The not-infrequent impulsive, saccharine statement to a patient that he may live for 10, 15, or 20 years should be avoided. This can lead only to disappointment and mistrust on the part of the patient and troubles in the future for the physician. Equally inadvisable is to hide behind intellectualized statements in terms of group survival expectations. Patients resent being thought of in terms of one of a group, as an average, or as a point on a survival curve. It is preferable to give the patient, as well as members of the family, a range of life expectancy rather than a specifically timed prognostication. Depending on the type of leukemia or lymphoma, estimations of 3 to 6 months, 1 to 2 years, or 3 to 5 years—perhaps all expressed in terms of months—are most satisfactory.

A single-duration prognosis such as 6 months, 2 years, 5 years may lead to complications which are difficult for both patient and physician. Many patients then pattern their expectations on this single time span. If they become sicker before that time they are disappointed and angry. Many deal with a specific life expectancy in such a way that when this time is up they may become very euphoric, feeling that they have beaten the system. They may then become disappointed with subsequent relapse of the disease. Other patients become very apprehensive and may become quite depressed, feeling that they are then living precariously or undeservedly on borrowed time. This reaction is frequently observed now with the prevalent focus on 5-year survivals in neoplasia in general which patients with these diseases, as well as other types of malignancy, come to know as an accepted end point of therapeutic success.

When He Will Die?

Predicting when a specific patient is going to die is not within the clairvoyant capacity of any physician, and most patients do not really ask such a question. Most patients do not want a specific answer but prefer to assume that this is indeterminate and that the physician cannot explicitly foresee or foretell the future. There is a rare patient, however, who has difficulty enduring the unpredictability of this possibility and insists on an answer. Recently a 22-year-old man with Hodgkin's disease could not tolerate not knowing exactly when the disease would lead to his death. Deciding this point for himself was a factor in his committing suicide. Suicide, however, is extremely rare among patients with leukemia or lymphoma. In my 20 years' experience, suicide has not occurred among several hundred patients with leukemia and in only two patients among many hundreds with lymphoma.

VARIABLES CONTRIBUTING TO A PATIENT'S PSYCHOLOGICAL ADJUSTMENT

The psychological problems of the patient with leukemia or lymphoma are a function of many factors. His particular disease manifestations, the methods available for treatment, and his individual personality makeup contribute to the intensity and type of his psychological distress. More important are his knowledge or understanding of the disease, his ancillary life circumstances or social resources, and his reaction to the individual attitudes and personality of his physician.

Knowledge and Understanding of Leukemia or Lymphoma

All patients and their families have apprehensions and misapprehensions about leukemia or lymphoma. It seems that everyone has known a neighbor or close friend or has heard of someone who has had such a disease. The patient and his family members usually equate his prospects in the light of their knowledge of the course of illness of an acquaintance, friend, or relative. Direct or hearsay knowledge about some other person usually engenders ominous expectations which may preclude realistic coping by the patient and family members. Since the patient may have some such ominous example on his mind, it is well to inquire of the patient and family members whether they have ever known of anyone sick with this disease. To talk about the known person with leukemia or Hodgkin's disease and the patient's apprehension and misinterpretations can be most effective in dissociating the patient's assumptions about his disease course from an inappropriate example. Verbalization in itself is of some benefit. Variations in the types of leukemia or lymphoma can be emphasized along with improvements in therapy over time, to facilitate the patient's dealing with his disease in the future by being less haunted by his recollection of someone else's course.

AVAILABLE SOCIAL RESOURCES

Whether or not the patient has supporting family members, parents, a spouse, or children may play an important role in the extent to which he is psychologically distressed with the development of leukemia or lymphoma and the course of the disease. A church affiliation and relationship with a clergyman can be very helpful. A job and the ability to continue with work or school are particularly important to patients, and they should be encouraged to stay at their work or studies as long as their disability permits.

Like any other person, patients with leukemia may become anxious, sad, or ashamed because of disappointments, concerns, and changes in relation to family members. This should be borne in mind as a possible source of psychological distress in the leukemic patient rather than assuming that his apparent emotional discomfort is related to having the disease. Such distress may occur with illness in a family member, disappointments in children, or conflicts at work. Often this develops in response to the withdrawal of a family member because of his or her anxiety and inability to communicate directly with the sick patient. The family members' obvious anxiety may lead to the patient's feeling guilty because the relatives' discomfort is engendered by his being sick. The situation frequently can be eased if the patient has the opportunity to voice these concerns to his physician and, at times, if the physician gives the family members an opportunity to talk about their concerns, generally by themselves with the physician or at times with other professional persons.

PERSONALITY AND APPROACH OF THE PHYSICIAN

Fortunately for everyone, physicians as well as patients vary in personality type. This is reflected in differences in physicians' approach to patients and perhaps particularly to the care of the patient with leukemia and lymphoma. Some self-selection takes place in this regard by the physician's chosen field of specialty practice. Hematologists or radiation therapists because of the nature of their work frequently take care of such patients, while other types of specialists, cardiologists or endocrinologists, never have to be concerned with this type of problem. Such screening is not available to general physicians or internists, who also differ appreciably in personality type and the relationships they develop with patients.

Patients, including those with leukemia or lymphoma, select their physician partly for his personality characteristics. Some patients will do better with a very organized, impersonal, controlled approach while others require a less structured, more direct personal relationship with the physician. Hopefully the physician can vary his approach in the conduct of the diagnostic appraisal and therapy to best suit the needs of the individual patient. Generally patients do better initially and over the course of the disease in a relationship with a physician which is mutual and affords the opportunity to voice concerns about the disease and about the ancillary factors in their lives which may be contributing to their degree of apprehension or depression.

Many patients recognize the futility the physician feels at times with the progress of the treatment and can share this concern with him. At the same time the patient should not have to feel sorry for the physician so that he is reluctant to share his own apprehensions with the physician. Occasionally patients know their diagnosis without being told directly or are aware of the futility of therapeutic measures or become uncomfortable with some symptom, but they are unable to talk about these matters because they feel it would be too distressing for the doctor. They are in a way sorry for the physician and his predicament with them, so they carry on by themselves. When this occurs it is usually due to the simple fact that the physician directly responsible for the care of the patient is the one who shoulders the responsibility for the success or, in these circumstances, the lack of success of treatment. It may be that the physician is realistically overextended in his practice, is dealing with other emotional problems himself, or has idiosyncratic emotional reactions to patients with leukemia or lymphoma.

There are patients who use the psychological defense mechanism of denial and are unable to appreciate consciously the significance of their disease. They do not seem to appreciate the seriousness of the illness and are apparently unrealistically optimistic or withdrawn. When the patient with leukemia or lymphoma expresses no concerns, it can be helpful both for the patient and for the physician to have a third person talk with the patient— another doctor, social worker, clergyman, or perhaps a psychiatrist who is at ease with the seriously physically sick. The patient may then be able to express his apprehensions and disappointments about treatment, matters which he is not able to do directly with his administering personal physician.

Whatever the approach of the doctor may be, it will likely be reflected in his seeing patients on a very regular basis or with irregularly spaced appointments. With either approach, it is preferable that appointments be scheduled so that patients are seen at times when they are quite comfortable as well as when sicker. Thus the relationship does not develop only on the basis of discomfort, or become dictated only by the patient's having to call the physician. Such an arrangement provides the patient the opportunity to associate with the physician when relatively well and not exclusively when sick. The physician is afforded the opportunity to relate to the patient on the basis of fulfilling successful activities at home and at work, rather than exclusively on the basis of disability and disease progression.

In the long run it is preferable to relate to patients with reference to their disease in terms of how they feel, how the physician finds their general physical status, and what they are and are not able to do. It is important not to let patients know, or at least not to focus on, levels of the white blood count, platelet count, or hematocrit. These figures may become the measure of the successful or unsuccessful course of the disease and the basis of pleasant or unpleasant feelings in the physician-patient relationship. If this suggestion is followed, it is important to caution nurses and technicians to refrain from telling patients their laboratory results and to leave this decision up to the physician. At times technicians and nurses, who get attached to these patients over the course of time, are distressed about the patient who has leukemia or lymphoma. They may tell patients laboratory findings, at times in response to the patient's request, when the results remain within normal limits and even more when results are approaching normal as a result of therapy. This can lead to some difficult impasses for nurses and technicians, and the physician, as well as patients, when the numbers change for the worse. For such information to come only from the doctor is the preferable policy in the long run.

A PERSPECTIVE FOR THE PHYSICIAN

This account suggests that there are several contributing factors in the variety of psychological problems for the physician and his patient with leukemia or lymphoma. From two decades of study focusing on psychological adjustments and maladjustments in the course of patients with these diseases, it has become evident that there are two main factors conducive to the emotional comfort of the patient and to the easing of his degree of distress. First is the extent of the physician's emotional comfort or confidence in diagnosing and treating the disease, which is mainly a function of his hematologic knowledge and experience. Secondly, and complementing this, is the fact that basic to the patient's degree of comfort throughout the course of the disease is the patient's inference that the physician has such self-confidence and "knows his leukemia" or "knows his Hodgkin's disease." He seems versatile in treatment measures both therapeutic and palliative. These two aspects of the physician-patient relationship in the course of the disease take priority over the physician's sophistication about psychological matters in general or his understanding of the particular psychological variables which have been discussed.

Even so, a mutual relationship in which the patient is able to express his concerns and the physician can give some help in dealing with psychological distress will lessen the patient's pain, both physical and psychological. In spite of the most experienced hematologic know-how and psychological acumen on the physician's part, the disease will be accompanied by anxiety and sadness, at times intense, for the patient and to some degree for the physician. Awareness of and perhaps attention to this distress also affords the physician the opportunity to appreciate better the courage, tenderness, and dignity with which patients live with these diseases and at times relate to the physician. These are matters which are difficult for the participant physician or observer truly to appreciate, much less describe, and are best expressed by a patient with leukemia such as Hans Zinsser, who was also a perceptive physician.

REFERENCES

Albertson, P. D., and Krauss, M. (Eds.). Second conference on psychophysiological aspects of cancer. *Ann. N.Y. Acad. Sci.* 164:307, 1969.

Chodoff, P., Friedman, S. B., and Hamburg, D. A. Stress, defenses and coping behavior: Observations in parents of children with malignant disease. *Amer. J. Psychiat.* 120:743, 1964.

Dameshek, W., and Gunz, F. *Leukemia* (2d ed.). New York: Grune & Stratton, 1964. P. 32.

Emanuel, E. Alone with your patient (letter to the editor). *Ann. Intern. Med.* 72:1, 1970.

Friedman, S. B., Chodoff, P., Mason, J. W., and Hamburg, D. A. Behavioral observations on parents anticipating the death of a child. *Pediatrics* 32:610, 1963.

Friedman, S. B., Karon, M., and Goldsmith, G. *Childhood Leukemia: A Pamphlet for Parents.* Washington: U.S. Public Health Service, Department of Health, Education, and Welfare, 1965. (Available from the Office of Information, National Cancer Institute, Bethesda, Md.)

Greene, W. A. Psychological factors and reticuloendothelial disease: I. Preliminary observations on a group of males with lymphomas and leukemias. *Psychosom. Med.* 16:220, 1954.

Greene, W. A. What the Cancer Patient Should Be Told About His Diagnosis and Prognosis. In *The Physician and the Total Care of the Cancer Patient.* New York: The American Cancer Society, 1962. Pp. 69–74.

Greene, W. A. The psychosocial setting of the development of leukemia and lymphoma. *Ann. N.Y. Acad. Sci.* 125:794, 1966.

Greene, W. A., Young, L. E., and Swisher, S. N.   Psychological factors and reticuloendothelial disease: II. Observations on a group of women with lymphomas and leukemias. *Psychosom. Med.* 18:284, 1956.

Hewitt, D.   Some features of leukemia mortality. *Brit. J. Prev. Soc. Med.* 9:81, 1955.

LeShan, L.   Psychological states as factors in the development of malignant disease: A critical review. *J. Nat. Cancer Inst.* 22:1, 1959.

LeShan, L., Marvin, S., and Lyerly, O.   Some evidence of a relationship between Hodgkin's disease and intelligence. *A.M.A. Arch. Gen. Psychiat.* 1:477, 1959.

LeShan, L., and Worthington, R. E.   Some recurrent life history patterns observed in patients with malignant disease. *J. Nerv. Ment. Dis.* 124:460, 1956.

Zinsser, H.   *As I Remember Him. The Biography of R. S.* Boston: Little, Brown, 1940.

24. BIOCHEMICAL THERAPEUTICS OF ACUTE LEUKEMIA

Thomas C. Hall

THE IDEAL therapeutic goal in acute leukemia is cure. However, with the exception of about 100 patients who have been free of disease for more than 10 years and may thus be "cured," a more realistic goal is the induction of a remission. Remissions may occur in peripheral blood with the disappearance of abnormal forms which, however, persist in the marrow. In marrow remissions, normalization of the peripheral blood picture is accompanied by improvement in the marrow differential. The degree of remission can be partial, involving a marked reduction in the total blast count and percentage of leukemic blasts infiltrating the blood or marrow; or it may be complete, with the abnormal blasts reduced to less than 5%, a level not distinguishable by microscopy from that seen in normal marrow and blood, and accompanied by disappearance of all other evidence of organ infiltration such as splenomegaly, lymphadenopathy, anemia, thrombocytopenia, or granulocytopenia. Remission must occur before a cure can be expected, and remissions are accompanied by increased length and quality of survival.

The total number of leukemic cells in the body that are required for a clinical or morphologic diagnosis to be made is approximately 1 kg, or 10^{12} cells. Patients who have had complete marrow remission and died of other causes have been found at autopsy to harbor colonies of leukemic cells in various organs to an estimated volume of 10 to 100 gm, or 10^{10} to 10^{11} cells. Hence a clinically "complete" remission can occur when the initial number of cells has been reduced to 1/10 to 1/100 or less of the initial volume, and the number of cells remaining as a "body burden" can vary

This work was supported by Grants Ca 11198 and 11083 and Contract pH 69-39 of the National Cancer Institute.

309

considerably. Patients in whom the remaining fraction is small—e.g., 10^6, or 0.0001%, of the initial volume—will continue in remission longer than those in whom a larger number of residual cells remains. A cure cannot be expected until the number of cells killed approaches 10^{11} or 10^{12}; and in order to decrease the number remaining at the time of clinical remission, continued therapy is necessary for periods of time which correlate with the rate at which clinical remission was induced. For example, if it takes 2 months for the body burden to be reduced by 4 logs from 10^{12} to 10^8, therapy should be continued for 6 additional months, the period needed for a further decrease from 10^8 to 10^0. After 10^9 cells have been killed, if the remaining cells are alive because they are relatively drug resistant, even longer therapy may be needed. However, it may not be necessary to use multiple drugs to cause the killing of the last few "logs" of cells. A single agent or several agents given one at a time during remission may also have the desired antileukemic effect as well as sparing the normal marrow blasts.

Bacteria, when reduced to a comparably small residual number, are destroyed by normal phagocytic and immunologic mechanisms. Unfortunately, leukemic cells are not similarly recognized and destroyed by the host. Various attempts have been made to stimulate immunologic recognition and rejection of leukemic cells experimentally, including the use of irradiated leukemic cells as antigens, BCG vaccination, and interferon inducers such as poly-inosinic-cytidylic acid (Poly-IC). None of these has yet been shown to have clinically exploitable benefits.

ACUTE LYMPHOBLASTIC LEUKEMIA

Acute lymphoblastic leukemia (ALL) accounts for four-fifths of the cases of acute leukemia in children and one-fifth of cases in adults. Agents which are effective in inducing remission include folic acid antimetabolite analogs such as methotrexate (MTX), antipurines such as 6-mercaptopurine (6MP), and pyrimidine analogs such as cytarabine (CA). Each of these used alone causes remission in about 40% of patients. The alkylating agent cyclophosphamide induces remission in about 20% of patients. Adrenal corticoids, such as prednisone, and vincristine, an alkaloid of the common garden periwinkle, also induce remission in about 40% of patients. The duration of single-drug-induced remissions is usually short, implying a restricted ability of these single agents to kill leukemic blasts. In addition, prednisone, vincristine, and cyclophosphamide appear to have a restricted capacity to maintain such remissions, suggesting rapid development of drug resistance. Hence multiple-drug therapy has been tried and has resulted in increased numbers of remissions of prolonged duration. The single-drug dosages, routes, and rate of complete drug response are shown in Table 24-1. Modes of action of the drugs are listed in Table 24-2. Sites of action are

Table 24-1. Drugs and Dosages Employed in the Therapy of Acute Myelogenous and Acute Lymphoblastic Leukemia

Name	Type	Dosage	Route	Schedule	Complete Responses Induced (%) ALL	AML	Principal Side Effects
Prednisone[a]	Corticoid	1–3 mg/kg	PO	Daily	40	—	Cushing's syndrome
Methotrexate	Antifol	0.5 mg/kg	IV or IM	Twice weekly	40	10	Myelosuppression, stomatitis
6-Mercaptopurine	Antipurine	3 mg/kg	PO	Daily	40	10	Myelosuppression
Vincristine[a]	Periwinkle alkaloid	50 µg/kg	IV	Weekly	40	—	Neurotoxicity, alopecia
Cytarabine	Antipyrimidine	25 mg/kg or 30–300 mg/m²	IV pulse IV infusion	Twice weekly Daily, days 1–4	40	25	Nausea, myelosuppression
Cyclophosphamide	Alkylating agent	20 mg/kg	IV	Weekly	20	—	Alopecia, myelosuppression, nausea
L-Asparaginase[a]	Enzyme	1000 units/kg	IV	Weekly	40	—	Bleeding, anaphylaxis, pancreatitis, myelosuppression
Daunorubicin	*Streptomyces* antibiotic	1–2 mg/kg (total 30 mg/kg)	IV	Twice weekly	25	60	Myelosuppression, cardiotoxicity, stomatitis
Thioguanine[b]	Antipurine	25 mg/kg	PO	Daily	—	40	Myelosuppression

[a] These drugs are not generally thought to be of use in the treatment of acute myeloblastic leukemia.
[b] AML only (in conjunction with cytarabine).
ALL = acute lymphoblastic leukemia; AML = acute myelogenous leukemia.

Table 24-2. Mode of Action of Antileukemic Drugs

Drug	Action
Prednisone	Impairs integrity of leukemic lymphocyte cell membrane; acts independently of mitotic cycle
Methotrexate	Inhibits dihydrofolic reductase; interferes with methylation of deoxyuridylate to thymidine; blocks incorporation of C_2 and C_8 into hypoxanthine skeleton, thus interfering with endogenous synthesis of purine and pyrimidine bases of DNA; may also affect thymidylate synthetase, RNA methylation, and protein synthesis; acts in G_1 and early S phase of mitotic cycle
Vincristine	Interferes with tRNA synthesis; blocks proper function of cytoplasmic microtubules; microtubules in mitotic spindle cell apparatus damaged; microtubules in nervous tissue also impaired; acts during late S and M phases
6-Mercaptopurine	Blocks conversion of phosphoribosylpyrophosphate to phosphoribosylamine; blocks conversion of inosinic acid to adenylate and guanylate; blocks new DNA synthesis; acts during S phase of mitotic cycle
Cytarabine	Inhibits DNA polymerase and ribotide reductase; blocks reduction of cytidine to deoxycytidine; blocks incorporation of nucleotides into new DNA; is incorporated into RNA; at high doses shows immediate cytocidal effects; acts primarily in S phase
Cyclophosphamide	Alkylates preformed DNA and forms covalent bonds between DNA helixes; alkylates sugar-phosphate links and disrupts lengths of DNA chains; alkylates RNA; at higher doses alkylates enzymes and interferes with energy production; acts relatively independently of mitotic cycle

diagrammatically shown in Figure 24-1. With a combination of 3 or 4 of the first 4 drugs listed in the two tables, virtually all patients with ALL experience a complete remission; with continued therapy, 30% of patients remain in remission for almost 4 years, during which time they are virtually normal in all respects.

Relapse usually occurs, however, accompanied by resistance to one or more of the drugs used in the combination. At this point the agents to which the patient is resistant should be withdrawn and new agents added. In the second echelon of drugs, cytosine arabinoside, cyclophosphamide, and L-asparaginase are currently used. The first has recently been released for marketing, but with it, as with the other two, short-lived remissions are the rule. L-Asparaginase is interesting in that it is the first enzyme to be used extensively in the induction of remissions in leukemia. However, remissions are confined to acute lymphoblastic leukemia, are short, and allergic reac-

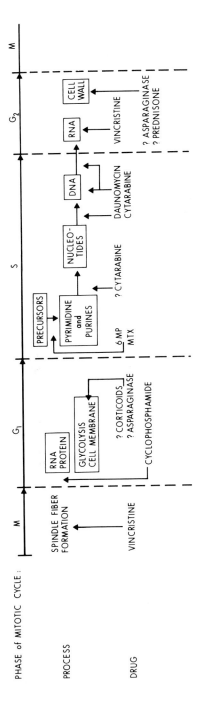

Figure 24-1. Possible sites of action of antileukemic drugs.

tions and drug toxicity are high; the drug therefore is currently of primarily theoretical and experimental interest. Table 24-3 summarizes the current status of chemotherapy for ALL using combinations of agents that induce or maintain remissions.

ACUTE MYELOGENOUS LEUKEMIA

The cells of acute myelogenous leukemia (AML) are markedly more resistant to drugs than are those of ALL. This may be because the myeloblasts are more "at home" in the marrow. They divide more slowly—5 days doubling time versus 1 day in ALL—and hence have a smaller fraction of the leukemic mass synthesizing DNA at any given instant. This results in less sensitivity to antimetabolites than is seen with leukemic lymphoblasts. The myeloblasts may produce rather differentiated, nonproliferating, long-lived daughter cells with a high tendency to pass from marrow to peripheral blood and circulate there, but which are not responsive to antimetabolites.

The drugs most commonly used in the therapy of ALL are also used for AML but with much less benefit. Prednisone may actually decrease survival; vincristine rarely shows any antileukemic effect when given alone; and L-asparaginase, even at high doses, only rarely has shown any effect. The remaining drugs have much lower response rates in AML than in ALL.

Table 24-3. Initial Remission Inductions with Combination Chemotherapy for Acute Lymphocytic Leukemia

Agents	Complete Response Rate (%)	Investigators
Prednisone + vincristine	84	Selawry et al. (1965)
Prednisone + 6-mercaptopurine	82	Frei et al. (1961), Freireich et al. (1963), Krivit et al. (1966)
Prednisone + methotrexate	80	Frei et al. (1961), Krivit et al. (1966)
Methotrexate + 6-mercaptopurine	45	Frei et al. (1965)
Methotrexate + 6-mercaptopurine + prednisone + vincristine	94	Freireich et al. (1964)
Prednisone + vincristine + daunorubicin	100	Henderson (1969), Mathé et al. (1970)

SOURCE: From G. Mathé (Ed.), *Advances in the Treatment of Acute (Blastic) Leukemias.* New York: Springer-Verlag, 1970.

Combinations have increased the response to 50% and have prolonged survival in responding patients.

Table 24-4 shows some of the reported experiences with chemotherapy of AML. It appears that cytarabine used with 6-thioguanine, cyclophosphamide, or with the combination of cyclophosphamide, vincristine, and prednisone is the best current regimen. We prefer to give the cytarabine in direct intravenous pulses once or twice weekly, since little advantage appears to be gained from prolonged infusions, and patients are able to remain ambulatory and with their families for a longer period of time on intermittent regimens. However, the duration of response is often short and maintenance therapy both necessary and difficult. One of the most pressing clinical problems associated with inducing remissions in AML is that of rapid death due to infection and hemorrhage: half the patients die within 3 weeks after institution of therapy, whereas therapy is needed for 4 to 6 weeks to induce a remission. Modern techniques of platelet and granulocyte transfusion and proper use of antibiotics may help keep these patients alive until a remission has time to occur. Even the discovery of a totally curative drug for AML could not contribute maximally to the care of these patients without all community resources for supportive therapy being simultaneously mobilized to carry the patient through the high-risk period required for remission induction.

When used alone, the currently available agents are not as effective in AML as they are in ALL. Therefore, when they are not given in combina-

Table 24-4. Reported Experience in Chemotherapy of Acute Myelogenous Leukemia

Agent	Complete Marrow Remissions in Adequate Trials (%)	Reference
Methotrexate	30	Huguley et al. (1965)
6-Mercaptopurine	20	Freireich et al. (1970), Henderson (1969)
MOAP [a]	35	Thompson et al. (1965)
Cytarabine	25	Henderson et al. (1968), Howard et al. (1968)
Cytarabine + 6-thioguanine	50	Gee et al. (1969)
Cytarabine + cyclophosphamide	50	Freireich et al. (1970)
COAP [b]	71	Freireich et al. (1970)

[a] MOAP = 6-mercaptopurine + vincristine + methotrexate + prednisone.
[b] COAP = cyclophosphamide + vincristine + cytarabine + prednisone.

tion, they are usually administered in doses of larger size, for longer periods before remission induction, and more aggressively. Because of this and because multiple-drug combinations are often finally needed to induce remissions, toxicity must be expected. With vincristine and cyclophosphamide, temporary alopecia may result and be psychologically disturbing to adult women, who therefore should always be informed of this possibility. Vincristine may give rise to troublesome neuropathy, manifested as constipation progressing to acroparesthesia and anesthesia after a month of therapy. Rarely, high doses (greater than 2 mg per week of vincristine) may affect the central nervous system with resultant convulsions. Hemorrhagic cystitis may occur following the prolonged use of cyclophosphamide or its intravenous administration to dehydrated patients. Hydration prior to therapy is of help in preventing this complication. Cytosine arabinoside can cause nausea —particularly when given in large, single, direct intravenous injections— and liberal use of antiemetics may be desirable. Daunorubicin may cause cardiac arrhythmias if infused too rapidly; a half-hour infusion is desirable. Late cardiac toxicity from daunorubicin can be prevented by not exceeding a total dosage of 40 mg per kilogram of body weight.

The acute myeloblastic leukemia that commonly occurs in the end stages of chronic myelocytic leukemia is often referred to as "blastic crisis" or "blastic transformation." The course is frequently very short and virulent, and this form of AML seems unusually unresponsive to chemotherapy. The reasons for this are not known. Table 24-5 shows the poor experience obtained in this condition with the same agents which are of use in ALL and in other forms of AML.

BIOCHEMICAL BASES FOR DRUG SENSITIVITY AND RESISTANCE

Effective chemotherapy depends upon the interrelation of factors in host, drug, and target cell. These factors are only partially understood for each of the several drugs involved, but utilization of what is known can enable more effective drug regimens to be set up.

METHOTREXATE

The drug methotrexate inhibits dihydrofolate reductase. When given in greater amounts than the usual therapeutic doses it also inhibits thymidylate synthetase, liver alcohol dehydrogenase, and might theoretically interfere with RNA and protein synthesis. The human host handles the drug largely by renal excretion, without catabolic changes; this is in contrast to other host species such as the rabbit, in which the drug is much less toxic

Table 24-5.   Chemotherapy for Blastic Crisis of Chronic Myelocytic Leukemia

Drug	Response Rate	Reference
Methotrexate	$< \frac{1}{10}$	Huguley et al. (1965)
6-Mercaptopurine	$< \frac{1}{10}$	Ellison & Burchenal (1960)
Prednisone	$\frac{1}{4}$	Bousser et al. (1970), Cattan et al. (1970)
Hydroxyurea	0	Carbone et al. (1970)
Vincristine	$\frac{3}{10}$	Cattan et al. (1970)
Cytarabine	$\frac{1}{9}$	Carbone et al. (1970), Cattan et al. (1970)
MOAP [a]	$\frac{3}{10}$	Thompson et al. (1965)
Cytarabine + bischloroethylnitrosourea	$\frac{1}{13}$	Carbone et al. (1970)
POMP [b]	$\frac{1}{13}$	Carbone et al. (1970)
Vincristine + prednisone	$\frac{3}{12}$	Carbone et al. (1970)
Methyl-GAG [c]	$\frac{2}{16}$	Carbone et al. (1970), Cattan et al. (1970)
GAG + prednisone	$\frac{1}{4}$	Bousser et al. (1970), Cattan et al. (1970)
GAG + rubidomycin	$\frac{1}{2}$	Bousser et al. (1970)

[a] MOAP = 6-mercaptopurine + vincristine + methotrexate + prednisone.
[b] POMP = prednisone + vincristine + methotrexate + 6-mercaptopurine.
[c] Methyl-GAG = methylglyoxalbisguanylhydrazone.

because of extensive hepatic degradation. The target tumor cell will be most sensitive to MTX if it has an active concentrative transport system for folinic acid, since MTX appears to share this uptake system. Mouse leukemia cells commonly can concentrate MTX intracellularly and are much more sensitive to the drug than are human cells, which permit only restricted entry of the drug.

Once inside the cell, MTX can work best in those leukemic cells which produce DNA thymidine from deoxyuridine, as opposed to those which depend more upon the "salvage" pathway in which thymidine, presumably from tissue breakdown, is reutilized preferentially to synthesize DNA for the chromosomes of new daughter leukemic cells. The amount of dihydrofolate reductase (dHFR), the target enzyme for methotrexate, contained in the leukemic cell is also a determinant of MTX sensitivity. This enzyme is usually, but not always, newly synthesized during the late G_1 and early S phases of mitosis, in quantities which are usually but not always just sufficient for the conversion of enough deoxyuridylate (UdR) to thymidylate (TdR) to permit the formation of the chromosomes of new daughter cells.

However, in some cells—e.g., polymorphonuclear leukocytes—an excess of enzyme is formed and stored, even though the cells are fully differentiated and nonmitotic. In addition, production of dHFR may be induced by exposure to MTX as well as other nontoxic pteridines such as the diuretic triamterene (2, 4, 7-triamino, 6-phenyl pteridine). Cells which have little dihydrofolic reductase because they use other pathways to provide the thymidylate necessary for DNA, as well as cells with a large excess of enzyme, may both show relative resistance to MTX. Fortunately, methods are available for measuring cell membrane transport of tritiated methotrexate, content of dihydrofolate reductase, and relative incorporation of UdR and TdR into DNA. In addition, one can measure the change in the rate of UdR and TdR incorporation into DNA as well as the percent inhibition of the initial level of dHFR after a single full therapeutic dose to the patient. Taken together, these values can give a very reasonable estimate of the degree of sensitivity of a particular human leukemia to methotrexate.

Studies carried out in our laboratory to date have indicated that leukemia cells which cannot take up MTX are not able to respond to the drug. Such transport-based resistance is found naturally in most acute myeloblastic leukemias, all chronic lymphocytic leukemias, but less than half of children with untreated acute lymphoblastic leukemia. When patients with acute lymphoblastic leukemia become resistant to methotrexate, loss of drug transport is invariably found, accompanied by high levels of dHFR which may not have been seen prior to the initiation of treatment.

Existence of drug transport and an intracellular level of dHFR is not enough per se to ensure the antileukemic action of MTX. The cell should also substantially depend upon the use of UdR as a precursor for DNA. Finally, when MTX is given and UdR incorporation inhibited, the cell should not have the ability to compensate by the use of TdR in place of UdR. This compensating phenomenon, probably related to an induction of thymidine kinase, usually presages the cell's ability to escape from methotrexate inhibition.

6-MERCAPTOPURINE

In the case of 6-mercaptopurine, entrance of the drug into the cell is by a process which resembles free diffusion. Although the cell membrane presents no barriers to the entrance of the drug, 6MP and most other antipurines and antipyrimidines must be converted into an active metabolite or nucleotide by phosphorylation. Such phosphorylated derivatives are charged and cannot be transported across mammalian cell membranes. Hence the active drug is retained within the cell and can act as a metabolic inhibitor of the processes shown in Figure 24-1. In the case of 6MP, ribose and phosphate are added in a single-step reaction catalyzed by the enzyme inosinic pyrophosphorylase. When this enzyme is deficient in intact leukemic cells, the patient's disease is unresponsive to 6MP. Inosinic pyrophosphorylase deficiency is found in about 60% of patients with acute lymphoblastic leukemia, 100% of those with chronic lymphocytic leukemia, 90% of those with acute myeloblastic leukemia, and 25% of those with chronic myeloid leukemia. These percentages closely parallel the known resistance rates of such patients to clinical treatment with 6MP.

As is the case with methotrexate, acquired resistance appears in most drug-sensitive patients who are treated with 6MP and lose this sensitivity with the passage of time. This form of resistance is also associated with the cell's loss of ability to retain the drug, presumably due to alteration or deletion of inosinic pyrophosphorylase or the acquisition of a phosphatase which breaks down the active metabolite 6MP ribose phosphate (6MPRP). For reasons at present poorly understood, intact cells must be used in order to do these correlative studies with 6MP. In patients whose cells show intermediate levels of phosphorylation not clearly falling into the ranges for clinical sensitivity or resistance, changes in the rate of DNA synthesis following a therapeutic pulse dose of 6MP can be used to identify sensitive cells. In these instances, DNA levels in blast cells fall to less than 25% of pretreatment values for periods of more than 24 hours, and both UdR and TdR are prevented from being incorporated.

CYTARABINE

With methotrexate, the target cell primarily contributes a variable level of transport as a determinant. In the case of 6MP the cell also contributes activating enzymes, possibly catabolic phosphatases, and a particular spatial arrangement found only in the intact cell. In the case of cytarabine, an analog of the nucleoside cytidine, the host assumes a more important role. This is because of the presence in the liver and other host tissues of a potent deaminating enzyme, cytidine deaminase, which converts CA into uracil arabinoside, an inactive metabolite. This enzyme is usually low at the institution of CA therapy and does not contribute to the determination of initial drug responsiveness, which is, as in the case of 6MP, related to the synthesis and retention of the phosphorylated and active metabolite. However, as time passes, initially sensitive patients develop drug resistance, which can be due to the deletion of deoxycytidine kinase or to the appearance in the serum of a deaminating enzyme, presumably of hepatic origin, which destroys CA before it can reach the target cells in amounts adequate for a therapeutic effect. This is accompanied by progressive shortening of the plasma half-life of a dose of administered CA. Oddly, the target cells' concentration of cytidine deaminase is not a factor in determining resistance, presumably because the deaminating enzyme is sequestered spatially or has an affinity for CA lower than that of the kinase. As with other drugs, however, retention of active drug within the cell is a necessary precondition of drug action, yet it does not guarantee drug effectiveness. Some greater precision in predicting drug efficacy, a measure of net effect, is needed. Since the primary action of cytosine arabinoside nucleoside is to inhibit DNA polymerase, an enzyme which uses TdR from whatever source, there should be uniform inhibition of both UdR and TdR incorporation into DNA in drug-sensitive cells following a clinical pulse dose.

PRESELECTION OF A DRUG REGIMEN

At least half the patients with acute lymphocytic leukemia develop drug resistance and relapse, and an even larger number of acute myelogenous leukemia patients are initially resistant to the usual drugs. It would therefore be helpful in establishing a therapeutic regimen to be able to select drugs to which the leukemic cells are sensitive. Conversely, if a patient could be identified as unable to respond to a specific agent, this could be omitted from his therapy. With current therapy, all patients are put on empirical drug combinations to which no more than half respond over a 4- to 6-week period. Since many die from hemorrhage or infection during this time, it would be very helpful to identify patients who are incapable of responding to traditional drugs and thus justify the earlier use in such patients of new and unusual therapies. As mentioned previously, workable methods for selecting possibly effective drugs can be based on either the uptake of the drug by whole cells in vitro or the inhibition of DNA synthesis upon the leukemic cells following test doses. The former methods are suitable for use with antimetabolite drugs for which patterns of uptake and metabolism are known and for which isotopically tagged forms are available. The pulse technique can also be applied to nonradioactive drugs, e.g., vincristine, daunorubicin, L-asparaginase, and drugs whose metabolic pathways are not known, e.g., prednisone, cyclophosphamide. By this technique, a sample of blood or marrow is examined for the rate of synthesis of a critical molecule —such as DNA, RNA, or cell membrane glycoprotein—before and at intervals after a single full clinical dose of a potentially useful drug. Inhibition of DNA synthesis by 75% for 24 to 48 hours following a single-drug dose often predicts a clinical response after 24 to 48 days of therapy. Lack of inhibition is almost always an index of clinical resistance to the drug being tested. Pulse test doses can be used to evaluate the clinical effectiveness of antimetabolites, singly or in combination, for which prior studies in vitro have shown levels of intracellular retention that lie in a "gray" or intermediate zone between the high uptakes usually associated with drug responsiveness and the low levels of drug resistance. Such pulses may also be used to clarify the significance of shortened plasma half-times of cytarabine and other drugs.

RESULTS OF IN VITRO PREDICTIVE BIOCHEMICAL STUDIES

Although Brockman found that the decrease of 6MP phosphorylation by mouse ascites leukemia extracts correlated well with the sensitivity of the whole leukemic cells to 6MP, Davidson and Winter failed to relate clinical responsiveness to 6MP to the levels of inosinic pyrophosphorylase in extracts of human leukemia. Adding drugs to cells cultured in vitro has not been valuable in helping to preselect effective drugs. Bertino found that changes in UdR incorporation into DNA by themselves were not always effective in predicting responses to MTX. By combining tests of drug uptake and retention with measurements of dihydrofolate reductase concentration and of relative utilization of UdR and TdR to the effects upon DNA synthesis within isolated cells in vitro of pulse doses of drugs given in vivo, we have been able to confirm or predict accurately the resistance or sensitivity to single drugs and combinations in 36 of 38 patients with acute myeloblastic leukemia and 13 of 14 patients with acute lymphocytic leukemia. Such studies are difficult to accomplish properly because of the difficulty of obtaining adequate amounts of representative leukemic cells, at the proper intervals, for all the analyses required. In addition the techniques are still difficult, painstaking, and expensive, so that at present they represent a method which has promise for the future rather than broad general applicability. It is to be hoped that precise selection of single drugs and combinations for positive benefits can be attained. However, even at present if drug-resistant patients can be identified with precision, the early use of new and experimental agents or of expensive and arduous gut-sterilization and environmental sterilization may be justified on such poor-risk patients to protect them during intensive therapy regimens for long periods of time and to enable greater degrees of bone marrow suppression to be achieved.

REFERENCES

Acute Leukemia Group B. Studies of sequential and combination antimetabolite therapy in acute leukemia. *Blood* 18:431, 1961.
Acute Leukemia Group B. The effect of 6-mercaptopurine on the duration of steroid-induced remission in acute leukemia. *Blood* 21:699, 1963.
Acute Leukemia Group B. The effectiveness of combinations of antileukemic agents in inducing and maintaining remission in children with acute leukemia. *Blood* 26:642, 1965a.

Acute Leukemia Group B. New treatment schedule with improved survival in childhood leukemia, *J.A.M.A.* 194:75, 1965b.

Bernard, J., Weil, M., Levy, J. P., Seligman, M., and Najean, Y. Étude de la rémission complète des leucémies aigues. *Nouv. Rev. Franc. Hemat.* 2:195, 1962.

Bertino, J., Hyrniak, W. M., and Capizzi, R. Prediction of Methotrexate Responsiveness of Tumors in Man. In T. C. Hall (Ed.), *Prediction of Response to Antitumor Therapies.* (Monograph No. 34.) Washington: National Cancer Institute.

Bodey, G. P., Luce, J. K., Harris, J. E., and Frei, E., III. The effect of cytosine arabinoside (CA) on metastatic cancer and acute leukemia (AL). *Int. Congr. Hemat.* 12:6, 1968.

Bousser, J., Bilski-Pasquiee, G., Briere, J., and Reyes, F. Blastic Crisis in Chronic Leukemia and Polycythemia Vera. In G. Mathé (Ed.), *Advances in the Treatment of Acute (Blastic) Leukemias.* New York: Springer, 1970.

Carbone, P. P., Canellos, G. P., and DeVita, V. T. Therapy of the Blastic Phase of Chronic Granulocytic Leukemia. In G. Mathé (Ed.), *Advances in the Treatment of Acute (Blastic) Leukemias.* New York: Springer, 1970.

Cattan, A., Mathé, G., Amiel, J. L., Schlumberger, J. R., Schwartzenberg, L., Schneider, M., and Berumen, L. Treatment of Blastic Crisis in Chronic Myelocytic Leukemia. In G. Mathé (Ed.), *Advances in the Treatment of Acute (Blastic) Leukemias.* New York: Springer, 1970.

Davidson, J. D., and Winter, T. S. Purine nucleotide phosphorylases in 6-mercaptopurine-sensitive and -resistant human leukemias. *Cancer Res.* 24:261, 1964.

Ellison, R. R., and Burchenal, J. H. Treatment of chronic granulocytic leukemia with the 6-substituted purines, 6-mercaptopurine, thioguanine and 6-chloropurine. *Clin. Pharmacol. Ther.* 1:631, 1960.

Freireich, E. J., Bodey, G. P., Hart, J., Rodriguez, V., Whitecar, J. P., and Frei, E., III. Remission Induction in Adults with Acute Myelogenous Leukemia. In G. Mathé (Ed.), *Advances in the Treatment of Acute (Blastic) Leukemias.* New York: Springer, 1970.

Freireich, E. J., Karon, M., and Frei, E., III. Quadruple therapy (VAMP) for acute lymphocytic leukemia of childhood. *Proc. Amer. Ass. Cancer Res.* 5:20, 1964.

Gee, T. S., Yu, K. P., and Clarkson, B. D. Treatment of adult acute leukemia with arabinosylcytosine and thioguanine. *Cancer* 23:1019, 1969.

Henderson, E., Serpick, A., Leventhal, B., and Henry, P. Cytosine arabinoside infusions in adult and childhood acute myelocytic leukemia. *Proc. Amer. Ass. Cancer Res.* 9:29, 1968.

Henderson, E. S. Treatment of acute leukemia. *Seminars Hemat.* 6:271, 1969.

Howard, J. P., Albo, V., and Newton, W. A., Jr. Cytosine arabinoside: Results of a cooperative study in acute childhood leukemia. *Cancer* 21:341, 1968.

Huguley, C. M., Jr., Vogler, W. R., Lea, J. W., Corley, C. C., Jr., and Lowery, M. E. Acute leukemia treated with divided doses of methotrexate. *Arch. Intern. Med.* (Chicago) 115:23, 1965.

Kessel, D., Hall, T. C., and Rosenthal, D. Uptake and phosphorylation of cytosine arabinoside by normal and leukemic blood cells in vitro. *Cancer Res.* 29:459, 1969.

Knospry, W. H., and Conrad, M. E. The danger of corticosteroids in acute granulocytic leukemia. *Med. Clin. N. Amer.* 50:1653, 1966.

Krivit, W., Brubaker, C., Hartmann, J., Murphy, M. L., Pierce, M., and Thatcher, G.   Induction of remission in acute leukemia of childhood by combination of prednisone and either 6-mercaptopurine or methotrexate. *J. Pediat.* 68:965, 1966.

Mathé, G., Amiel, J. L., Schwartzenberg, L., Cattan, A., Hayat, M., deVassal, F., and Schlumberger, J. R.   Methods and Strategy for the Treatment of Acute Lymphoblastic Leukemia. In G. Mathé (Ed.), *Advances in the Treatment of Acute (Blastic) Leukemias*. New York: Springer, 1970.

Mathé, G., Schwartzenberg, L., Mery, A. M., Cattan, A., Schneider, M., Amiel, J. L., Schlumberger, J. R., Poisson, J., and Wajcner, G.   Extensive histological and cytological survey of patients with acute leukemia in "complete remission." *Brit. Med. J.* 1:640, 1966.

Roberts, D., and Hall, T. C.   Enzyme activities and deoxynucleoside utilization of leukemia leukocytes in relation to drug therapy and resistance. *Cancer Res.* 29:166, 1969.

Roberts, D., Hall, T. C., and Rosenthal, D.   Coordinated changes in biochemical patterns: The effect of cytosine arabinoside and methotrexate on leukocytes from patients with acute granulocytic leukemia. *Cancer Res.* 29:571, 1969.

Thompson, I., Hall, T. C., and Moloney, W. C.   Combination therapy of adult acute myelogenous leukemia: Experience with the simultaneous use of vincristine, amethopterin, 6-mercaptopurine and prednisone. *New Eng. J. Med.* 273:1302, 1965.

25. POLYCYTHEMIA VERA

Arthur W. Bauman

THE MYELOPROLIFERATIVE DISORDERS: A UNIFYING CONCEPT

The many similarities shared by polycythemia vera, chronic myelogenous leukemia, and myelofibrosis with myeloid metaplasia have led to proposals that they may have a single origin and that they may be classified under the general term *myeloproliferative disorders.* It has been suggested that neoplastic proliferation of a multipotential stem cell capable of differentiating along multiple lines is the primary defect. The eventual clinical disorder is determined by the pattern taken by the particular lines of proliferation that follow (Fig. 25-1). In polycythemia vera, erythroid proliferation is dominant; in chronic myelogenous leukemia, granulocytes proliferate. In myelofibrosis, extramedullary hematopoiesis (myeloid metaplasia) is a prominent feature early in the disease, and it is often present early in polycythemia vera. In all these disorders other marrow elements, including the megakaryocytes, are capable of excessive proliferation. Fibroblastic activity in the marrow, and to some extent in the reticuloendothelial system elsewhere, occurs in varying degrees in both polycythemia vera and chronic myelogenous leukemia. Osteoblastic and osteoclastic proliferation usually is not so obvious in these disorders but occasionally may be the presenting problem rather than myelofibrosis.

It is well to keep in mind that fibroblasts are essentially incapable of leaving the site of production, as opposed to the other cellular products of marrow proliferation; hence replacement of marrow will occur secondary to fibroblastic activity but not secondary to proliferation of the other precursor cells, and the clinical significance of fibroblastic activity depends on the degree of such proliferation. This view makes it easier to understand why fibrosis may be the initial problem in some myeloproliferative disorders, the end stage in others, and an insignificant postmortem finding in still others.

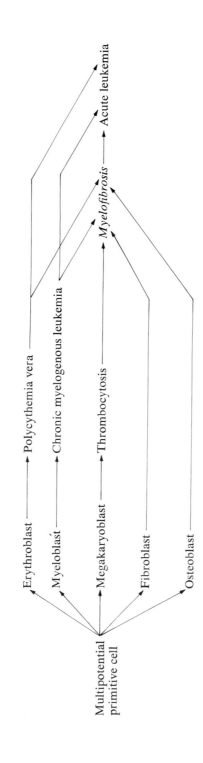

Figure 25-1. The myeloproliferative disorders. The clinical disorder reflects the pattern of proliferation taken primarily by the undifferentiated stem cell. Proliferation of more than one cell line is common in these diseases, however. Myelofibrosis occurs frequently, and acute myeloblastic leukemia may be the terminal event. (Adapted from H. N. Robson, *Aust. Ann. Med.* 2:170, 1953.)

The common pathway often followed by the myeloproliferative disorders is the development of varying degrees of myelofibrosis and extramedullary hematopoiesis (myeloid metaplasia). Terminally acute leukemia may occur. Otherwise these disorders, particularly chronic myelogenous leukemia and polycythemia vera, do not evolve into each other. That is, patients with an established diagnosis of one disorder do not develop the other, although features of one disorder may be present in the other. Marked erythrocytosis is almost never seen in chronic myelogenous leukemia. Patients with polycythemia vera and myeloid metaplasia, while their condition may appear superficially to resemble a "chronic leukemic" phase at some point in their disease, do not usually meet the other criteria for chronic myelogenous leukemia.

The possible contribution of radioactive phosphorus (^{32}P) to the evolution of acute leukemia in polycythemia vera has recently received much attention. The incidence of acute leukemia is significantly higher in patients with polycythemia vera who have been treated with ^{32}P, but it has also been emphasized that patients who have received ^{32}P live longer than those who have not received it. Resolution of this controversy may be achieved through treatment studies which are being carried out at several centers at the present time.

POLYCYTHEMIA VERA: THE CLINICAL PICTURE

Polycythemia vera usually develops in middle age. It is more common in men than women in a ratio of 1.5 to 1 and is rare in Negroes. The symptoms of polycythemia vera at the outset are usually attributable to the high hematocrit level and the accompanying increased blood viscosity and volume. Increasing splenic enlargement and left upper quadrant discomfort may be initial findings. Thromboembolic phenomena and excessive bleeding following minor trauma or surgery may also be presenting signs and are attributable to increased blood volume and viscosity or to the thrombocytosis. White blood cell proliferation causes still other symptoms. Excessive pruritus, particularly after a hot bath, correlates with increased numbers of basophils, which are rich in histamine. The high incidence of peptic ulcer and hemorrhagic gastritis in these patients may also be related to excessive histamine release. Attacks of gout or of nephrolithiasis may be presenting complications secondary to increased urate production caused by the increase in nucleoprotein turnover. Splenomegaly is present in about 70% of affected patients and hepatomegaly in about half. Lymph node enlargement is not seen.

The most common laboratory finding is erythrocytosis, reflected by a hematocrit level greater than 55%. The white cell count is usually elevated, ranging between 10,000 and 30,000 per cubic millimeter. The dominant cell is the polymorphonuclear leukocyte, but increases in the absolute number of eosinophils, basophils, and monocytes are also frequently present. Platelets generally are increased, ranging from greater than normal to as high as a million per cubic millimeter. At the outset of the disease the red cells in the peripheral blood smear are usually normochromic and normocytic, although fragmentation tends gradually to become more prominent as time goes on. Erythroid and myeloid immaturity can often be demonstrated early in the disease in buffy coat preparations.

Iron kinetic studies and assessment of hemoglobin production with ^{15}N glycine, coupled with observations that the red cell survival is normal or only slightly decreased in polycythemia vera, indicate that the rate of production of red cells is increased in this disorder. The marrow hypercellularity and high white cell and platelet counts, coupled with the data obtained with red cells, imply that the rate of production of these cells is also increased. Erythropoietin levels are normal or diminished, and neither a stimulus for nor the lack of a normal inhibition of proliferation in this disease has been detected.

COURSE OF THE DISORDER

The course of this disease may be quite variable. Subtle symptoms such as vague left upper quadrant discomfort and pruritus may antedate the clinical diagnosis for from 2 to 7 years. After the diagnosis is established the disease may persist for up to 12 years, offering various therapeutic challenges, depending on the symptoms and complications. Eventually the spleen becomes increasingly large, and anemia often develops. During this phase of the disease, the diagnosis of myeloid metaplasia and myelofibrosis is usually apparent and can be established by careful evaluation on the peripheral blood smear and by bone marrow biopsy. Late in the course of the disease, with or without myeloid metaplasia and myelofibrosis but more commonly when these changes have developed, acute leukemia evolves as the terminal disorder.

About 50% of patients with polycythemia vera die of some disorder not necessarily related to the disease. Cardiovascular diseases and their complications, even in treated polycythemia vera patients, are the most common cause of death.

DIFFERENTIAL DIAGNOSIS

Differentiating polycythemia vera from secondary polycythemia does not present a problem in the majority of cases. Occasionally, when the only finding is an increase in red cell mass indicated by the hematocrit level, differentiation becomes a significant challenge. A good history and physical examination should eliminate most of the obvious causes of secondary polycythemia; the major causes are listed in Table 25-1. Some of the more subtle means of differentiating polycythemia vera and secondary polycythemia include an elevated leukocyte alkaline phosphatase, an elevated serum vitamin B_{12} or serum vitamin B_{12}–binding capacity, and increased blood and urine histamine levels in polycythemia vera, all these measurements being normal in secondary polycythemia. Conversely, erythropoietin levels are increased in secondary polycythemia and are normal or decreased in polycythemia vera. The serum uric acid may be increased in both disorders, and the red cell mass and blood volume are increased in both disorders. Perhaps the most difficult problem of differential diagnosis lies in separating out patients with so-called stress polycythemia who have a normal red cell mass but a decreased plasma volume.

MANAGEMENT

Polycythemia vera is a myeloproliferative disorder of unknown etiology in which the predominant initial abnormality is erythrocytosis in the absence of any increase in erythropoietin level. While it is true that most patients have an excessive red cell mass as the dominant feature, many of the other problems encountered in this disease are not affected and may actually get worse if treated by phlebotomy alone. These include the complications of increased myeloid activity, such as increased urate production and

Table 25-1. Causes of Secondary Polycythemia

Hypoxemia with increased erythropoietin
    Congenital heart disease
    Chronic lung disease
    High altitude
    Hypoventilation
    Reduced O_2-carrying capacity (hemoglobin M, DPNH diaphorase deficiency, deficient synthesis of glutathione)
    Increased O_2 affinity (hemoglobin Ranier, etc.)

Increased erythropoietin
    Renal disease (usually characterized by fluid-retaining lesions and/or local hypoxia)
    Carcinoma of liver, cirrhosis
    Cerebellar hemangioblastoma
    Uterine myomas

---

excessive histamine production, and increased megakaryocytic activity with resultant thrombocytosis and either bleeding or thrombotic tendencies. The white cell count alone is not an indication for treatment. The platelet count may be, particularly for levels above one million per cubic millimeter, at which thrombotic and bleeding episodes are more likely to be encountered. The mechanisms of both these phenomena are complex and poorly understood at this time. The spleen usually increases slowly in size, but symptomatic splenomegaly generally does not develop until myeloid metaplasia and myelofibrosis are evident. In a few patients hypermetabolism may dictate therapeutic intervention.

Over the years various modes of therapy, particularly radioactive phosphorus, have been introduced in the management of this disorder and clearly have lengthened survival from a mean of 5 to 7 years, when phlebotomy alone was being used, to about 13 years at the present time.

PHLEBOTOMY

Phlebotomy is still the treatment of choice early in the course of polycythemia vera. As the hematocrit level rises above 60%, the blood viscosity increases substantially. This occurs because at a hematocrit level above 60%, the blood viscosity becomes a reflection of erythrocyte deformability, since at that concentration red cells must deform to occupy the space that each fills. Such elevated hematocrit values enhance the likelihood of spontaneous thrombosis, which is more likely to occur anyway in this age group. Thus hematocrit readings over 55% indicate the need for phlebotomy, and it is advised that 500 ml of blood be removed daily or every other day until the hematocrit reaches a level of approximately 40 to 45%. Subsequent phlebotomy requirements are dependent on the rate of elevation of the hematocrit level. Repeated phlebotomies eventually may result in iron deficiency, and the patient may develop symptoms of lethargy and fatigue out of proportion to the level of his hematocrit under such circumstances. If this develops, iron may have to be administered and another approach employed to keep the hematocrit level down.

It is our practice to use phlebotomy alone in those patients in whom it is possible to control the hematocrit level by bleeding them once every 2 to 3 months, or in patients in whom the other complications of this disease are not playing a dominant role. Sooner or later, however, phlebotomies are not enough and other measures have to be introduced.

IRRADIATION

For many years radioactive phosphorus has been used and has been a most effective means of treating polycythemia vera. Its main advantage has been that it induces remissions lasting anywhere from 6 months to several years, during which the patient need not be followed continually. The radioactive phosphorus is concentrated in the nucleoprotein of the proliferating cells and later in the phosphate of the bone cells, so that the maximum effects of the beta radiation are exerted at these selected sites. The recommended dose is usually 3 to 5 millicuries intravenously, and 4 to 28 weeks may be required before the maximum effect of this treatment is noted. Treatments are usually repeated in about 12 weeks if the desired effect has not been achieved, with a limit of 6 to 7 millicuries administered in any 6-month period. ^{32}P has also been given by mouth, but its absorption is irregular and unpredictable, and this approach is not recommended. With each treatment there may be a progressive drop in the platelets and white cells, but this is not necessarily a contraindication to ^{32}P unless these cellular elements drop to dangerously low levels.

Because ^{32}P may contribute to the development of acute leukemia late in the course of polycythemia vera, we tend to reserve ^{32}P therapy for patients who are over the age of 40 or whose disease is refractory to other measures.

Splenic irradiation is discussed in the chapter on myeloid metaplasia. It rarely is necessary early in the management of polycythemia vera.

CHEMOTHERAPY

Alkylating agents have been found to be effective in the control of polycythemia vera, and favorable reports have been made by Wasserman and Gilbert. In view of the controversy concerning ^{32}P it may be advisable to use these drugs as the first line of therapy beyond phlebotomy, although insufficient data are available to exclude any possible influence of alkylation in the development of leukemia. Of all patients receiving alkylation therapy, 80 to 85% have had a remission regardless of the choice of alkylating agent. The dosages of these drugs and the complications of their use are summarized in Table 25-2.

It is well to note that the dosages of all these preparations are somewhat lower for polycythemia vera than for other proliferative disorders. These low dosages reflect the increased sensitivity of patients with polycythemia vera to marrow suppressants in general, which may in part be explained by marrow replacement by fibrous tissue and by varying degrees of hypersplenism, if the spleen does not respond as sensitively as the marrow.

Uracil mustard may be effective in some patients in whom the dominant problem is thrombocytosis. Pipobroman (Vercyte), another alkylating agent, does not appear to have any distinct advantages, though an occasional patient might benefit from it, particularly if he is unable for one reason or another to take the other drugs mentioned. Melphalan (Alkeran), still another alkylating agent, has been found to be effective and has a low incidence of side effects.

In addition to becoming depleted of iron secondary to phlebotomy, some

Table 25-2. *Alkylating Agents for the Treatment of Polycythemia Vera*

Dosage and Complications	Agent		
	Busulfan	Chlorambucil	Cyclophosphamide
Initial dosage	4–6 mg/day for about 4–6 weeks	6–8 mg/day for about 20 weeks	100–150 mg/day for about 14 weeks
Maintenance regimen	Repeat initial dosage after 4 weeks off therapy; or 2 mg q.d. or q.o.d.	Same as busulfan	Repeat initial dosage after 4 weeks off therapy; or 50 mg q.d. or q.o.d.
Complications (% of patients)			
Thrombocytopenia ($< 100{,}000/mm^3$)	27	13	6
Leukopenia ($< 3{,}000/mm^3$)	5	4	2
Hemorrhagic cystitis	—	—	13
Gastrointestinal (anorexia, nausea, vomiting)	—	—	10
Alopecia	—	4	4
Skin rash, increased pruritus	2.5	4	4

NOTE: The white cells and platelets usually decrease before the red cells; hence phlebotomies are required during the initial phase of treatment. Busulfan may be preferable for patients with initially high platelet counts. Cyclophosphamide is the agent of choice if the pretreatment platelet counts are only slightly elevated or normal.
SOURCE: Adapted from L. R. Wasserman and H. S. Gilbert, *Med. Clin. N. Amer.* 50:1501,1966.

patients, because of the increased proliferative turnover of marrow precursor cells and concomitant hypersplenism, may become folate-depleted. This complication should be kept in mind with any patient who does not seem to be responding to therapy as might have been predicted or who has become excessively sensitive to an alkylating agent. Megaloblastic changes in the marrow are essential to establish the diagnosis, which can usually be corroborated by a low serum folate level, although a low serum folate level per se does not invariably mean that the folate stores are depleted (see Chap. 2).

The hyperuricemia of polycythemia vera is usually managed by administration of allopurinol in doses of 100 mg three times a day. This approach need not necessarily be continued if the disease is being brought under control concomitantly by the use of alkylating agents or ^{32}P but may have to be used continuously if only phlebotomies are being employed and there is hyperuricemia.

TREATMENT OF ACUTE LEUKEMIA

No effective means of managing the acute leukemia that develops late in the course of polycythemia vera has been demonstrated. The same supportive measures discussed in Chapter 22 are recommended. If symptoms of hypermetabolism are present and proliferation of blast cells is a prominent feature, chemotherapy should also be considered when acute leukemia does develop. However, the marrow is usually largely replaced by fibrous tissue, and it is doubtful that aggressive chemotherapy to ablate both the leukemic and residual normal marrow cells will be followed by a return of many normal marrow cells. Indeed, the age at which most patients with antecedent polycythemia vera develop acute leukemia is such that aggressive chemotherapy and its complications pose major problems, in themselves, for most patients.

SURGERY IN POLYCYTHEMIA VERA

The enormous risks from hemorrhage and thrombosis during and particularly following surgery in untreated patients with polycythemia vera have been reported by Wasserman and Gilbert. Their observations make it clear that no patient with untreated polycythemia vera should be subjected to major surgery unless it is absolutely essential, and even then attempts should be made to reduce the red cell mass to approximately normal levels before surgery is undertaken. Prolonged control of polycythemia vera (greater than 4 months) affords the best chance for avoidance of hemorrhagic or thrombotic complications postoperatively.

REFERENCES

Glasser, R. M., and Walker, R. I. Transitions among the myeloproliferative disorders. *Ann. Intern. Med.* 71:285, 1969.

Jepson, J. H. Polycythemia: Diagnosis, pathophysiology and therapy. Parts I and II. *Canad. Med. Ass. J.* 100:271, 327, 1969.

Lawrence, J. H., Winchell, H. S., and Donald, W. G. Leukemia in polycythemia vera. *Ann. Intern. Med.* 70:763, 1969.

Logue, G. L., Gutterman, J. U., McGinn, T. G., Laszlo, J., and Rundles, R. W. Melphalan therapy of polycythemia vera. *Blood* 36:70, 1970.

Modan, B., and Lilienfeld, A. Leukaemogenic effect of ionizing-irradiation treatment in polycythemia. *Lancet* 2:439, 1964.

Osgood, E. Polycythemia vera: Age relationships and survival. *Blood* 26:243, 1965.

Wasserman, L. R., and Gilbert, H. S. Surgery in polycythemia vera. *New Eng. J. Med.* 269:1226, 1963.

Wasserman, L. R., and Gilbert, H. S. The treatment of polycythemia vera. *Med. Clin. N. Amer.* 50:1501, 1966.

26. MYELOID METAPLASIA: MEDICAL MANAGEMENT AND ROLE OF SPLENECTOMY

Arthur W. Bauman
Seymour I. Schwartz

MYELOID METAPLASIA is a disorder of unknown etiology that occurs most frequently in middle-aged and older adults and, like polycythemia vera, is unusual in Negroes. Many different terms such as *agnogenic myeloid metaplasia* and *chronic nonleukemic myelosis* have been used over the years to signify this disorder, but generally they have all referred to the same disease, namely, *myeloid metaplasia with myelofibrosis*. The disorder is characterized by increased connective tissue proliferation in both the marrow and the extramarrow sites and, in many cases, increased production of white cells and platelets in both the marrow and the extramedullary sites. Nucleated red blood cells are also common in the extramedullary sites.

CLINICAL FEATURES

The presenting symptoms are usually secondary to anemia and increasing splenomegaly (Fig. 26-1). Occasionally hypermetabolism, pruritus, and complications of hyperuricemia are the presenting features. The most common physical findings are pallor and splenomegaly. At least 95% of the patients have palpable splenomegaly at the time of the initial diagnosis, and in many of them the spleen may be very large. Hepatomegaly is quite common; lymph node enlargement is not common.

The laboratory hallmark of myeloid metaplasia is the peripheral blood smear. Red cell fragmentation, nucleated red cells, and immature white cells ("a leukoerythroblastic picture") are the most common abnormalities (Fig. 26-2). Anemia is common but is usually not severe early in the dis-

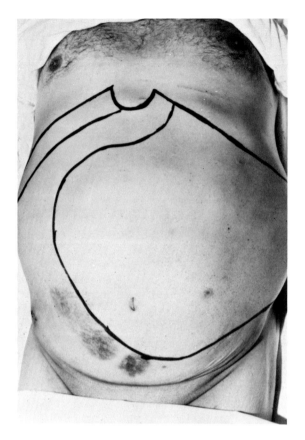

Figure 26-1. Abdomen of a 51-year-old man with myeloid metaplasia. Poly-cythemia vera was first diagnosed when he was 35. Myeloid metaplasia was diagnosed at age 43 (see Fig. 26-3). After this photograph was taken, the spleen was removed and was found to weigh 6000 gm. (Lines indicate outlines of liver and spleen on the right and left, respectively.)

ease. Leukocytosis with a shift to the left and a total white count in the range of 10,000 to 30,000 are common, and occasionally counts up to 50,000 are encountered. The platelet count may be low, normal, or high. Variations in platelet morphology accompanied by megakaryocyte frag-ments are frequently found in the peripheral blood smear. The leukocyte alkaline phosphatase is usually high, and hyperuricemia is frequently pres-ent. Liver function studies usually show little or no abnormality. X-rays of the bones show diffusely increased density in about 50% of the patients, particularly in the pelvic region. Focal sclerotic changes may also be pres-ent. Early in the disease the bone marrow on routine aspiration may be hypercellular or hypocellular. Bone marrow biopsy usually discloses the fibrotic changes, but islands of normal marrow may also be present. Occasionally, late in the disease, increased numbers of bizarre megakaryocytes may be noted in the marrow biopsy (Fig. 26-3). The Philadelphia chromosome (Ph[1]) is not present in myeloid metaplasia, permitting a distinction from those cases of chronic myelogenous leukemia in which myelofibrosis has developed.

DIFFERENTIAL DIAGNOSIS

Disorders that cause "leukoerythroblastic" changes in the peripheral blood are occasionally difficult to distinguish from myeloid metaplasia. Tuberculosis of the bone marrow is usually accompanied by less marked splenomegaly and more clinical toxicity. Red cell fragmentation tends to be less prominent, and there may be monocytosis in the peripheral blood smear. Marrow biopsy with demonstration of a granulomatous focus and tubercle

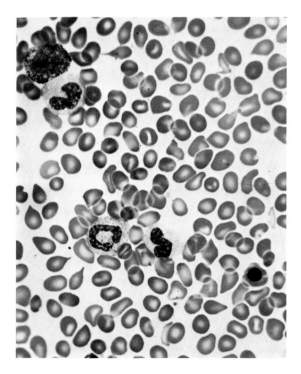

Figure 26-2. Peripheral blood smear of myeloid metaplasia. The red cells show numerous fragmented forms, particularly "teardrop" cells. Myeloid immaturity, nucleated red cells, and basophils are other characteristics. (× 1120, before 35% reduction.)

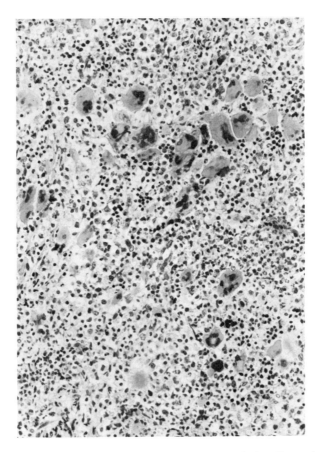

Figure 26-3. Bone marrow biopsy in myeloid metaplasia. Hyperplasia of all elements is present, particularly of reticulum cells and megakaryocytes. Many of the latter are atypical. (× 200, before 35% reduction.)

bacilli may be the only means of establishing the diagnosis. Malignancy involving the marrow and causing marrow fibrosis, especially Hodgkin's disease, is usually accompanied by much less splenomegaly and by pancytopenia—if the process is generalized in the marrow. Other clinical and laboratory features of Hodgkin's disease tend to make the differential diagnosis apparent. Chronic myelogenous leukemia may be difficult to separate from myeloid metaplasia at a specific point in the course of either disease. The history is usually sufficient to make the differentiation. Nucleated red cells and red cell fragmentation are much more prominent in the peripheral blood smear in myeloid metaplasia, whereas the white count tends to be much higher and leukocyte alkaline phosphatase low or absent in chronic myelogenous leukemia.

COURSE AND COMPLICATIONS

The course of myeloid metaplasia is quite variable. Length of survival has varied from 1 to 20 years with an average of about 5 to 7. Approximately 25% of patients with polycythemia vera develop myeloid metaplasia, and about 15% of all patients with myeloid metaplasia have a previous history of polycythemia vera. The common presenting problems of anemia and splenomegaly are also the commonest management problems. Portal hypertension often develops and may be complicated by the development of bleeding esophageal varices. The explanation for the portal hypertension in some patients appears to be a markedly increased blood flow through the large spleen into the portal system without accompanying significant intrahepatic or extrahepatic obstruction. Other patients may have significant fibrosis in the liver or a combination of fibrosis and increased portal blood flow as the explanation for their hypertension. Hyperuricemia and pruritus as well as hypermetabolism are other features.

Eventually acute leukemia develops in about 35% of patients with myeloid metaplasia and constitutes the terminal phase of the disease. The white count may not rise appreciably when the acute leukemia develops, but rather there may be a subtle increase in the percentage of blast forms accompanied by increasingly severe anemia and thrombocytopenia. The percentage of blasts does not often reach more than 50%.

EVALUATION OF THE PATIENT

Evaluation of the disease requires a broad understanding of the disorder and of the multiple complications that each patient may present. Some patients show little progression of their disease for a matter of years, and little or no treatment is required in these except to watch for evidence of increasing and troublesome splenomegaly or deterioration of the hematologic parameters.

The anemia requires careful evaluation. It is usually due to a combination of marrow failure and splenic sequestration or destruction (or both) of red cells. The degree of pooling of red cells in the spleen tends to correlate with its size and has approximated 33% of the red cell mass in some patients. On the other hand, splenic destruction of red cells does not correlate well with spleen size. Another factor related to splenomegaly, and possibly to shunting around the liver, is increased plasma volume, which may be much greater than what might be expected from the degree of anemia present. Reticulocytes in this disease are often prematurely released from the marrow and presumably also from the extramedullary sites of erythropoiesis. Hence reticulocyte counts may not accurately reflect the capacity of the marrow to produce red cells. Indeed, even routine marrow aspirates are not always useful, as the marrow cellularity may be quite variable from site to site until late in the disease. Red cell survival studies with ^{51}Cr tagging with assessment of the degree of splenic sequestration are consequently important. If the red cell survival is not markedly shortened and marrow failure is therefore implicated, a trial of male hormone therapy may be of value.

Other reasons for anemia warrant consideration. Blood loss from esophageal varices, gastritis, or peptic ulcer is always possible, and secondary iron deficiency is a complication. Folate depletion may develop as in polycythemia vera. Proliferation of other cell lines, as in chronic myelogenous leukemia, may be at the expense of the erythroid cells, and the early phases of transformation into acute leukemia may accentuate the anemia.

THERAPY

Treatment of myeloid metaplasia usually focuses on efforts to manage the splenomegaly and the anemia. The various approaches may be used singly or in combination.

HORMONAL TREATMENT

Male hormone preparations may be of value in patients whose anemia seems to be due more to marrow failure than to splenic sequestration and destruction of the red blood cells. Erythropoietin release from the kidneys (and other sites) is enhanced by male hormones, with a resultant increased number of marrow red cell precursor cells and their accelerated maturation. Our practice has been to give 600 mg of testosterone enanthate (Delatestryl) intramuscularly weekly for at least 2 months, and usually 3 or 4 months, before deciding that this approach will not be effective. Alternatively, oral administration of fluoxymesterone (Halotestin) or oxymetholone may be tried. The advantages and complications of the various male hormone preparations are discussed in Chapter 12, which deals with therapy of aplastic anemia. It should be recognized, however, that male hormones occasionally have been noted to accentuate the generalized proliferative activity of myeloid metaplasia.

Corticosteroids occasionally are effective in patients who have evidence of hypersplenism. As in immune hemolysis, the mechanism of action of the steroids is not well understood, but splenic destruction may be decreased. Occasionally marrow function also improves with corticosteroids, for reasons that are not understood.

CHEMOTHERAPY

Alkylating agents may be effective in reducing the transfusion requirement in patients with myeloid metaplasia, particularly if there is considerable proliferation of the white cells and platelets or if hypersplenism, rather than marrow failure, is playing the dominant role. Great caution must be exercised with the alkylating agents because of reduced marrow reserves and the possibility that more marrow suppression than splenic shrinkage will be achieved with the alkylating agents. Most of our experience has been with busulfan in small doses, although other alkylating agents may well be useful in this disorder. The potential advantage of an agent such as cyclophosphamide is that it is less likely to suppress megakaryocyte activity. The dose of busulfan is usually 2 to 4 mg daily for 2 to 3 weeks, and then maintenance doses of 2 mg 3 times a week for an indefinite period.

Busulfan is particularly useful in the occasional patient whose predominant clinical problem is hypermetabolism.

RADIOTHERAPY

Radioactive phosphorus is rarely indicated in the treatment of myeloid metaplasia, particularly in view of its potential to produce long-term marrow suppression. If it is employed, it probably should be reserved for those patients with a reasonably good hematocrit level and high platelet and white counts, and even then it should be used cautiously. Splenic irradiation, if used with caution, is effective in reducing the size of the spleen and symptoms associated with splenomegaly. Occasionally hypersplenism may become much more pronounced when the spleen is irradiated initially, but this rarely becomes a problem unless the leukopenia and thrombocytopenia were already present prior to splenic irradiation. The most disappointing aspect of splenic irradiation, even when there is marked reduction in the size of the spleen, is the rapidity with which the splenomegaly recurs. A reprieve of several months is a good result.

Transfusions may become necessary and have been used over prolonged periods for a number of patients with myeloid metaplasia. Our practice is to give packed red cells at such intervals as are required either to keep the patient asymptomatic or to keep his hematocrit level in the range of 25% or better. If prolonged transfusion requirements are anticipated—and they can be in this disease—it is well, prior to giving any transfusion, to type the patient's red cells as extensively as possible. Knowing the patient's own red cell type may make the detection of specific isoantibodies much easier at some later date. If severe buffy coat reactions develop, the use of frozen red cells should be considered.

SPLENECTOMY

For many years splenectomy was considered to be contraindicated in myeloid metaplasia because the extramedullary sites of hematopoiesis, particularly in the spleen, were considered to be compensatory on account of the fibrous replacement of the bone marrow. There is no evidence that the spleen in myeloid metaplasia contributes more formed cells to the circulation than it removes, although the degree of hypersplenism does not bear a direct relationship to spleen size. Splenectomy in this disease can be regarded as potentially beneficial from a hematologic point of view if there is significant splenic destruction of one or more of the formed cellular elements and *if some functioning bone marrow is still demonstrable.* Clearly, if the marrow is totally fibrotic—and this is generally reflected by marked pancytopenia—removal of the spleen is not likely to result in sustained significant hematologic improvement. In general, it can be assumed that significant marrow function persists even in the presence of fibrosis at the time of marrow biopsy, if the white count and platelet count are only modestly reduced.

The indications for splenectomy include the following:

1. *Increasing splenomegaly with resultant mechanical problems.* Removal should be considered in the case of the increasingly large spleen which is causing digestive difficulties, such as early satiety and epigastric distress after meals, or which is symptomatic because of recurrent infarctions. Splenectomy should not be entertained until other measures such as chemotherapy have been tried and have failed, or unless chemotherapy appears to be too dangerous because of pancytopenia and a hypocellular marrow.

2. *Hypersplenism.* This complication of the disease is one of the more frequent indications for splenectomy and is most often reflected by markedly increased transfusion requirements with clear-cut shortening of the red cell half-life and evidence of splenic sequestration of the red cells. The only absolute indication for splenectomy in the presence of anemia is hypersplenism with red cell destruction and development of such combinations of isoantibodies as to make cross-matching virtually impossible.

3. *Bleeding esophageal varices.* Portal hypertension is probably common in myeloid metaplasia, and some of these patients develop bleeding esophageal varices.

Surgical Considerations

In 1937 Hickling first called attention to the high mortality associated with splenectomy in patients with myeloid metaplasia. This and subsequent affirmations led to the conclusion that splenectomy is generally contraindicated in this disorder. In 1953 Green and associates carefully reviewed the individual case histories and could provide no support for the concept of harmful results being attributed to splenectomy.

In our own review of 200 cases in which splenectomy was performed for hematologic disorders, there were 12 patients with myeloid metaplasia. The in-hospital mortality (2 patients in this group) was considerably higher than that noted with other diseases. However, one of the deaths was related to progression of disease and general inanition, while the second death was due to infection.

The complications associated with surgery are also higher in this disease and include wound hematoma and subphrenic abscess. As a consequence of anticipated complications, certain principles are adhered to in performing the splenectomy. In view of the size of the organ and the amount of collateral circulation, leading to the potential for increased bleeding, a large incision is mandatory; we prefer the subcostal incision. At the time of laparotomy it is appropriate to measure splenic pulp pressure in order to define the presence of portal hypertension and also to inspect the liver for evidence of involvement. If indicated, wedge biopsy of the liver should be performed. In patients without a history of bleeding varices, splenectomy alone is performed; whereas if bleeding varices complicate the picture, a concomitant splenorenal shunt should be carried out. The operative procedure requires deliberate interruption of the collaterals so that an ultimate pedicle of splenic artery and vein remains and ligation of these vessels permits removal of the organ. In view of the propensity for infection, the large dead space resulting from removal of a markedly enlarged organ, and the extensive collaterals which provide an opportunity for increased bleeding, we believe that routine drainage of the left subphrenic space is indicated. In none of the surviving 10 patients in our series was there an adverse hematologic effect related to removal of the organ.

Course and Management after Splenectomy

The course that myeloid metaplasia follows after splenectomy is usually a reflection of the proliferative status of the disease prior to operation. As there is always a component of splenic sequestration and destruction of the blood cells, the blood counts usually rise after splenectomy. Indeed phlebotomy may again be necessary from time to time, particularly in those patients whose myeloid metaplasia was preceded by polycythemia vera. The white cell and platelet counts may rise abruptly and markedly to ranges of 100,000 and one million per cubic millimeter, respectively, depending on the amount of normal marrow function still present. These changes usually may be anticipated by the counts prior to splenectomy. If the marrow is generally replaced by fibrous tissue, there may be little change in the blood counts except usually a decrease in transfusion requirements.

Liver enlargement, due to extramedullary hematopoiesis and connective tissue proliferation, will progress following splenectomy, but there is little basis for the claim that splenectomy enhances the rate of liver enlargement. Portal hypertension develops eventually in most patients and may make subsequent abdominal surgery hazardous because of difficulty in controlling bleeding from collateral blood vessels.

The treatment of myeloid metaplasia after splenectomy is based on the same principles that are followed before splenectomy. If proliferation of white cells or platelets or both is prominent, particularly at the expense of red cell production, alkylation is advised. Marrow failure because of fibrosis and accompanied by pancytopenia may be alleviated by male hormones. Transfusions are usually necessary eventually.

The management of terminal acute leukemia is discussed in Chapter 25.

REFERENCES

Bouroncle, B. A., and Doan, C. A. Myelofibrosis: Clinical, hematologic and pathologic study of 110 patients. *Amer. J. Med. Sci.* 243:697, 1962.

Donaldson, G. W. K., McArthur, M., Macpherson, A. I. S., and Richmond, J. Blood volume changes in splenomegaly. *Brit. J. Haemat.* 18:45, 1970.

Gardner, F., and Pringle, J., Jr. Androgens and erythropoiesis: II. Treatment of myeloid metaplasia. *New Eng. J. Med.* 264:103, 1961.

Rosenbaum, D. L., Murphy, G. W., and Swisher, S. W. Hemodynamic studies of the portal circulation in myeloid metaplasia. *Amer. J. Med.* 41:360, 1966.

Sanchez-Medal, L., Gomez-Leal, A., Duarte, L., and Rico, M. G. Anabolic androgenic steroids in the treatment of acquired aplastic anemia. *Blood* 34:283, 1969.

Silver, R. T., Jenkins, D. E., Jr., and Engle, R. L., Jr. Use of testosterone and busulfan in the treatment of myelofibrosis with myeloid metaplasia. *Blood* 23:341, 1964.

27. CHRONIC MYELOGENOUS LEUKEMIA

Paul F. Griner

CHRONIC MYELOGENOUS LEUKEMIA (CML) accounts for approximately 20% of all forms of leukemia. The incidence of this disease appears to be uniform throughout the Western hemisphere. Slightly over 1 new case per 100,000 population per year can be expected. A somewhat lower figure has been reported for Negroes and Indians in this country; this difference may be more apparent than real. As is the case for all leukemias, the reported incidence of CML has risen steadily since 1920. Whether this reflects a true increase in the frequency of the disease or simply more accurate diagnosis remains conjectural. Men and women are affected with about equal frequency. In the great majority of patients the disease appears between the ages of 30 and 70 with a median age of about 50 years. The illness has been described at both extremes of life, however, including a number of cases in newborns. Chronic myelogenous leukemia has been reported in multiple family members, including identical twins. Such cases are rare.

In this chapter the discussion of CML is directed to the practicing internist. Etiologic considerations, although important in themselves, are not reviewed. Aspects of granulocyte kinetics and function which pertain to diagnosis and therapy are discussed. The natural history of the disorder and its treatment and prognosis are reviewed with particular attention to recent advances.

THE GRANULOCYTE IN CHRONIC MYELOGENOUS LEUKEMIA

Leukocytes from patients with CML are morphologically indistinguishable from normal leukocytes. Studies of the metabolism, physiology, and cytogenetics of these cells, however, have revealed important differences from the normal. A consistent chromosomal abnormality (Philadelphia chromosome) has been identified in the majority of patients. The activity of at least one enzyme (leukocyte alkaline phosphatase) is reduced in a high proportion of patients. Kinetic studies have revealed a greatly expanded granulocyte mass and an interchange of these cells between splenic, blood, and bone marrow compartments. The significance of some of these observations remains unclear, but many have contributed to the understanding of the disease. Some are of distinct value to the clinician in the diagnosis and management of CML; these are discussed in these pages. The references cited at the end of the chapter provide a more in-depth review of these and other leukocyte abnormalities found in CML.

PHILADELPHIA CHROMOSOME

The Philadelphia chromosome (Ph[1]), a cytogenetic abnormality found in most patients with CML, is discussed in detail in Chapter 21. When patients with CML are grouped according to the presence or absence of the Ph[1] chromosome, significant differences in the clinical picture and response to therapy are apparent. Ph[1]-negative patients often present with atypical features. Splenomegaly may be minimal or absent. The white blood cell and platelet counts tend to be lower than in typical CML. Fewer basophils are noted. The bone marrow may reveal normal or reduced cellularity. In addition, Ph[1]-negative patients, as a group, respond less predictably to therapy. Some are totally refractory. The median survival is considerably shorter for these patients than for those who demonstrate the Ph[1] abnormality.

As indicated in Chapter 21, the identification of the Ph[1] abnormality has raised an important issue concerning diagnostic criteria for CML. Some now restrict this diagnosis to those patients who demonstrate the Ph[1] phenomenon. Nevertheless the practicing physician must base decisions concerning therapy on the overall clinical picture rather than on the presence or absence of the Ph[1] phenomenon per se. The treatment of Ph[1]-negative patients whose clinical features resemble those of CML does not differ from that of their Ph[1]-positive counterparts.

LEUKOCYTE ALKALINE PHOSPHATASE

The enzyme alkaline phosphatase is a normal constituent of human granulocytes. Its role in leukocyte metabolism remains obscure. The enzyme appears to bear no relationship to serum alkaline phosphatase. Appropriate histochemical staining of blood smears permits a semiquantitative estimate of leukocyte alkaline phosphatase (LAP). The majority of patients with CML reveal reduced or absent LAP levels. By contrast, elevated levels are the rule in disorders most often confused with CML (i.e., polycythemia vera, myeloid metaplasia, and leukemoid reactions). The LAP test has thus become a helpful adjunct in the diagnosis of CML. In about 15% of CML patients, however, the values are normal or increased. Also, a low LAP reading is not specific for CML. Occasional patients with myeloid metaplasia have low or absent levels. Other disorders which may reveal low LAP values include paroxysmal nocturnal hemoglobinuria, idiopathic thrombocytopenic purpura, infectious mononucleosis, pernicious anemia, aplastic anemia, and congenital hypophosphatasia. Abnormal LAP determinations in CML may represent a qualitative rather than quantitative abnormality. Complete hematologic remission in CML may be accompanied by a return of the LAP to normal. This has been interpreted by some as a favorable prognostic sign.

Although both the Ph^1 abnormality and low LAP values are present in most patients with CML, the two are not dependent. The distribution of LAP levels is about the same for both Ph^1-positive and Ph^1-negative patients.

Muramidase (lysozyme), a hydrolytic enzyme found in granulocytes and monocytes, has recently been shown to be present in the urine of some patients with CML. Muramidasuria was present in Ph^1-negative but not Ph^1-positive patients. If a consistent relationship between muramidase and the Ph^1 phenomenon is confirmed, the determination of urinary muramidase levels could become a practical substitute for cytogenetic studies in the evaluation of patients with CML.

VITAMIN B_{12} BINDING

Plasma vitamin B_{12} levels are increased, often strikingly, in patients with CML. This observation can be explained by an increase in the capacity of plasma to bind B_{12} through a rise in the carrier protein, transcobalamin I. The significance of this observation remains unknown. The utility of this test in helping to differentiate CML from other disorders has been restricted by the finding that B_{12} levels may be elevated in polycythemia vera and myeloid metaplasia as well.

URIC ACID

Serum and urine uric acid levels are consistently increased in patients with CML. Studies with radioactive purine precursors indicate that exaggerated nucleic acid turnover is the explanation for hyperuricemia in these subjects. Despite the hyperuricemia in CML, clinical gout is not common. Of greater concern is the potential for urolithiasis and uric acid nephropathy after successful treatment. A rapid reduction in granulocyte mass following treatment is accompanied by a marked increase in nucleic acid breakdown and uric acid production. Serum uric acid levels exceeding 30 mg per 100 ml have been reported. Transient or irreversible renal failure from urate nephropathy has occurred despite high fluid intake and urinary alkalinization in these patients.

The introduction of allopurinol [4-hydroxypyrazolo (3,4-d) pyrimidine] has completely revolutionized the treatment of hyperuricemia in CML. This agent reduces the production of uric acid from its precursors hypoxanthine and xanthine by inhibiting the enzyme xanthine oxidase. When allopurinol is administered to patients with CML, the uric acid level almost invariably returns to normal and remains normal during therapy. Morbidity from hyperuricemia is thus eliminated.

THE CLINICAL PICTURE

Early in the course of CML the patient is without symptoms. The diagnosis may be made by serendipity following a routine blood count, an annual physical examination, or treatment of an unrelated minor illness. Over the past 5 years, approximately one-third of the patients referred to the University of Rochester Medical Center for diagnosis and treatment of CML were discovered in this fashion. Persistent and unexplained neutrophilic leukocytosis may be the only manifestation of the illness. On rare occasions the white cell count is normal at the time of diagnosis. The spleen may not be palpably enlarged. The hematocrit level is normal or slightly elevated. Platelets are often increased in number, only rarely reduced. The presence of a few immature granulocytes or increased numbers of basophils, or both, on the blood smear may be the only clue to the disease. In contrast to chronic lymphocytic leukemia, it is not common for this quiescent phase to persist for long periods. An occasional patient, however, may show no progression of disease for up to 2 years.

The majority of patients are well into the "proliferative" phase of their illness by the time the diagnosis is established. Symptoms and signs develop insidiously and are the consequence of a greatly expanded granulocyte mass. The most consistent symptoms are fatigue and a sensation of fullness in the left upper quadrant. The latter is often increased after meals and may lead to early satiety. Mild heat intolerance and sweating are common. Splenic enlargement is the most consistent and often the only physical finding. In atypical cases, the spleen may not be palpable. Most commonly it is easily felt 8 to 10 cm below the left costal margin. Occasionally the spleen is massively enlarged. Slight to moderate enlargement of the liver is an almost invariable accompaniment of splenomegaly. Pallor, tachycardia, and weight loss are inconstant observations. Mild bone tenderness may be noted. Lymphadenopathy is rare. Unexplained fever and susceptibility to infection are unusual at this stage of the illness. Splenic infarction or perisplenitis is an occasional complication of splenic infiltration. Left upper quadrant pain (usually pleuritic), pronounced tenderness over the spleen, low-grade fever, and a transient increase in the white blood count are hallmarks of this complication. A friction rub may be heard over the spleen. Symptoms and signs usually subside within 7 to 10 days. Renal colic (due to urate calculi), priapism, and nodular skin lesions may also complicate CML.

The hematocrit level may be normal; more often it is moderately reduced. Severe anemia is the exception. White cell counts of 100,000 to 250,000 per cubic millimeter are the rule in patients with untreated CML. On occasion the count may exceed one million. The majority of leukocytes are mature neutrophils. Variable numbers of immature myeloid forms are present. Myelocytes predominate. A small proportion of cells are promyelocytes and myeloblasts. Typically the latter do not exceed 5% of the total count. An increase in basophils (2 to 5%) is a consistent observation. This feature is often helpful in differentiating CML from other disorders. Eosinophils may be increased as well. Red blood cell morphology is either normal or minimally disturbed. Nucleated red cells may be present in the anemic patient. The platelet count is normal or elevated. Levels of 800,000 to one million per cubic millimeter are not uncommon. Thrombocytopenia is distinctly unusual in untreated CML. Platelet morphology is usually normal. Mild bleeding or thrombotic manifestations may be noted in patients with greatly increased platelet counts.

Typically the bone marrow is extremely cellular and can be aspirated without difficulty. It is common to see complete replacement of fat by marrow elements. The myeloid to erythroid ratio is markedly increased (i.e., as much as 100 to 1). Myeloid maturation is orderly. The predominant cell is the myelocyte. Blasts and promyelocytes generally account for less than 10% of cells. Erythroid maturation is normal. Megakaryocytes are usually present in normal to increased numbers.

Eventually the character of the illness changes. After months or years of successful control, the patient becomes refractory to treatment. The hematocrit level can no longer be maintained. Thrombocytopenia tends to develop. Therapy is no longer effective in reducing the leukocyte count or the enlarged spleen. Increasing numbers of myeloblasts and promyelocytes appear in the peripheral blood. The marrow may be difficult to aspirate; "dry taps" are common. Bone marrow biopsy may be necessary. The marrow may be hypocellular, packed with myeloblasts, or replaced by fibrous tissue. Erythroid and megakaryocytic elements are almost always reduced. These features characterize the so-called blast crisis of chronic myelogenous leukemia. They may appear abruptly; more often they develop insidiously. They occur in approximately 70% of all patients, cannot be prevented by prior treatment, appear to be independent of the type of treatment used, and indicate a dire prognosis.

Karanas and Silver have suggested more inclusive criteria to define the onset of the terminal phase of CML since features of myeloblastic transformation are not always present. They noted that the development of one or more of the following characteristics predicted death within 6 months in 87% of their patients with CML: (1) myeloblasts and promyelocytes in excess of 30% in the peripheral blood, (2) fever not clearly related to infection, and (3) the combination of anemia (hemoglobin less than 10.5 gm per 100 ml), thrombocytopenia (platelet count less than 100,000 per cubic millimeter), and persistent leukocytosis (white cell count exceeding 30,000 per cubic millimeter), despite adequate therapy.

DIAGNOSIS

Chronic myelogenous leukemia in its classic form presents little difficulty in diagnosis. The syndrome of splenomegaly, marked leukocytosis, immature granulocytes and an increase in basophils in the peripheral blood, thrombocytosis, and extreme myeloid hyperplasia of the marrow are characteristic if not pathognomonic of the disorder. A low LAP reading lends empirical support to the diagnosis. Demonstration of the Ph[1] abnormality is a diagnostic luxury that is not often required. Difficulties in diagnosis may be encountered when these features are less clear-cut. Such may be the case early in the course of the disease or in the elderly patient with multiple illnesses. Leukemoid reactions, chronic liver disease, polycythemia vera, and myeloid metaplasia may be confused with CML.

Granulocytic leukemoid reactions may accompany Hodgkin's disease, tuberculosis, carcinoma, and certain inflammatory disorders such as polyarteritis. In such reactions, myeloid immaturity is often present in the peripheral blood and the platelet count may be elevated. Basophilia is not common, however, and the white blood count only rarely approaches the levels commonly seen in CML. The marrow is usually less cellular than in CML. Splenomegaly, if present, is not often pronounced.

Patients with chronic active liver disease may present features suggestive of CML, namely, marked splenomegaly and leukocyte counts as high as 30,000 to 40,000 per cubic millimeter. Thrombocytosis is unusual, however; more often the platelet count is reduced. Basophilia is not present. Hepatic function studies or liver biopsy, or both, are sufficient to clarify the diagnosis.

Polycythemia vera has been confused with CML. Early in the course of CML, a modest increase in the hematocrit value may be noted in addition to leukocytosis and thrombocytosis. Differentiation is usually possible by marrow examination. Neither extreme cellularity nor marked myeloid hyperplasia is present in polycythemia vera.

Myeloid metaplasia and CML are often confused. The clinical features of both disorders overlap to a considerable degree. Individual cases of myeloid metaplasia may reveal one or more of the following characteristics suggestive of CML: white blood count in excess of 50,000 per cubic millimeter, minimal disturbance in red cell morphology, pronounced thrombocytosis, cellular marrow aspirate, low or negative LAP and, rarely, the Ph[1] abnormality. Conversely, in otherwise typical CML, extramedullary hematopoiesis may be demonstrated in the spleen and liver, patchy myelofibrosis may be present, the LAP may be normal or elevated, and the Ph[1] abnormality may be absent. Every attempt should be made to clarify the diagnosis in confusing cases since treatment of these disorders often differs.

TREATMENT

Most of the symptoms and signs in CML (e.g., abdominal discomfort, fatigue, sweating, hepatosplenomegaly, anemia) are the consequence of a greatly expanded granulocyte mass. The objective of treatment is to reduce the granulocyte mass to or toward normal and thereby eliminate symptoms. Patients in the early phase of their illness may be totally free from symptoms. In these patients the hematocrit is usually normal, the white blood count is only moderately elevated, and splenomegaly is not marked. Such patients are the exception rather than the rule. They do not require treatment at the time of diagnosis. The average patient with CML develops mild symptoms together with a reduction in hematocrit reading when the leukocyte count exceeds 100,000 to 150,000 per cubic millimeter. Thus although the white count per se is not an indication for treatment, its level correlates reasonably well with the total leukocyte mass and therefore with the presence or absence of symptoms and the need for therapy. Effective treatment is followed by the disappearance of most if not all manifestations of the illness. The leukocyte count, hematocrit reading, and platelet count return to normal. The spleen regresses or disappears above the costal margin. Marrow cellularity is reduced, sometimes to normal. The patient is returned to a state of good health. Persistence of the Ph[1] abnormality and the continued presence of basophils in the peripheral blood may constitute the only residuum of disease.

Remissions in CML can be regularly induced by either irradiation or chemotherapy. The former is effective whether delivered as splenic or as total-body irradiation. Chemotherapy has been limited primarily to the use of the alkylating agent busulfan (Myleran). Treatment with this agent has been so successful that there has been little need to evaluate other chemotherapeutic agents. Busulfan has gradually replaced irradiation as the preferred treatment for CML because of its ease of administration. In addition, many hematologists have considered this drug superior to irradiation in controlling the disease. This suggested superiority was recently confirmed by the results of a cooperative study initiated in Great Britain in 1959. Busulfan was more effective than irradiation in raising and maintaining hematocrit levels. Of greater importance was the observation that patients treated with busulfan survived significantly longer than those receiving irradiation. Based upon these findings, the greater convenience of this agent, and its ability to induce remissions in some patients who are refractory to irradiation, busulfan must now be considered the treatment of choice in CML.

BUSULFAN THERAPY

Busulfan is supplied in 2 mg tablets. Treatment is initiated in doses of 4 to 10 mg per day. Concurrent administration of allopurinol in doses of 300 to 400 mg daily is recommended to prevent hyperuricemia and its complications. The rate of fall of the white blood count is determined by the daily dose of busulfan. Remission may be induced within 3 to 6 weeks using doses of 8 to 10 mg daily. More commonly, smaller doses are employed and remission can be anticipated within 6 to 10 weeks. It is only rarely necessary to induce a rapid remission in patients with CML. Symptoms due to the disease are not usually severe. For this reason a gradual remission induced by a daily busulfan dose of about 6 mg is generally preferred. When larger doses are employed, the potential for bone marrow toxicity is greater and weekly monitoring of blood counts is necessary. The effects of therapy persist for some time after the drug has been discontinued. Thus a further reduction in the leukocyte and platelet counts can be anticipated for an additional 1 to 6 weeks. Continuation of therapy until the leukocyte count is well within the normal range may lead to irreversible marrow aplasia. For this reason, therapy should be terminated when the white blood count has fallen to 10,000 to 15,000 per cubic millimeter. The cutoff level is decided upon empirically. The upper level should be used for patients receiving a larger dose of busulfan whose leukocyte count is dropping rapidly. It is often safer to reduce the dose of busulfan as treatment proceeds, to permit a more gradual reduction in the white count.

During treatment the white blood count falls in an exponential fashion. Figure 27-1 demonstrates the relationship between the leukocyte count (plotted on a logarithmic scale) and time in a patient receiving a fixed daily dose of busulfan. After a few points have been established on such a graph, one can estimate when the leukocyte count is likely to drop within the normal range. For patients who must travel some distance for treatment, such graphs are helpful in determining the frequency of visits as well as in predicting when therapy should be discontinued.

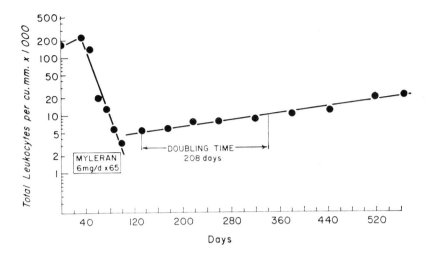

Figure 27-1. Changes in the leukocyte count of a patient with chronic myelo-cytic leukemia treated with busulfan. (From D. E. Bergsagel, *Canad. Med. Ass. J.* 96:1615, 1967.)

The resolution of symptoms and reduction in the size of the spleen and liver parallel the effects of busulfan on the leukocyte count. Modestly en-larged spleens usually regress completely. The reduction in size may be less striking in patients with massive splenomegaly. Effective therapy results in sequential changes in the differential leukocyte count. Myeloblasts disap-pear first, followed by promyelocytes and then myelocytes. After comple-tion of therapy, the differential count may be perfectly normal with the possible exception of persistent basophilia. A reduction in the platelet count from elevated to normal levels generally parallels the leukocyte response. As a rule, patients whose platelet counts are normal before therapy do not develop thrombocytopenia. The hematocrit level almost invariably im-proves with treatment. In the British study previously quoted, 47 of 48 patients treated with busulfan demonstrated a rise in hematocrit reading. On occasion an increase to polycythemic levels may be noted.

The great majority of patients with CML respond to initial treatment with busulfan in the manner just described. Those who do not more often present with atypical clinical features including absence of the Ph[1] abnor-mality. Attempts have been made to eliminate the leukemic stem cell by continuing to administer busulfan until the leukocyte count has fallen to 2000 to 3000 per cubic millimeter. Such therapy may result in a prolonged remission. On at least one occasion, it has been accompanied by a partial reversal of the Ph[1] abnormality. Because of the potential for marrow apla-sia, however, treatment of this nature cannot be considered routine.

FURTHER TREATMENT

Following the initial remission, it is customary to observe the patient at periodic intervals and reinstitute therapy when symptoms warrant. Patients may be treated effectively with intermittent courses of busulfan for many years. On the other hand, one may elect to maintain the remission by administering small doses of this agent for an indefinite period. For many patients such therapy is effective in eliminating the "ups and downs" of their disease. To date there is no information to suggest that either method is superior in terms of reducing complications, affecting the development of blast crises, or prolonging life. Maintenance therapy is not known to accelerate the development of resistance to busulfan.

Whether any one patient should receive intermittent versus maintenance therapy is best determined by the duration of good health between remissions. This can be gauged by evaluating the rate at which the leukocyte count rises after a course of therapy. Just as the leukocyte count falls exponentially during treatment, its rise in the treatment-free interval is also exponential (Fig. 27-1). By plotting serial white blood counts, one can determine the leukocyte doubling time and predict about when another course of treatment will be required. Patients who reveal a long doubling time (i.e., 150 to 200 days) are ideal candidates for intermittent therapy. Those in whom the doubling time is short (i.e., 30 to 60 days) should be considered for maintenance therapy. Busulfan in doses of 2 to 4 mg daily is usually effective in maintaining such patients in good health until the character of the illness changes.

With repeated courses of therapy, the doubling time between remissions tends to become progressively shorter. The explanation of this phenomenon is not clear. Eventually the character of the disease changes, and therapy with busulfan is no longer effective. Usually this heralds the terminal phase of the illness either with or without manifestations of blast crisis. The failure of the spleen or leukocyte count to regress satisfactorily, the persistence of anemia, and the development of thrombocytopenia or an increase in myeloblasts all indicate resistance to busulfan and the futility of continued therapy with this agent. The treatment of patients entering the terminal phase of their illness in blast crises is similar to that of those with acute myeloblastic leukemia (see Chap. 24). Unfortunately these patients are usually refractory to the drugs employed in the treatment of acute myeloblastic leukemia.

BUSULFAN TOXICITY

For some patients with CML, it is necessary to discontinue busulfan because of troublesome side effects rather than drug resistance. The major limiting side effects are hematologic toxicity, the development of a syndrome resembling Addison's disease, and pulmonary interstitial fibrosis. Other side effects include amenorrhea, impotence, and the development of cataracts.

Bone marrow hypoplasia following busulfan excess is well recognized and requires no additional comment. The occasional patient with thrombocytopenia prior to or during therapy may be unable to tolerate doses of busulfan sufficient to induce a remission. In such cases one should resort to another agent.

Skin pigmentation per se is a rather common and innocuous side effect of busulfan therapy. The pigment is melanin, and it may or may not have a distribution suggesting Addison's disease. Of greater concern is the peculiar but rare pseudo-addisonian syndrome that may accompany pigmentation. The syndrome develops insidiously, usually after long-term treatment with busulfan. It is characterized by anorexia, weight loss, and weakness in addition to the hyperpigmentation. Hypotension may be present. Adrenal function is usually normal. A few instances of decreased adrenal responsiveness to stress have been reported, however. It is essential that this syndrome be recognized. Continuation of therapy with busulfan may lead to severe wasting and death.

Interstitial pulmonary fibrosis is another rare but potentially lethal complication of busulfan treatment. Like the wasting syndrome, this illness usually develops after some years of therapy. Its clinical features are indistinguishable from those of idiopathic pulmonary fibrosis (Hamman-Rich syndrome). Exertional dyspnea and a nonproductive cough develop insidiously. The lungs are usually clear to auscultation. Chest x-ray reveals a diffuse, fine pulmonary infiltrate. Pulmonary function studies demonstrate a diffusion block. Pulmonary fibrosis and atypical epithelial hyperplasia are noted on lung biopsy. Vasculitis may be present. A case of bronchiolar cell carcinoma has been reported in association with the other changes just described. Discontinuation of busulfan and treatment with corticosteroids may reverse the illness. Unfortunately, for many patients the disease is well advanced before the diagnosis is suspected, and therapy is ineffectual.

Cytologic dysplasia has been demonstrated in many other organs in patients treated with busulfan (as well as other alkylating drugs). For this reason, it has been suggested that the long-term complications of busulfan represent the cumulative cytotoxic effects of this drug rather than hypersensitivity.

OTHER DRUGS

When busulfan must be discontinued because of nonhematologic side effects, other alkylating agents such as chlorambucil and cyclophosphamide may be effective substitutes. Chlorambucil, also supplied in 2 mg tablets, should be administered in doses slightly larger than busulfan for a comparable effect. Cyclophosphamide has received little attention in the treatment of CML. This agent should be considered particularly when thrombocytopenia precludes the use of busulfan. The efficacy of these drugs as substitutes for busulfan in patients with nonhematologic side effects can be challenged on the grounds that these side effects may not be unique to busulfan, but rather may be a function of alkylating agents per se.

Recently, dibromannitol and hydroxyurea have shown promise in the treatment of CML. Dibromannitol is also an alkylating agent but has properties of an antimetabolite as well. Treatment with this agent in doses of 125 to 250 mg daily is followed by predictable clinical improvement. Maintenance therapy is necessary, however, and the development of thrombocytopenia often limits its effectiveness. Hydroxyurea, an antimetabolite, is an inhibitor of DNA synthesis. Its specific site of action remains to be clarified. In daily doses of 30 to 50 mg per kilogram of body weight, it has been equally successful in inducing remissions in patients with CML. As with dibromannitol, maintenance therapy is required. Gastrointestinal side effects are more pronounced than with dibromannitol, but thrombocytopenia may be less marked.

Demecolcine and 6-mercaptopurine have been used in the treatment of CML with variable success. Of the two, demecolcine is clearly superior.

Comparative studies are necessary to define the relative merits of dibromannitol, hydroxyurea, and demecolcine. At present they can be considered as second-line drugs. Resistance to busulfan appears to be the major indication for their use.

PROGNOSIS

Most patients with CML die within the first few years following diagnosis and relatively few survive for prolonged periods. Thus an estimate of survival based upon the overall average gives a falsely optimistic expectation of life. It is more informative to determine the time at which 50% of patients have died. For this reason, survival of patients with CML is generally expressed in terms of *median* rather than *mean* duration of life.

Tivey compared the life expectancy of untreated patients with CML to those receiving irradiation. The median survival of untreated patients (1898–1923) was 2.4 years. Patients treated with irradiation (1898–1940) survived 2.7 years. More recent data indicate a median survival of about 3.5 years for patients treated with busulfan. Despite an impressive record in controlling symptoms, treatment has thus accomplished little in prolonging the life of patients with CML.

Approximately 20% of patients with CML are alive at 5 years, and occasional patients survive 10 or more years. The presence of the Ph[1] abnormality and a long leukocyte doubling time tend to be favorable prognostic indicators. Poor prognostic signs include absence of the Ph[1] chromosome, a short leukocyte doubling time, and either thrombocytopenia or an unusually high proportion of myeloblasts, basophils, or both at the time of diagnosis.

Improved survival in CML cannot be anticipated unless the development of blast transformation can be delayed or aborted and effective treatment of blast crises introduced. Remissions following blast transformation may now be possible with the availability of newer chemotherapeutic agents and combination chemotherapy.

REFERENCES

Bergsagel, D. E. The chronic leukemias: A review of disease manifestations and the aims of therapy. *Canad. Med. Ass. J.* 96:1615, 1967.

Craddock, C. G. The physiology of granulocytic cells in normal and leukemic states. *Amer. J. Med.* 28:711, 1960.

Cronkhite, E. P. Kinetics of Leukemic Cell Proliferation. In W. Dameshek and R. M. Dutcher (Eds.), *Perspectives in Leukemia.* New York: Grune & Stratton, 1968.

Dameshek, W., and Gunz, F. *Leukemia* (2d ed.). New York: Grune & Stratton, 1964.

Galton, D. A. G. Chemotherapy of chronic myelocytic leukemia. *Seminars Hemat.* 6:323, 1969.

Karanas, A., and Silver, R. T. Characteristics of the terminal phase of chronic granulocytic leukemia. *Blood* 32:445, 1968.

Kennedy, B. J., and Yarbro, J. W. Metabolic and therapeutic effects of hydroxyurea in chronic myeloid leukemia. *J.A.M.A.* 195:162, 1966.

Krakoff, I. H. Use of allopurinol in preventing hyperuricemia in leukemia and lymphoma. *Cancer* 19:1489, 1966.

Perillie, P. E., and Finch, S. E. Muramidase studies in Philadelphia-chromosome-positive and chromosome-negative chronic granulocytic leukemia. *New Eng. J. Med.* 282:456, 1970.

Perry, S., Moxley, J. H., Weiss, G. H., and Zelen, M. Studies of leukocyte kinetics by liquid scintillation counting in normal individuals and in patients with chronic myelocytic leukemia. *J. Clin. Invest.* 45:1388, 1966.

Ramanan, C. V., and Israel, M. C. G. Treatment of chronic myeloid leukemia with dibromannitol. *Lancet* 2:125, 1969.

Tivey, H. The prognosis for survival in chronic granulocytic and lymphocytic leukemia. *Amer. J. Roentgen.* 72:68, 1954.

Valentine, W. N. The metabolism of the leukemic leukocyte. *Amer. J. Med.* 28:699, 1960.

Wintrobe, M. M. *Clinical Hematology* (6th ed.). Philadelphia: Lea & Febiger, 1967.

Witts, L. J., et al. Chronic granulocytic leukemia: Comparison of radiotherapy and busulfan therapy. (Report of The Medical Research Council's Working Party in Therapeutic Trials in Leukemia.) *Brit. Med. J.* 1:201, 1968.

IV
DISORDERS OF THE LYMPHATIC SYSTEM

28. LYMPHOCYTES AND PLASMA CELLS: NEWER VIEWS OF THEIR RELATIONSHIPS, LIFE CYCLES, AND FUNCTIONS

Lawrence N. Chessin

HISTORICAL ASPECTS

From a historical point of view, William Hewson in 1770 in his studies on the structure of the lymphoid organs first described the "round cells," or lymphocytes. In 1838 Müller called attention to the fact that the lymph contained lymphocytes and that these cells made their appearance in lymph after they had passed through a lymph node. Subsequently, Fleming in 1885 noted the presence of large numbers of mitotic figures in the germinal centers of lymph nodes and first described the site and mode of origin of the lymphocyte. With the development of methods for differentially staining fixed smears, Ehrlich identified what he called the lymphoid parenchyma as a group of cells present throughout the body, in both the solid tissues and in the circulation, with a distinctive pattern of cytodifferentiation. The first modern, detailed morphologic study of the development of lymphocytes was that of Downey and Weidenreich in 1912. While such prominent investigators as Maximow, Bloom, Dominici, Pappenheim, and Naegli were primarily concerned with the origin, derivation, and cytodifferentiation of lymphocytes, little was known about the functions of these cells.

The first description of the plasma cell is credited to Ramón y Cajal in 1894, although its precise relationship to the lymphocyte was not recog-

This work was supported by National Institutes of Health Grant AI 09030-01.

361

nized for many years. Wright first associated the plasma cell with multiple myeloma. With the development of improved bone marrow techniques in the 1940's, Waldenström described several clinical situations in which he began to correlate the proliferation of plasma cells, lymphocytes, and their distinctive morphologic intermediates, the lymphocytoid-plasma (LP) cells, with the appearance of increased gamma globulins in the serum. While in the 1950's there was mounting evidence from clinical, experimental, and morphologic studies that plasma cells were the major source of antibodies, a number of investigators presented compelling evidence that lymphocytes also possessed the capacity to synthesize antibody. In his recent treatise *Cellular Immunity,* Sir MacFarlane Burnet comments:

Before 1960 it is fair to say that the function of the lymphocyte was unknown although many felt that it must be primarily immunological, and at one period there had been strong claims that it was the antibody-producing cell. In 1958 I wrote that the only cellular basis for a clonal selection theory must be the lymphoid cells comprising in a single series both lymphocytes and plasma cells.

In this section I consider the current evidence that the lymphocytes and plasma cells are *immunologically competent cells* that are a part of an integrated *lymphoid complex* in which structure, development, and function are intimately related. The term *immunologically competent cells* was introduced at a meeting devoted to the cellular aspects of immunity, held in Prague in June, 1959, to refer to the complex of cells involved in immunity. While lymphocytes, plasma cells, and macrophages are considered immunologically competent cells, in this chapter I am primarily concerned with the lymphocyte–plasma cell system.

THE LYMPHOID COMPLEX

Lymphocytes are present in the circulation (peripheral blood, lymphatics, and thoracic duct) and in the solid organs. A variety of observations and experimental laboratory models have attested to the fact that the lymphoid complex is composed of a heterogeneous population of differentiating cells with multiple origins, life-spans, fine-structural features, and capabilities for mediating several immunologic functions. The sequential embryologic development of the lymphopoietic organs is seen in Table 28-1. In man, the first lymphoid tissue to develop is the thymus. Lymphocytopoiesis in the thymus is first recognizable at the ninth week of gestation. Subsequently, lymphocytopoiesis develops in the spleen, lymph nodes, and bone marrow.

The significance of the sequential appearance of the lymphoid organs in terms of embryologic development and function was first clearly appreci-

Table 28-1. Ontogeny of the Lymphopoietic Organs in Man

Organ or Tissue	Time of Appearance (week)
Blood islands from embryonic mesoderm of the yolk sac	Third
Circulation	Fourth
Thymus[a]	
3rd and 4th pharyngeal pouches—endoderm	Fourth to sixth
Hassall's corpuscles—mesoderm	Sixth to twelfth
Spleen—mesoderm	Sixth
Lymph nodes—mesoderm	Sixth to eighteenth
Association between lymphoid tissue and buccal, pharyngeal, and gastrointestinal epithelium	
1. Lingual tonsils[b]	
2. Pharyngeal tonsils[b]	
3. Peyer's patches[b]	
4. Appendix	
Bone marrow	Twelfth

[a] The thymus is the "central" lymphoid organ responsible for the development of cell-mediated immunities.

[b] The appendix, Peyer's patches, and tonsils have been suggested as the "central" lymphoid organs for the development of humoral immunity.

ated in 1954, when Dr. Robert Good and his colleagues were impressed by the association of acquired agammaglobulinemia with thymoma and first suggested a relationship between the thymus and the immune system. Subsequently, Gitlin and Janeway, in studying congenital sex-linked agammaglobulinemia, noted the absence of small lymphocytes and Hassall's corpuscles in the thymus of these patients. The significance of these clinical observations was explored further in a variety of studies on the ontogeny and phylogeny of the immune response in experimental animals. From these studies it was learned that both a developmental and a functional hierarchy exists within the lymphocyte complex which could be operationally divided into the central lymphoid organs and the peripheral lymphoid tissues. A lymphoid organ is *central* or *primary* in type if its removal during embryogenesis would interfere with or compromise further development of the *secondary* or *peripheral* lymphoid tissues—the spleen, lymph nodes, and circulating lymphocytes. The central lymphoid organs are derived from epithelial *anlagen*—the epithelial thymus and the epithelial bursa. The epithelial bursa in birds develops into the bursa of Fabricius. The equivalent of the epithelial bursa in the rabbit is the sacculus rotundus, and in man it appears to be the appendix, Peyer's patches, and tonsils.

Thymic-dependent functions have been shown to be associated with the cell-mediated immunities (delayed hypersensitivity, graft-versus-host (GVH) reactivity, transplantation immunity, tumor immunity, resistance to certain pathogens, and autoallergy), whereas the bursal-dependent functions are associated with the expression of humoral or antibody-mediated immunity. In studying the ability of the peripheral lymphoid tissues to mediate specific immunologic functions, Peterson and co-workers have recently presented experimental evidence for the existence of the morphologic counterpart of the central lymphoid tissue in the secondary structures of the spleen and lymph node. They have shown that in lymph nodes, the immunocompetent cells located in the deep cortical areas and splenic white pulp are *thymus dependent* for their development, expansion, and maintenance. These cells are functionally involved in the cell-mediated immunities, whereas in the extreme cortical and hilar areas of the node are the *bursa-dependent* lymphoid cells, which give rise to germinal centers and plasma cells. There is additional experimental evidence to suggest that as a central lymphoid organ, the thymus is concerned with the development, expansion, and maintenance of the peripheral lymphoid tissues. Although the precise mechanism by which the thymus acts as a "regulator" is not as yet fully defined, it appears that both humoral and cellular factors and mediators are involved.

In 1963 Dr. William Dameshek first proposed a functional nomenclature of *immunologically competent cells* or *immunocompetent cells,* based on the cytodynamics of the immune response, in which he defined the interrelationships between morphologically identifiable cells in the lymphocyte–plasma cell series (Table 28-2). He introduced the term *immunoblasts* to refer to the undifferentiated stem cells observed in the immune response derived from histiocytes of reticuloendothelial origin. He referred to those cells having the morphologic appearance of small lymphocytes and plasma cells as *immunocytes* or the differentiated *effector cells* involved in either the cell-mediated or humoral immune reactions. It is from this basic understanding that the immune response can be viewed from both a structural and functional level in which the hematopoietic stem cell, the *hemocytoblast,* under the appropriate stimulus differentiates into a series of immunologically competent effector cells.

HUMORAL IMMUNE SYSTEM

Plasma cells, lymphocytes, and the morphologic intermediates, the lymphocytoid-plasma (LP) cells, are the immunocytes, or effector cells, of humoral immunity. They synthesize the globular protein macromolecules, the immunoglobulins, which possess antibody activities (agglutination, precipi-

Table 28-2. Cytodynamics of the Immune Response

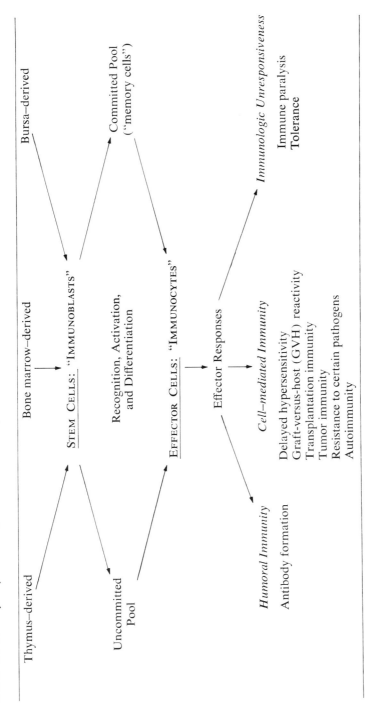

tation, neutralization, lysis, and opsonization). The system of nomenclature presently includes five major classes of immunoglobulins: IgG or γG, IgA or $\gamma\alpha$, IgM or $\gamma\mu$, IgD or $\gamma\delta$, and IgE or $\gamma\epsilon$. Each molecule of these globulins is thought to consist of two heavy (H) and two light (L) polypeptide chains (Table 28-3). The heavy polypeptide chains, which have a molecular weight of 53,000 each, determine the biologic properties of each immunoglobulin class and are designated as γ, α, μ, δ, and ϵ chains for the IgG, IgA, IgM, IgD, and IgE classes, respectively. The light polypeptide chains occur in only two antigenic types: κ (kappa) chain, corresponding to Type K immunoglobulin chain, and λ (lambda) chain, corresponding to Type L immunoglobulin chain.

Studies on the biosynthesis, assembly, and secretion of immunoglobulins have revealed that the heavy polypeptide chains are synthesized on large 270S polyribosomes composed of 7 to 8 subunits. The size of these polysomes is such as to suggest synthesis of each chain as a single unit; however, there is some controversy whether, under normal conditions, synthesis of H and L chains is balanced or if there is an excess synthesis of L chains. The detection of L chains in association with the polysomes synthesizing H chains makes it likely that the L chains combine with H chains on the polysomes and thus initiate their orderly release.

Table 28-3. Human Serum Immunoglobulin Nomenclature

	IMMUNOGLOBULINS				
Proposed Symbols[a]	IgG [b]	IgA	IgM	IgD	IgE
	γG	γA	γM	γD	γE
Other notations	γ_2	β_2A	γ_1M	γ_1J	IgND
	γ_{ss}	γ_1A	β_2M		
	6.6Sγ	(6.6S–13S)	18S		8S
	7Sγ				
	POLYPEPTIDE CHAIN COMPOSITION				
Types					
Kappa (κ)—Type K	$\gamma_2\kappa_2$	$(\alpha_2\kappa_2)$n	$(\mu_2\kappa_2)5$	$\delta_2\kappa_2$	$\epsilon_2\kappa_2$
Lambda (λ)—Type L	$\gamma_2\lambda_2$	$(\alpha_2\lambda_2)$n	$(\mu_2\lambda_2)5$	$\delta_2\lambda_2$	$\epsilon_2\lambda_2$

[a] The system of nomenclature of human immunoglobulins recommended by a committee of the World Health Organization in 1964 and extended in 1966.

[b] Subclasses of the IgG have been identified on the basis of specific antigenic determinants detectable by the use of simian and rabbit antisera. The following subclasses are known: IgG (We, gamma-2B or -2C); IgG2 (Ne, gamma-2a); IgG3 (Vi, gamma-2c); and IgG4 (Ge, gamma-2D).

Immunofluorescent studies employing class- and type-specific reagents have revealed that individual immunoglobulin-producing cells secrete molecules containing one type of light chain, heavy chain, and allotypic determinant. It has also been demonstrated that single cells from animals injected with multiple immunogens produce antibody against only one of the immunogens, clearly indicating that the antibody secreted by a single cell is homogeneous. Thus the observed heterogeneity of serum antibody—that is, the isotype variation, allotypic variation, idiotypic variation, and charge heterogeneity—appears to be related to differences among antibody-producing cells in the individual.

CELL-MEDIATED IMMUNITY

In contrast to humoral immunity, cell-mediated immunity is a form of immunity characterized by the delayed-type hypersensitivity (DH) response. The cell-mediated immunities are concerned with a mechanism of *immunologic surveillance,* that is, a cellular immune mechanism that serves to protect the host against certain infectious agents and foreign, mutant, and neoplastic cells. The delayed-type hypersensitivity response is characterized by the arrival of lymphocytes to the test site where antigen has been introduced; the antigen reacts with or upon the sensitized cell, and this interaction between a product synthesized by the lymphocytes and other mononuclear cells produces the characteristic local lesion. Since these reactions can be transferred passively from sensitized to normal individuals with cells but not with serum antibody, they are distinguished from the humoral immune reactions. The common histopathologic characteristic of all delayed-type hypersensitivity reactions, regardless of the nature of the antigen, is vascular stasis, edema, and perivascular mononuclear infiltration. There is abundant evidence to suggest that delayed hypersensitivity involves the reaction of a few sensitive lymphocytes with antigen, a large number of nonsensitive mononuclear cells, and several other factors that may include the clotting mechanism. A variety of effector macromolecules released from antigen-stimulated lymphocytes have been identified as mediators in this type of response (Table 28-4).

Recent studies have shown that the cellular immune responses are characterized by a high degree of specificity, that is, that the recognition of antigen by immunologically committed cells involves a specific receptor system which can distinguish between closely related antigens on the basis of structural complementarity. While there is evidence that the binding site on the sensitized lymphocyte or processing cell differs from the binding site for humoral antibody, and that the antigen receptor on the cell differs in both kind and degree from conventional antibody, the chemical nature of the

Table 28-4. Effector Macromolecules Released by Sensitized Lymphocytes in Cellular Immune Reactions

Effector Macromolecules	Chemical Properties	Biologic Properties
Transfer factor (TF)	Soluble; dialyzable; lyophilizable; polypeptide-polynucleotide; mol. wt. 10,000	Immunologically specific recruiting factor, nonimmunoglobulin; non-immunogenic; converts normal lymphocytes in vitro and in vivo to antigen-responsive state; transformation and clonal proliferation of converted lymphocytes exposed to antigen; informational molecule that acts as a derepressor of a select population of small lymphocytes predestined to become antigen-sensitive
Macrophage-inhibitory factor (MIF)	Protein; mol. wt. 70,000	Specific inhibitor of macrophage migrations; MIF causes skin reactions similar to delayed hypersensitivity reactions; probable role of stabilizing macrophages in immunologic surveillance
Lymphotoxic factor (LTF)	Protein; mol. wt. 80,000	Acts to preserve the natural state of affairs by eliminating altered cells, e.g., somatic cell mutants or neoplastic cells
Chemotactic factor	Protein; mol. wt. 60,000	Attracts macrophages
Mitogenic factor	—	Transforms small lymphocytes to large pyroninophilic "blastlike" cells
Interferon	Protein; mol. wt. 25,000	Species specific; macromolecule that confers upon unaffected cells resistance to virus infection
Cytophilic antibody	Protein; mol. wt. 140,000	Specific antibodies that fix to cell surfaces; may be valuable in guiding activated macrophages in effector cytotoxic processes

receptor and the means by which this receptor reacts with antigen to initiate the biosynthetic and proliferative cellular immune responses remain undefined. It is currently thought that specific antigen interacts at the cell surface receptors and induces conformational changes on the plasma membrane to produce a signal for activation of the immunocompetent cell. Subsequently, multiplication and differentiation take place with the production of *memory* and *effector cells*. The antigen–cell interactions proceed on a specific, thermodynamically driven basis. The concept that two types of antigen-sensitive cells are operative in the cellular immune reactions has been suggested by several workers. The X cell is the first antigen-sensitive cell in the lymphocytic series; upon stimulation it is converted into a Y or memory cell. Triggering of Y cells by antigen results in division and irreversible maturation to a plasmacytic series of Z cells, whose terminal member is the mature, antibody-producing plasma cell.

KINETICS, FATES, AND LIFE-SPANS OF LYMPHOCYTES

Based on in vitro studies of the incorporation of tritiated thymidine into DNA, it is estimated that only 0.06% of the circulating small lymphocytes in the peripheral pool can synthesize DNA. Thus circulating lymphocytes have been referred to as *resting cells.* Kinetic studies have revealed that there are at least two classes of lymphocytes with respect to their rate of formation and circulating life-span. The first class is *short-lived,* rapidly labeled, and bone marrow–derived, while the second class is *long-lived,* slowly labeled, and thymus-derived. The latter cells appear to be the basis for immunologic memory and long-term immunity. Mature plasma cells, on the other hand, appear to be fully differentiated, mature secretory cells of immunoglobulins.

From a variety of studies, there is evidence that two distinct physiological processes control the "traffic" of lymphocytes in the circulating pool. There is a migrating stream of proliferating cells from the bone marrow that travel via the thymus to lymph nodes, where they undergo a sequence of maturation within a matter of weeks. There is also evidence for the recirculation of long-lived, small lymphocytes, whereby small lymphocytes delivered to lymphoid tissue leave the intravascular compartment through the venous end of the lymph node capillary bed and pass through the tissue to efferent lymphatic channels. The thoracic duct then delivers the lymphocytes back to the circulation. Thus small lymphocytes may be exchanged between the blood and lymphoid tissue within a matter of hours very many times during their lifetime. In addition to the regulatory effect of specific antigens, it appears that the effector macromolecules produced by activated lymphocytes also control the "traffic" of cells in the lymphoid pool.

SMALL LYMPHOCYTE: FUNCTIONAL CONSIDERATIONS

Small lymphocytes are capable of producing antibody, transferring delayed hypersensitivity, eliciting the graft-versus-host reactions (homograft rejection), preventing the neonatal thymectomy wasting syndrome, repopulating the lymphoid tissues of irradiated animals and, in some situations, preventing the effects of lethal irradiation. There is also evidence that in vivo these cells are capable of undergoing further differentiation to lymphoblasts. Small lymphocytes can be stimulated to synthesize RNA, DNA, and protein and to transform into immature pyroninophilic "blast" cells, similar to those seen in the lymph node following antigen administration, by exposure in vitro to (1) nonspecific mitogenic agents, e.g., phytohemagglutinin (PHA), pokeweed mitogen (PWM), streptolysin S (SLS), filtrates from cultures of *Staphylococcus aureus* (SF); (2) specific antigens; (3) tissue antigens; (4) antiallotype sera; and (5) antilymphocyte sera. This process, referred to as *lymphocyte transformation,* has been used as a convenient clinical means of assessing an individual's immunocompetence (cf. Table 28-5).

LYMPHOCYTES AND PLASMA CELLS: STRUCTURAL CONSIDERATIONS

Although countless systems have been proposed to classify lymphocytes on the basis of cell size, number of mitochondria, nucleolar size, and cytoplasmic granules, no system based on morphologic criteria alone has been adequate for meaningful classification of this heterogeneous population of cells. While it is unclear whether small lymphocytes are the only major class of cells involved in immunologic reactions, there is evidence that there are distinct subpopulations of lymphocytes which may be morphologically identical but are functionally distinct. Physiologic, biochemical, enzymatic, and radioisotopic labeling studies have further emphasized this heterogeneity (Fig. 28-1).

At the ultrastructural level small lymphocytes have a double nuclear membrane; a centriole; a defined Golgi apparatus which, when stained with neutral red, includes a vacuole; and a nucleolar apparatus (Fig. 28-2). In addition, there are free, as well as aggregated, polyribosomes with varying degrees of development of rough-surfaced endoplasmic reticulum (Fig. 28-3). The association of the rough-surfaced endoplasmic reticulum of the mature plasma cell with the synthesis of the heavy polypetide chains α, γ, μ, δ, ϵ, and light polypeptide chains κ and λ, has been demonstrated both by immunofluorescence and the ferritin-labeled antibody techniques. Cell types such as the *lymphocytoid-plasma* (LP) cells and the *plasmacytoid-lymphocytes* observed in cellular immune responses appear to be fine-structural intermediates that display varying degrees of development of polyribosomes and rough-surfaced endoplasmic reticulum (Fig. 28-4). Mature plasma cells distinguish themselves from small lymphocytes and the

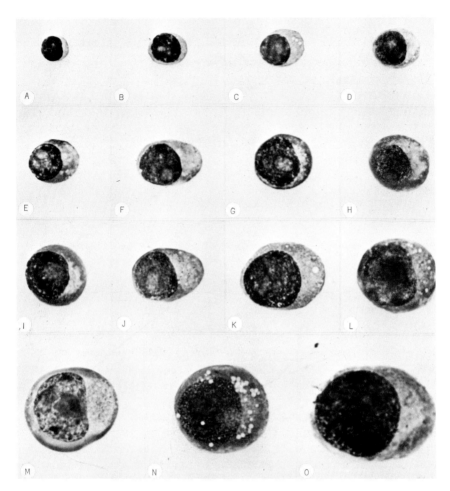

Figure 28-1. Morphologic transformation of human peripheral blood lympho-cytes by the pokeweed mitogen (PWM). Composite photomicrograph of the spectrum of PWM-transformed human peripheral blood lymphocytes; time course study. (Stained with Giemsa; × 1600, before 40% reduction.) (A) Un-incubated small lymphocyte. (B–D) Transformed lymphocytes seen after 24 hours. (E–L) Transformed lymphocytes seen from 24 to 72 hours. (M–O) Large blastlike cells seen at 72 hours. Immunofluorescent studies have indicated that some of these transformed cells contain immunoglobulins. (From L. N. Chessin et al., *J. Exp. Med.* 124:873, 1966.)

lymphocytoid–plasma cell intermediates by the presence of a well-developed Golgi zone in association with the rough-surfaced endoplasmic reticulum. These structures are extensively developed, since they are associ-ated with the secretion of immunoglobulins.

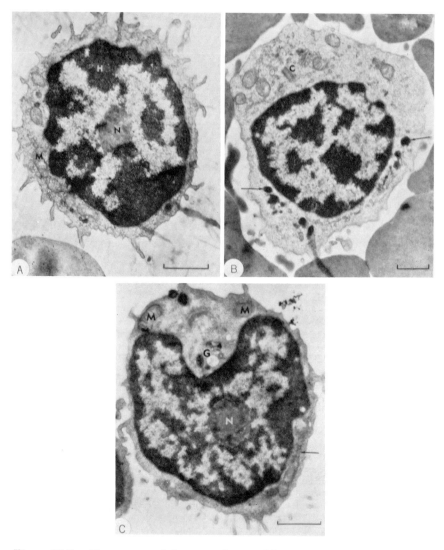

Figure 28-2. Fine-structural features of normal human peripheral blood small lymphocytes (⌣ = 1μ). (A) Electron-dense clumped heterochromatin (*H*), nucleolus (*N*), mitochondria (*M*), and uropods (cell membrane projections) are seen. (× 18,400, before 18% reduction.) Cells were fixed in glutaraldehyde osmium and embedded in araldite. All sections are stained with uranyl acetate–lead citrate. (B) Features similar to those of the cell shown in (A). A centriole (*C*) is prominent and several electron-dense lysosome-like bodies are present (*arrows*). (× 13,000, before 18% reduction.) (C) Nucleolus (*N*), mitochondria (*M*), and Golgi apparatus (*G*) are labeled. Note the sparse rough-surfaced endoplasmic reticulum (*arrow*). (× 1700, before 18% reduction.) (From S. D. Douglas et al., *J. Immun.* 98:17, 1966. © 1966, The Williams & Wilkins Co., Baltimore, Md. 21202, U.S.A.)

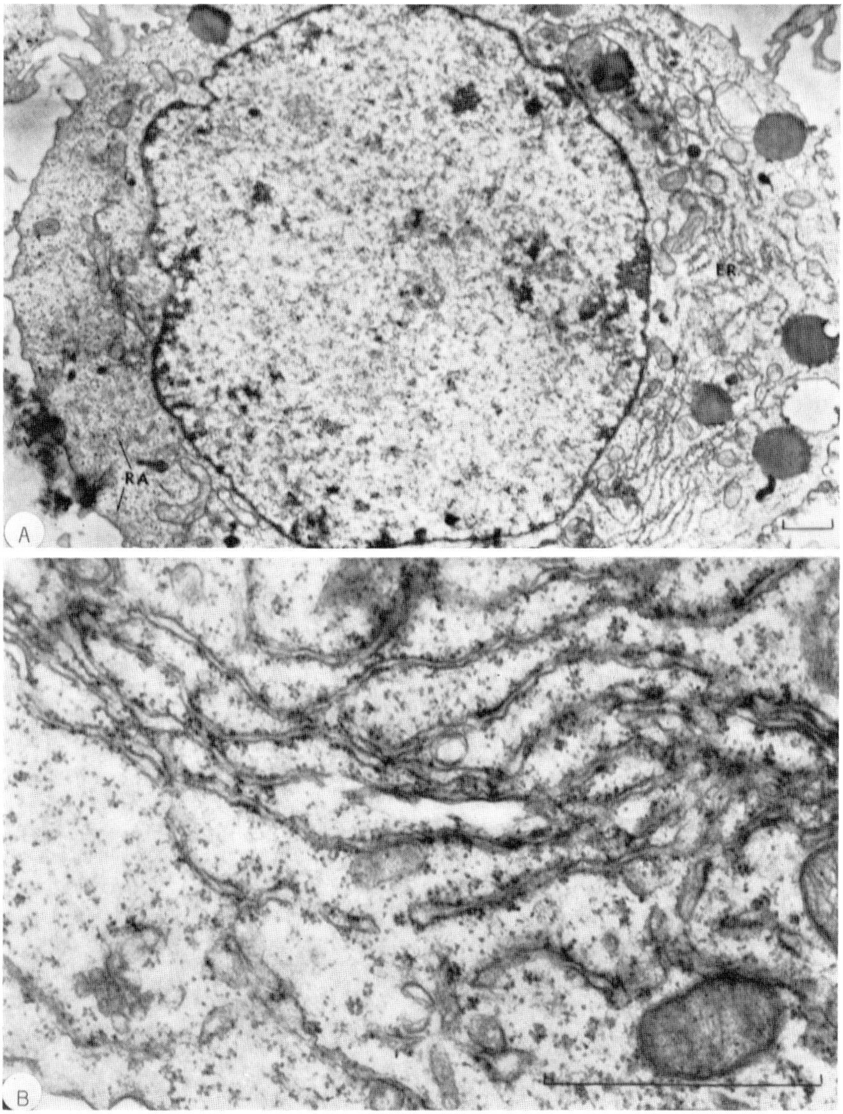

Figure 28-3. Polyribosome structure and endoplasmic reticulum development in lymphoid cells (⌴ = 1μ). (A) The nucleus shows much diffuse chromatin (euchromatin). Cytoplasm shows many ribosomal aggregates (*RA*) and well-developed, rough-surfaced endoplasmic reticulum (*ER*). (× 10,300, before 18% reduction.) (B) Higher power electron micrograph of a portion of the cell shown in (A). Rough-surfaced endoplasmic reticulum is seen with attached ribosomes. (× 58,000, before 18% reduction.) (From S. D. Douglas et al., *J. Immun.* 98:17, 1966. © 1966, The Williams & Wilkins Co., Baltimore, Md. 21202, U.S.A.)

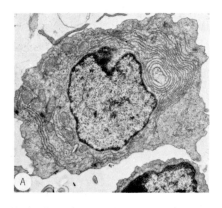

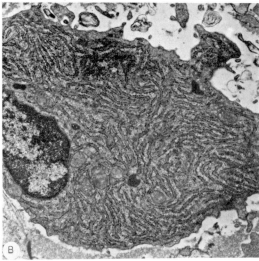

Figure 28-4. Lymphocyte–plasma cell morphologic intermediate: lympho-cytoid plasma (LP) cells and plasmacytoid lymphocytes. (A) LP cell from the peripheral blood of a patient with Waldenström's macroglobulinemia. (× 7000, before 15% reduction.) (B) Extensive development of rough-surfaced endo-plasmic reticulum in a plasma cell. (× 12,000, before 25% reduction.) (Cour-tesy Steven D. Douglas, M.D., Mt. Sinai Hospital School of Medicine, New York.)

CLINICAL DISORDERS OF PLASMA CELLS AND LYMPHOCYTES

Based on our recent understanding of the cellular and humoral immune responses, it is possible to classify diseases of lymphocytes and plasma cells in terms of function. The immunologic deficiency disorders (underproduction states) are a group of conditions, sometimes referred to as the "experiments of nature," which are called to clinical attention because of the appearance of serious infections. A classification of the congenital immunologic deficiency disorders, based on our current thinking regarding cellular immune responses, is seen in Table 28-5. The immunoglobinopathies or hyperglobulinemias (overproduction states) can be further subdivided into those syndromes associated with the increased synthesis of normal immunoglobulins (Table 28-6) and the dysproteinemias, those syndromes associated with the synthesis of abnormal immunoglobulins (Table 28-7). In these syndromes the normal cellular immune responses may also be altered.

There is growing evidence that basic defects of the immune system may be important underlying factors in the etiology of the autoallergic diseases. Cited as supportive of this concept have been such observations as the frequent occurrence of rheumatoid arthritis with immunologic deficiencies, the morphologic abnormalities in the thymus and in other lymphoreticular tis-

Table 28-5.   Functional Classification of the Congenital Immunologic Deficiency Disorders

---

I. *Stem cell defects:* absent or decreased humoral and cell-mediated immunity
   A. Reticular dysgenesis (DeVaal syndrome with aleukocytosis): absent stem cells
   B. Lymphopenia with agammaglobulinemia: abnormal stem cells
      1. Autosomal recessive (Swiss type)
      2. Sex-linked recessive

II. *Disorders of the thymus:* normal humoral immunity with absent or diminished cell-mediated immunity
   A. Thymic aplasia (DiGeorge syndrome): absent thymus
   B. Thymic dysplasia (Nezelof syndrome): abnormal thymus, lymphopenia with normal immunoglobulins

III. *Disorders of the bursa equivalent:* absent or diminished humoral immunity with normal cell-mediated immunity
   A. Nonlymphopenic agammaglobulinemia: absent bursa
      1. Sex-linked recessive (Bruton type)
      2. Non-sex-linked
   B. Dysgammaglobulinemia: deficient synthesis of specific immunoglobulins, abnormal bursa
   C. Specific antibody deficiency syndrome with normal concentrations of immunoglobulins, abnormal bursa

IV. *Disorders of the thymus and bursa equivalent (mesenchymal defect)*
   Ataxia-telangiectasia: abnormal thymus, absent or diminished cellular immunity, diminished or absent IgM and IgG

Table 28-6. Immunoglobinopathies, I

Clinical states with increased synthesis of normal immunoglobulins: hyperglobulinemias, benign gammopathies

  A. Collagen diseases
     1. Lupus erythematosus
     2. Rheumatoid arthritis
     3. Sjögren's syndrome
     4. Scleroderma
  B. Chronic infections
     1. Tuberculosis
     2. Subacute bacterial endocarditis
     3. Leprosy
     4. Trypanosomiasis
     5. Malaria
     6. Kala-azar
     7. Infectious mononucleosis
     8. Fungus diseases
     9. Bartonellosis
     10. Lymphogranuloma venereum
     11. Actinomycosis
  C. Liver diseases
     1. Infectious hepatitis
     2. Laennec's cirrhosis
     3. Biliary cirrhosis
     4. Lupoid hepatitis
  D. Sarcoidosis
  E. Cold agglutinin disease
  F. Hyperglobulinemic purpura

sues seen in systemic lupus erythematosus (SLE), the clinical improvement in some patients with myasthenia gravis following thymectomy, and the appearance of autoimmune diseases in neonatally thymectomized experimental animals. There is also growing evidence that the lymphoreticular malignancies (lymphatic leukemia, lymphosarcoma, Hodgkin's disease, and reticulum cell sarcoma) occur together with the immunologic deficiency syndromes and the autoallergic diseases, suggesting that there may be some basic defect at the stem cell, thymus-dependent, or bursa-dependent levels. Extending this concept, Dr. Robert Good has suggested that the same cellular defect that underlies the immunologic deficiencies may also predispose the patient to develop lymphoreticular malignancies. In more general biologic terms, it appears that in the immunologically competent individual, malignancies develop as a result of the loss of immunologic surveillance. Conceptually, it is intuitively clear how intricately related development, structure, and function are in maintaining immunologic homeostasis.

Table 28-7.   Immunoglobinopathies, II

Clinical states with increased synthesis of abnormal immunoglobulins: dysproteinemias, monoclonal gammopathies, M-component disorders

A. *Idiopathic dysproteinemic states*
   1. Multiple myeloma (IgG, IgA, IgD, IgE)
   2. Waldenström's macroglobulinemia (IgM)
   3. H(heavy)-chain disease (μ-chain, α-chain, γ-chain)
   4. L(light)-chain disease (Bence Jones proteinemia and proteinuria)

B. *Dysproteinemias associated with other clinical conditions*
   1. Myeloproliferative disorders
      a. Chronic myelogenous leukemia
      b. Polycythemia vera
      c. Myelofibrosis
      d. Myeloid metaplasia
      e. Erythroleukemia
   2. Lymphoreticular neoplasia
      a. Chronic lymphocytic leukemia
      b. Lymphosarcoma
      c. Hodgkin's disease
      d. Reticulum cell sarcoma
   3. Collagen diseases
      a. Rheumatoid arthritis
      b. Systemic lupus erythematosus
      c. Sjögren's syndrome
   4. Carcinoma
   5. Amyloidosis
   6. Idiopathic cryoglobulinemia
   7. Idiopathic pyroglobulinemia

REFERENCES

Bergsma, D., and Good, R. A. (Eds.).   *Immunologic Deficiency Diseases in Man*. New York: The National Foundation, 1968.

Bloom, W.   Lymphatic Tissue; Lymphatic Organs. In H. Downey (Ed.), *Handbook of Hematology*. New York: Hafner, 1965.

Brenner, S., and Milstein, C.   Source of antibody variation. *Nature* (London) 211:242, 1966.

Burnet, F. M.   *Cellular Immunology*. New York: Cambridge University Press, 1969.

Chessin, L. N., Glade, P. R., Kasel, J. A., Moses, H. L., Herberman, R. B., and Hirshaut, Y.   The circulating lymphocyte: Its role in infectious mononucleosis. *Ann. Intern. Med.* 69:333, 1968.

Dameshek, W.   "Immunoblasts" and "immunocytes": An attempt at a functional nomenclature. *Blood* 21:243, 1963.

Fagraeus, A.   Nomenclature of Immunologically Competent Cells. In G. E. W. Wolstenholme and M. O'Connor (Eds.), *Cellular Aspects of Immunity* (A Ciba Foundation Symposium). Boston: Little, Brown, 1959.

Ford, W. L., and Gowans, J. L.   The traffic of lymphocytes. *Seminars Hemat.* 6:67, 1969.

Good, R. A., and Gabrielson, A. E. *The Thymus in Immunobiology.* New York: Hoeber Med. Div., Harper & Row, 1964.

Gowans, J. L., and McGregor, D. D.   The immunological activities of lymphocytes. *Progr. Allerg.* 9:1, 1965.

Lennox, E. S., and Cohn, M.   Immunoglobulins. *Ann. Rev. Biochem.* 36:365, 1967.

Meuwissen, H. J., Stutman, O., and Good, R. A.   Functions of the lymphocytes. *Seminars Hemat.* 6:28, 1969.

Nomenclature for human immunoglobulins. *Bull. W.H.O.* 30:447, 1964.

Notation for human immunoglobulin subclasses. *Bull. W.H.O.* 32:953, 1966.

Peterson, R. D. A., Cooper, M. D., and Good, R. A.   The pathogenesis of immunologic deficiency diseases. *Amer. J. Med.* 38:579, 1965.

Van Furth, R.   The formation of immunoglobulins by circulating lymphocytes. *Seminars Hemat.* 6:84, 1969.

Waldenström, J.   Monoclonal and polyclonal gammopathies and the biological system of gamma globulin. *Progr. Allerg.* 6:320, 1962.

Zucker-Franklin, D.   The ultrastructure of lymphocytes. *Seminars Hemat.* 6:4, 1969.

29. MULTIPLE MYELOMA AND DYSPROTEINEMIC STATES

Roger S. Hill

IMMUNOGLOBULINS AND MONOCLONAL PROTEINS

Immunoglobulins are an extremely heterogeneous group of gamma globulins, closely related in their biologic activity and, as their name implies, associated with antibody activity. Detailed discussions of the structure and properties of the immunoglobulin molecule have been presented in recent reviews by Martin and Putman. Suffice it to say here that all immunoglobulins are known to have a common basic structural unit consisting of four covalently linked polypeptide chains, two heavy (H) and two light (L) (Fig. 29-1). The heavy chains are different in structure and antigenic properties for each immunoglobulin class. The light chains, on the other hand, are shared by all the immunoglobulin classes. They are of two types, kappa (κ) and lambda (λ). The major structural and antigenic differences in the heavy polypeptide chain have allowed the immunoglobulins to be classified into major classes now referred to as IgG, IgA, IgM, IgD, and IgE.

The synthesis of immunoglobulins by plasma cells and certain lymphocytes has been discussed in Chapter 28. In the normal individual a variety of antigens stimulate many different clones of immunoglobulin-producing cells (immunocytes) to synthesize gamma globulin. The immunoglobulins produced reflect the heterogeneity of the immunoglobulin population (Fig. 29-2A). Two-thirds of the IgG gamma globulin molecules, for instance, have κ and one-third have λ light chains, and all the antigenic and allotypic variants of IgG are represented. Similar heterogeneity can be demonstrated for the other immunoglobulin classes. A typically broad-banded or polyclonal increase of gamma globulin is seen on serum electrophoresis.

On the other hand, several lines of evidence indicate that normal individ-

This work was aided by Grant IN-18K from the American Cancer Society.

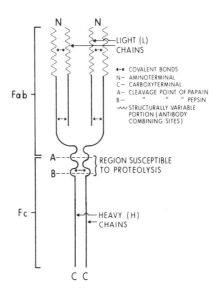

Figure 29-1. Basic structure of immunoglobulin molecule (IgG). The two Fab fragments are structurally variable. There is one antigen-combining site per fragment. The single Fc fragment is structurally invariable. It is the determinant for such things as complement fixation, skin sensitization, placental transfer, degradation rate, ?rate of secretion. The light chains may be bonded to each other.

ual immunocyte clones are probably restricted at any point in time to synthesizing single structural variants of heavy and light polypeptide chains. If one such restricted cell clone synthesizes excess globulin, a homogeneous, narrow-banded, myeloma-like or M gamma globulin increase appears on serum electrophoresis as a sharp, discrete protein peak (Fig. 29-2B). Despite the distinctive electrophoretic appearance of M protein bands, the proof of the monoclonal nature of an increased gamma globulin component rests with the demonstration that it is constituted by a single heavy and light chain type. If the plasma cell clone synthesizing this protein behaves in a malignant fashion, multiple myeloma develops.

Recent studies of the monoclonal proteins produced in multiple myeloma and macroglobulinemia suggest that in most cases they are normal synthetic products, as judged by structural criteria. When zone electrophoresis of M proteins from a large number of myeloma patients is compared with the heterogeneous gamma globulin population of normal serum, a remarkably similar distribution of gamma globulin is seen. In the same group of myeloma patients, the distribution of antigenic and allotypic markers is approximately the same as in the normal population, providing further support for the idea that myeloma cell clones occur randomly in the spectrum of immunocyte proliferation.

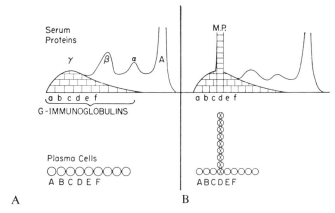

Figure 29-2. The possible relationship between (A) normal plasma cells and normal G immunoglobulins, and between (B) a malignant plasma cell clone and the corresponding myeloma protein (MP). (From E. F. Osserman, *Amer. J. Med.* 44:256, 1968.)

As a group, myeloma proteins differ from normal gamma globulins in one important respect, namely, their lack of antibody activity. Recently, however, several M proteins obtained from human and mouse myelomas and from Waldenström's macroglobulinemia have been described which resemble true antibodies by most presently available criteria. A number of other monoclonal proteins have also been observed to exhibit antibody-like activity to a variety of antigens. Thus some myeloma proteins have a high affinity for certain polynitrophenyl ligands, while others bind bacterial enzymes or neutralize bacterial viruses. Certain macroglobulins have high titers of antistreptolysin O, rheumatoid factor, or cold agglutinin activity, or exhibit antibody-like activity to lipoprotein. The complex problems of defining and demonstrating antibody activity in monoclonal proteins, and the unresolved questions raised by the described properties of certain of these proteins, have been excellently discussed in a recent review by Metzger.

Gradually accumulating evidence consistently confirms the idea that most myeloma and other monoclonal proteins represent the massive production of one structurally and antigenically restricted globulin derived from a single clone of proliferating immunocytes.

MONOCLONAL PROTEINS: BENIGN OR MALIGNANT?

If a monoclonal protein is detected in the serum of a person without other evidence of disease, the important question is whether the clone of cells synthesizing that protein will behave in a malignant or a benign fashion. The incidence of monoclonal proteins in large population samples of persons over the age of 25 years is 0.9%, increasing to more than 5% by the eighth decade. About one-half will be considered to have a benign condition 3 to 5 years after detection. Of those remaining, most will have developed a diagnosed malignant disease.

Waldenström has given the name *benign essential hypergammaglobulinemia* to a condition in which the patient has had a monoclonal protein peak for a period of 10 years or more without associated evidence of disease. This group is clearly distinct from those patients with a transient M protein very occasionally seen on electrophoresis during the course of acute infections, particularly in children, liver disease, and connective tissue disorders. Criteria characterizing the entity are (1) a quantity of monoclonal protein not exceeding 2 gm per 100 ml; (2) a persistence, but no increase, in the monoclonal protein component with time; (3) no quantitative decrease of normal polyclonal gamma globulin (IgG); (4) the absence of Bence Jones proteinuria; (5) the absence of clinical and radiologic evidence of disease; (6) the absence of abnormal (qualitative and quantitative) plasma cells or lymphoid cells (or both) infiltrating the bone marrow; and (7) a minimum follow-up period without change.

These criteria contrast sharply with the situation of most myeloma patients, in whom the serum M component shows a progressive and often rapid increase, a reduction of normal gamma globulin is usual, and Bence Jones proteinuria and histologic and radiologic evidence of disease are typically found. In the early stages the differentiation between benign and malignant disease is very often impossible. There is no characteristic of the benign condition which is absolute, allowing the diagnosis to be made with certainty. Correct evaluation is frequently dependent on careful follow-up over many years.

The crucial question, whether all patients with so-called benign hypergammaglobulinemia will ultimately be shown to have myeloma or some other malignant condition, is not answered at the present time. It is now clear that a good number of the idiopathic group ultimately go on to develop multiple myeloma or some other malignancy. A number of Waldenström's original patients, for instance, who fulfilled the criteria for the benign condition, have subsequently developed myeloma. The recent reports of persons developing myeloma up to 18 years after the onset of a condition of benign essential hypergammaglobulinemia further underline the need for extended follow-ups to settle this question, and also raise serious doubts whether such a benign condition exists.

It seems prudent to anticipate a potential for malignancy with all monoclonal proteins and to institute careful and regular follow-up of affected patients, with the appropriate hematologic, urinary, and serum protein studies. These should include hematocrit, blood film, sedimentation rate, serum protein electrophoresis, and quantitative estimation of monoclonal serum protein concentration. In addition, testing for and quantitative estimation of urinary Bence Jones protein are mandatory and should be pursued until concentration by dialysis and electrophoresis of not less than 3 voided early morning urine specimens or, alternatively, 3 urine collections (24-hour) have been shown to be negative. This laboratory data should be augmented by a careful history, thorough clinical examinations, and periodic x-rays of chest, skull, and pelvis.

MULTIPLE MYELOMA

The clinical manifestations of multiple myeloma have been frequently reviewed. In most patients with the disease, protein abnormalities are detected more frequently than conclusive histologic evidence is obtained. The frequency, however, with which monoclonal proteins are detected in the serum, and less often in the urine, from a variety of diseases (Table 29-1) has detracted from their usefulness in securing the diagnosis when other tests are inconclusive. Bone marrow cytology in myeloma, on the other

Table 29-1.   Diseases Reported with M Proteins

Association proved
   Primary (?benign) essential hypergammaglobulinemia
   Multiple myeloma (IgG, IgA, IgD, IgE)
   Waldenström's macroglobulinemia (IgM)
   Cold agglutinin disease
   Franklin's disease (IgG) ⎤
   α-Chain disease (IgA) ⎬ Heavy chain–Fc fragment disease
   μ-Chain disease (IgM) ⎦
   Malignant lymphoma—diffuse
      (chronic lymphatic leukemia, lymphocytic lymphoma, reticulum cell sarcoma)
   Primary amyloidosis

Association not proved
   Nodular lymphoma, Hodgkin's disease
   Nonreticular tumors
      (e.g., carcinoma of breast, gastrointestinal tract, biliary tract, lung)
   Gaucher's disease
   Lichen myxedematosus
   Pyoderma gangrenosum
   Chronic reticuloendothelial stimulation
      (e.g., bronchiectasis, chronic sepsis, liver disease)
   Collagen disease
   Miscellaneous
      (e.g., polycythemia, ankylosing spondylitis)

hand, can be difficult to interpret, and similar appearances are occasionally seen in diseases as varied as lymphoma, carcinoma, tuberculosis, collagen diseases, serum sickness, and certain infections including endocarditis and typhoid. There are unfortunately no morphologic features which distinguish the reactive from the malignant plasma cell. The appearances seen in the bone marrow or from localized bony lesions of infiltration by immature or atypical plasma cells, however, are generally indicative of multiple myeloma, and histologic evidence obtained from one or both of these sites remains the best single test for securing the diagnosis.

Since the application of immunoelectrophoresis to the detection and classification of myeloma proteins, it has become evident that a characteristic monoclonal protein is detected in the serum or urine, or both, in the great majority of cases (Table 29-2). About 1% of patients have no serum or urinary abnormality. Of interest is the IgD myeloma protein described for the first time in 1965 by Rowe and Fahey. Noteworthy in these cases have been the relatively low serum levels and the electrophoretically inconspicuous nature of the M protein. The high frequency (90%) of λ light chains is in interesting contrast to their lower frequency in other myeloma proteins. Bence Jones (BJ) protein has been a striking feature of most but not all of the cases.

Recently a fifth unique immunoglobulin class, IgE, has been described. The evidence available suggests that it is the carrier of reaginic antibody related to allergic states. The report of a second case of IgE myeloma has heightened interest in this entity. Both patients presented with increased numbers of plasma cells in the peripheral blood, associated λ BJ proteinuria, and absence of osteolytic lesions. Several reports suggest that increased

Table 29-2. Serum and Urinary M Proteins in Multiple Myeloma

Class of M Protein	Incidence (%)	Frequency of Bence Jones Proteinuria (%)	Bence Jones (Light chain) Type
IgG	55–65	Approx. 30	$\kappa \gg \lambda$
IgA	18–25	Approx. 30	$\kappa \equiv \lambda$
Bence Jones protein only	15–23	100 [a]	$\kappa > \lambda$
IgD	0.6–2	95	$\lambda \ggg \kappa$
IgE	Rare	Two cases, both positive	λ (in both cases)
No abnormality	1		

[a] In very rare cases, Bence Jones protein is not associated with proteinuria.

numbers of plasma cells can be found in the peripheral blood of at least 50% of patients with proved myeloma by careful examination of buffy coat smears. Plasma cell leukemia, however, is rare, constituting no more than about 2% of all cases of multiple myeloma.

BENCE JONES PROTEIN

Bence Jones proteins are the light chains of an immunoglobulin molecule excreted in the urine or detected in the serum. They are identical with the single type of light chain of the serum monoclonal protein from the same patient. They have the unique and characteristic property in solution of precipitating upon being heated to between 40° and 60°C, redissolving on boiling, and reprecipitating on further cooling. These events, occurring within a restricted pH range, have been the basis for the classic heat test performed to detect BJ proteinuria. Using this method, the overall incidence in myeloma patients has been reported as about 35 to 50%. It is clear, however, that in using the heat test a significant number of cases of BJ proteinuria will be missed. In recent years more sensitive methods of concentration dialysis and electrophoresis of urine have proved far superior for the detection of urinary light chains in patients with multiple myeloma, macroglobulinemia, and a variety of other conditions.

It has been conclusively demonstrated that BJ protein is not a breakdown product of serum immunoglobulins. Rather immunoglobulin light chains appear to be synthesized separately, and on different ribosomes, from the heavy chain and can be detected as a small intracellular pool of free light chains prior to the appearance of heavy chains. In normal immunoglobulin-forming cells, and probably in well-differentiated myeloma plasma cells, this process and interaction of protein chains is balanced, and virtually no light chains escape free from the cell. In those myeloma patients presenting with BJ protein as well as serum myeloma protein, it appears that the cells synthesize light chains in excess of heavy chains, so that the characteristic low-molecular-weight protein is then detected in the urine, serum, or both. This imbalance may proceed further so that no heavy chains are synthesized and only BJ protein is detected. Finally, the myeloma cell may be unable to synthesize any heavy or light chains. As cited later, Hobbs and others believe that the lack of capacity to synthesize intact immunoglobulin molecules may be correlated with clinicopathologic worsening, earlier appearance of myeloma, and more rapid growth of the tumor mass.

The survival of BJ protein in man is exceedingly short. Catabolic breakdown is rapid and probably takes place in the substance of the kidney within about 2 hours. Most of its disappearance can be attributed to endogenous kidney metabolism, and not more than perhaps 25% is due to loss in the urine as proteinuria. Furthermore, the presence of renal disease and uremia impairs this catabolic process and may contribute to the development of detectable serum levels and increased urinary excretion in myeloma patients. Thus only a small and variable portion of the BJ protein filtered by the kidney glomerulus may be excreted in the urine. This is in contrast to intact gamma globulin and certain gamma globulin chain fragments which do not appear to be catabolized to any significant degree in the substance of the kidney despite free renal glomerular filtration.

The increasingly important and often ominous significance attributed to the presence of BJ protein in the urine and serum of persons suspected of having malignant disease, particularly multiple myeloma, requires further comment. Waldenström considered the absence of BJ protein an important criterion of benign hypergammaglobulinemia, and significant BJ proteinuria as suggestive evidence of malignant transformation. It has become evident that up to 40% of patients with monoclonal serum protein spikes, fulfilling the criteria of the benign condition, will have detectable BJ proteinuria as judged by sensitive electrophoretic techniques. This is compared with an 80% incidence or more in malignant conditions. The degree of concentration of the urine as well as the sensitivity of the electrophoretic method are critical in this context. Even more significant than the actual frequency has been the quantitative difference in protein excretion between the benign and the malignant states. In most benign cases, patients with detectable BJ proteinuria have shown less than 20 mg per 100 ml, whereas patients with macroglobulinemia and myeloma in which BJ protein is found have values far in excess of this. The evidence from several large series suggests that virtually all patients presenting with monoclonal serum spikes in whom significant ($>$ 20 mg per 100 ml) BJ proteinuria is detected ultimately develop a malignant condition.

Recent reports indicate that BJ proteinuria can be detected in 80 to 90% of cases of macroglobulinemia which subsequently follow a malignant clinical course. This high incidence of increased urinary light chain excretion in macroglobulinemia is much more than the 15% positive incidence previously documented and can probably be attributed to the more sensitive methods for detecting BJ protein.

The presence of light chains in the urine is not in itself proof that the condition is malignant. Rather the quantitative determination of the protein appears to be the important parameter in the differential diagnosis of benign versus malignant disease. Detection is made more difficult because of the number of patients who appear to excrete small quantities intermittently. Approximately two-thirds of patients with IgG myeloma and BJ proteinuria have κ light chains in their urine. Kappa light chains also predominate in BJ myeloma patients. The exceptions, however, are those persons presenting with IgD myeloma. Of the two dozen or so reported up to 1969, virtually all had significant BJ proteinuria, and of these, 90% were of the λ variety. Similarly, both patients reported to have IgE myeloma excreted λ light chains.

BJ proteinuria probably never occurs without BJ proteinemia, although the quantity may be so small that it is not detected by the routine electrophoretic methods. On the other hand, BJ proteinemia has been reported without proteinuria, the serum component being tetrameric and nonfilterable through the kidney glomerulus. This, however, is a rare exception, not the rule. Free light chains have been described in plasma from normal individuals (the calculated level being approximately 0.005 to 0.008 mg per milliliter of normal serum) and in diseases as varied as collagen disease and serum sickness. Previous estimates suggest that the incidence of significant BJ proteinemia in multiple myeloma is about 10%. Light chain disease without detectable intact myeloma protein occurs in 15 to 23% of cases. The significance of the presence of these various proteins will be discussed in a later section.

OTHER DISEASES ASSOCIATED WITH MONOCLONAL PROTEINS

MACROGLOBULINEMIA

IgM monoclonal proteins, referred to as *macroglobulins* because of their high molecular weight (850,000 to 900,000), account for about 10% of serum monoclonal proteins and are detected in 1% of the population over 50 years of age. About one-third of these persons suffer symptoms directly attributable to the excess of high-molecular-weight protein and are admitted to the hospital. Macroglobulins are present in normal serum, usually constituting less than 3% of the total protein (50 to 200 mg per 100 ml). They have generally been regarded as quantitatively abnormal when present in excess of 5 to 10%. The amount of macroglobulin in the serum does not in itself distinguish the primary macroglobulinemia of Waldenström from secondary varieties, though the serum level is generally a useful clinical pointer in distinguishing between the two.

Waldenström's macroglobulinemia is generally associated with massive amounts of a monoclonal protein having a sedimentation constant of about 19S. The disease generally presents with macroglobulin levels greater than 3 gm per 100 ml, and most patients (75%) suffer symptoms as a direct consequence of the elevated serum globulin component. The macroglobulin exists mostly as a pentamer made up of five monomeric gamma globulin subunits, arranged in a ring configuration. Each subunit consists of two heavy and two light polypeptide chains. There is recent evidence from several laboratories to suggest that IgM exists also as a monomer and as an incidental finding in about 20% of cases of primary macroglobulinemia. A recent report, for instance, detailed the case of a 67-year-old woman with a disease resembling malignant lymphoma. A serum M protein band was detected, despite a normal total serum protein. The M protein was approximately the same molecular weight as normal monomeric IgG immunoglobulin but gave a positive reaction of identity with IgM. No excess of high-molecular-weight IgM was detected in the serum. The patient appeared to be suffering from IgM monomer disease. Several other, similar, cases have been studied in which the monomer appeared to be the prominent atypical protein. It is as yet too early to assess the pathophysiologic relationship between these two structural variants, however.

HEAVY CHAIN (F_c-FRAGMENT) DISEASES

The splitting of the immunoglobulin molecule by papain and pepsin into various heavy and light chain fragments (Fig. 29-1) in the early 1960's led to the prediction that diseases involving these immunoglobulin chain fragments would subsequently be found. Since 1964 several rare new disease entities involving heavy chain (F_c) fragments have been described. These include Franklin's disease (IgG–F_c fragment disease), α-chain disease (IgA –F_c fragment disease), and μ-chain disease (IgM–F_c fragment disease). The conditions will be alluded to briefly here. More detailed accounts are given by Zawadski, Seligman, and Ballard (see references).

Both Franklin's disease and α-chain disease belong in the category of malignant proliferative lymphoplasmacytic disorders, representing variants of malignant lymphoma. Indeed the strikingly similar pleomorphic cell infiltration seen in α-chain disease, Franklin's disease, some cases of Waldenström's macroglobulinemia, certain other variants of lymphoma, and some instances of cold agglutinin disease suggest a very close pathophysiologic relationship among these diseases. Approximately 10% of cases of cold agglutinin disease, for instance, terminate in lymphoma. Lymphocytic lymphoma as a terminal event in patients who initially present with classic primary macroglobulinemia is well recognized and has led to the suggestion that Waldenström's macroglobulinemia represents a stage in the development of malignant lymphoma. Cases have been reported of apparent viral infections associated with the development of a serum cold agglutinin which persisted in very high titer, the patient ultimately going on to develop a disease indistinguishable from Waldenström's macroglobulinemia.

LYMPHOMA AND MONOCLONAL PROTEINS

The occurrence of monoclonal proteins in lymphoproliferative disorders is not surprising in view of the fact that the lymphocyte occupies a key position in the immunocompetent cell compartment. Considering the degree of disordered immunity demonstrated in malignancies of the reticuloendothelial system, the elaboration of monoclonal proteins by lymphomas is a relative rarity, occurring in about 3% of cases. Most, but by no means all, are macroglobulins (IgM). Occasionally IgG, IgA, and even diclonal gammopathies occur. Most patients are asymptomatic, and unlike the situation with Waldenström's macroglobulinemia, the protein spike is usually detected unexpectedly. Typical 19S macroglobulins are, however, present in a high proportion of cases in which IgM proteins are found and occasionally constitute as much as half of all gamma globulins present in individual patients. Monoclonal proteins are rarely associated with Hodgkin's disease or nodular lymphoma. No patient with coexisting nodular lymphoma and IgM M protein has yet been reported. Whereas the incidence of IgM monoclonal proteins in a random population is about 0.07%, and in persons over 50 years of age, 1%, this incidence increases in patients with diffuse lymphoma (chronic lymphatic leukemia, well-differentiated and poorly differentiated lymphocytic lymphoma, and reticulum cell sarcoma) to 3 to 4%, significantly greater than the incidence of macroglobulinemia in random surveys and in cancer which is not of the myeloma-lymphoma group. On the other hand, the incidence of IgG monoclonal proteins is not significantly different from that found in population samples of random and cancer patients (0.6 to 1%).

The frequency of IgM monoclonal proteins increases with age in lymphoma patients, as in the normal population, and is reported to be more commonly found in patients demonstrating lymph node masses as their major clinical manifestation. Hobbs has noted generally massive regional lymph node involvement in cases of lymphoma with associated monoclonal proteins, and he describes this as a rapidly progressive disease with death usually occurring within 1 year. Others also have implied that lymphoma associated with an M component has a poor prognosis. This is easily understood in certain situations. Occasional cases of lymphoma are recorded in which acceleration of the disease coincides with the appearance of an M protein and a new line of malignant lymphoid cells, distinct from those present at the onset of the patient's illness. The emergence during or after treatment of a resistant, more malignant clone of lymphoid cells provides a plausible biologic explanation for the deterioration which is seen in such cases. It still remains to be demonstrated conclusively, however, that the natural history of most untreated and treated lymphoma patients with monoclonal serum protein spikes differs from that of patients without M proteins.

MONOCLONAL PROTEINS AND NONRETICULAR TUMORS

In contrast to lymphomas, in which the association of M protein is generally well established, the association of monoclonal protein and nonreticular malignancies remains controversial. When found, the monoclonal protein is mostly IgG. The occurrence of myeloma or myeloma-like disease in people who have or ultimately develop cancer is well recognized. Whether this is a chance association is not known. Numerous case reports have suggested an association between nonreticular malignancy and M protein, some implying a cause-and-effect relationship. Recent comparative studies of large groups of carcinoma patients and normal populations show a strikingly similar age incidence of monoclonal proteins in both groups, leading to the conclusion that the association is probably fortuitous. The failure of treatment to influence the protein concentration in large numbers of carcinoma patients is held as further evidence against the cause-and-effect relationship suggested by some writers. There are rare though well-documented cases of the disappearance of the M protein following treatment or removal of a malignant tumor and its reappearance with clinical relapse. These suggest that large population samples may overlook a small but significant group of patients in whom the M protein reflects a reactive benign monoclonal immunocyte reaction to the tumor.

The marked increase in the incidence of M proteins with advancing age in both tumor and normal population samples nevertheless remains to be adequately explained. The suggestion that many if not all of these patients will go on to develop myeloma is debatable. The incidence of myeloma in persons past the age of 25 years is about 1 or 2 per 10,000 population (0.01%). The total incidence of M proteins in persons more than 25 years of age is 0.9%. In the eighth decade the incidence of monoclonal proteins is 5.7%, and this increasing incidence with age far exceeds the predicted incidence of myeloma in the same age group.

CHEMOTHERAPY OF MULTIPLE MYELOMA

Two alkylating agents, phenylalanine mustard (Pam, Melphalan) and cyclophosphamide (Cytoxan) have proved to be the most effective chemotherapeutic agents for treating multiple myeloma. The overall response rate of 33% and 36%, respectively, for the two drugs, obtained from a number of reported series up to the present time, and their strikingly similar median survival figures (24 months) indicate that the agents are comparable in terms of efficacy when given individually in a variety of regimens.

Prior to 1968, the reported remission rates and the survival data for multiple myeloma had remained static for about 5 years. A number of factors including differing drug regimens, selection of patients, and changing criteria for assessing response have added to the confusion in assessing the results of therapy and influencing the outcome of studies. The choice of one or another agent has frequently rested, therefore, on other considerations; for instance, the platelet-sparing action of cyclophosphamide balanced against the frequency of hemorrhagic bladder complications and alopecia, or in the case of PAM the relative unpredictability of action and profound bone marrow hypoplasia which may be induced by the drug.

Bruce's important studies showing differential killing patterns of malignant cells and normal stem cells by a range of cytotoxic agents, including cyclophosphamide, have provided a rationale for intermittent chemotherapy in malignant diseases, including multiple myeloma, and have been exploited recently with initially hopeful results. The recent report by Alexanian of a much improved remission rate (61 to 65%) in myeloma patients treated with intermittent combined courses of PAM and prednisone is very promising but requires further confirmation. The addition of prednisone to intermittent courses of PAM seems to enhance the efficacy of the alkylating agent and to increase the remission rate from approximately 35% (the response rate of single agents used daily or intermittently) to over 60%.

The practice in many centers at present is to administer PAM together with prednisone for 4 consecutive days every 6 weeks in doses of 0.25 mg and 2.0 mg, respectively, per kilogram of body weight per day. Despite the very large dose of alkylating agent given in the combined regimen (a 70-kg man would receive 70 mg of PAM in each 4-day course), no significant increase in toxicity has been apparent to date. This observation serves to underline the most important potential advantage, predicted from Bruce's work, of intermittent over continuous alkylation, namely, being able to give very large loading doses of drug to ensure maximal myeloma cell kill without prohibitive hematologic toxicity. The interval between doses allows normal stem cell recovery to occur, unlike continuous therapy in which dose levels are clearly restricted by continuing stem cell kill and bone marrow toxicity.

The question of the interval separating successive therapeutic courses of alkylating agents remains to be settled, and the 6-week interval has been called into question. Occasional patients with myeloma clearly develop clinical and hematologic relapse between courses. Evidence from human and animal work shows that stem cell and bone marrow recovery following short-term, high-dose administration of cyclophosphamide is very rapid and, depending on the schedule, is probably complete 2 to 3 weeks after the drug is stopped. The pattern of hematologic recovery in man following combined intermittent chemotherapy has still to be studied in detail, but the courses may ultimately be shown to exert maximal benefit when the interval between them is reduced.

Long-term prednisone therapy has also been given on alternate days together with the intermittent PAM schedule. In Alexanian's series, however, serious toxicity necessitating drug withdrawal occurred in 10% of myeloma patients who were given more prednisone than 0.5 mg per kilogram of body weight on alternate days. In the remainder, less troublesome toxicity (for instance, cushingoid changes) was avoided when the steroid dose was reduced to 0.5 mg per kilogram or less. On the other hand, no serious toxicity was associated with concurrent high-dose intermittent prednisone therapy. PAM or cyclophosphamide and corticosteroid, given together as high-dose intermittent therapy, constitute a very effective treatment in multiple myeloma. Daily low-dose alkylation therapy continues to be a satisfactory regimen for patients demonstrating responsiveness and tolerance, as confirmed recently by McArthur and associates. Daily or alternate-day corticosteroids may be preferable in certain specific situations including bleeding, purpura, or thrombocytopenia.

RESPONSE TO TREATMENT

The need for careful and critical evaluation of therapeutic response has prompted the use of a variety of criteria for the evaluation of drug efficacy in inducing response and remission. The following arbitrary criteria can provide the clinician with helpful guidelines for assessing these parameters in multiple myeloma.

1. A decrease of serum myeloma protein to less than 50% of pretreatment levels and less than 4.0 gm per 100 ml
2. A decrease of urinary BJ protein to less than 50% of pretreatment levels and to less than 0.5 gm per 100 ml
3. Greater than 50% regression for a minimum period of 2 months in the product of the two largest diameters of plasmacytomas.
4. No response accepted unless the hemoglobin level rises 2 gm per 100 ml and is greater than 9 gm per 100 ml

Of particular interest has been the small but significant group of persons previously refractory to PAM alone (given continuously or intermittently) who have responded to combined intermittent therapy (alkylation plus steroids). In Alexanian's series, 6 of 14 patients unresponsive to daily PAM and 3 of 15 unresponsive to intermittent PAM responded to intermittent PAM and prednisone combined. There is no reason to believe that cyclophosphamide, similarly administered in combination with corticosteroids, would not induce an equally impressive remission rate. Ultimately, the choice of chemotherapy and dose schedule rests on the consideration of a number of factors, not the least of which is the comparative drug toxicity balanced against the patient's age, degree of debility, stage of the disease, and hematologic status.

The mean survival time obtained in continuing trials with combined intermittent regimens is about 24 months, considerably better than the 9 months obtained in untreated cases or the 11 months in patients treated with urethan, but not as yet significantly better than the median survival figures obtained by other established modes of administration of these agents. The demonstrated advantage of combined intermittent therapy at present lies in the increased percentage of patients able to obtain remission. Improved longevity has yet to be demonstrated by extended studies of large groups of patients.

In most cases a fall in serum myeloma protein concomitant with chemotherapy is indicative of response and will be accompanied by clinical improvement. Rarely, however, patients with myeloma die of progressive disease during chemotherapy despite a progressive reduction of serum M protein until death. The importance of careful and repeated urine testing for BJ protein is best exemplified by this small group of patients, constituting considerably less than 1% of cases. They are found to excrete considerably increased quantities of BJ protein despite falling serum myeloma protein levels and stable renal function. Their progressive deterioration is most likely explained by the proliferation of a second, resistant, more malignant clone of plasma cell synthesizing only light chains.

Patients with multiple myeloma who respond to treatment with a rapid reduction of monoclonal protein component may represent a poor prognostic group. Hobbs's recent data suggesting a significant difference in survival and relapse rate between so-called fast (39% alive at 2 years) and slow (78% alive at 2 years) responders is interesting but requires confirmation. A rapid responder would be expected to show approximately a 50% decrease of monoclonal protein by 6 to 8 weeks after the initiation of treatment. A typical slow responder would have a 50% decrease in from 6 to 12 months after commencing chemotherapy.

Although myelomonoblastic leukemia has evolved in a few myeloma patients treated with PAM, the therapeutic value of alkylating agents far outweighs any possible leukemogenic effect, based on present evidence.

CHEMOTHERAPY OF MACROGLOBULINEMIA

The treatment of macroglobulinemia has been unpredictable, inconsistent, and generally disappointing. Complete, incomplete, and transitory responses, as well as failures, have occurred with a variety of chemotherapeutic agents including nitrogen mustard, cyclophosphamide, and chlorambucil. Taken overall, the most optimistic therapeutic efforts have occurred with the use of chlorambucil (Leukeran). The starting dose has been mostly from 6 to 12 mg per day with maintenance therapy in the range of 2 to 3 mg per day after an initial period, usually 3 to 4 weeks. In general, longer remissions have been obtained in those patients given continuous maintenance chemotherapy. It has been suggested that discontinuation of the drug invariably leads to relapse and that the response to a second course of the drug is disappointing. On the other hand, those patients receiving continuous chemotherapy generally appear to remain in remission as long as the drug is continued (up to 5½ years). These last conclusions, mostly from single sources, have yet to be substantiated in large treatment groups and over extended periods.

Many of the most dramatic manifestations of the disease—for instance, circulatory impairment, bleeding, and deterioration of vision—are more often related to the level of high-molecular-weight macroglobulin, with or without cryoglobulin activity, than to the effects per se of progressive malignancy. These problems are best dealt with acutely by plasmapheresis. The improvement following this procedure is generally prompt and dramatic, and this form of therapy can be performed repeatedly and safely. Further, elderly patients have been described as having high levels of serum globulin (over 7 gm per 100 ml) and marked symptoms directly attributable to the effects of excess IgM macroglobulin who, 6 or 7 years later, were found to be fit and well without treatment and with no evidence of persisting macroglobulin in the serum. Well-documented cases such as these make it difficult to give an accurate overall assessment of the real value of cytotoxic agents such as chlorambucil. It is clear that in some patients primary macroglobulinemia may stay indolent for years. In others the disorder may present as a rapidly progressive malignant process, terminating in lymphoma and death in a year or less. It should be emphasized that Waldenström's macroglobulinemia is a disease of middle and old age, most commonly found in males over 50 years of age. Cytotoxic drugs have their own risks, which may be serious or fatal for the old and debilitated patient.

PROGNOSIS IN MULTIPLE MYELOMA

The immunologic class of myeloma protein, the quantity of BJ proteinuria, and the type (κ or λ) of light chain synthesized by the malignant plasma cell clone have been among the primary variables used in assessing the prognosis of multiple myeloma at the time of diagnosis. Of the patients with myeloma who survive more than 3 months, about two-thirds of those excreting more than 1 gm per day of BJ protein will be complicated by renal failure. While the actual incidence of BJ proteinuria is about the same for IgG and IgA myeloma protein classes (approximately 30%), the quantity excreted is frequently considerably more in patients with IgA myeloma. As has been commented on earlier, BJ proteinuria is present in virtually all patients with IgD myeloma, and renal failure is common. Recently, the level of serum albumin has been linked statistically with survival in multiple myeloma.

Recent analysis of large groups of myeloma patients suggests that those synthesizing κ light chains may have a longer survival than those synthesizing λ chains. Hobbs and Alexanian, for instance, have separated the BJ myeloma group from other myeloma classes. Their data suggest that patients having λ BJ myeloma show a poorer response to chemotherapy and a generally shorter survival (with small numbers of cases) than either κ BJ myelomas or other groups synthesizing κ chains as the light chain component of their myeloma protein.

It is clear that patients with IgG myeloma are in a better-risk category because of the reduced incidence of uremia and hypercalcemia. Alternatively, the proportion of patients with IgA, IgD, or BJ myeloma who have an unfavorable clinical course is relatively higher. The unfavorable correlation relating to uremia is of particular importance. The most common cause of death in myeloma patients surviving the first 3 months of treatment is renal failure (about 50% of all deaths), which is clearly related to the quantity of BJ proteinuria. A second important renal complication of myeloma, amyloidosis (occurring in about 10% of cases), is reported as being more frequently seen in BJ myeloma and relatively rarely seen with the IgG immunoglobulin class, an observation which, however, remains disputed.

Hobbs believes that the rare cases of myeloma without demonstrable serum or urinary monoclonal proteins are the most malignant and carry the worst prognosis of the myeloma groups. IgG myelomas are generally associated with greater increases of serum myeloma proteins, more reduction of normal immunoglobulins, and more frequent infections than other myelomas. Nevertheless malignant plasma cell clones synthesizing IgG myeloma proteins in general show the slowest growth rate and the best overall prognosis of all the myeloma classes.

REFERENCES

Alexanian, R., Haut, A., Khan, A. U., Lane, M., McKelvey, E. M., Migliore, P. J., Stuckey, W. J., and Wilson, H. E.   Treatment of multiple myeloma. *J.A.M.A.* 208:1680, 1969.

Ballard, H. S., Hamilton, L. M., Aaron, J. M., and Illes, C. H.   A new variant of heavy-chain disease (μ-chain disease). *New Eng. J. Med.* 282:1060, 1970.

Bergsagel, D. E., Griffith, K. M., Haut, A., and Stuckey, W. J.   The treatment of plasma cell myeloma. *Advances Cancer Res.* 10:311, 1967.

Bruce, W. R., Meeker, B. E., and Valeriote, F. A.   Comparison of the sensitivity of normal hemopoietic and transplanted lymphoma colony–forming cells to chemotherapeutic agents administered in vivo. *J. Nat. Cancer Inst.* 37:233, 1966.

Carbone, P., Kellerhouse, L. E., and Gehan, E. A.   Plasmacytic myeloma. *Amer. J. Med.* 42:937, 1967.

Cohen, S.   The nature of myeloma proteins. *Brit. J. Haemat.* 15:211, 1968.

Hobbs, J. R. Immunochemical classes of myelomatosis. *Brit. J. Haemat.* 16: 599, 1969.

Hobbs, J. R. Growth rates and responses to treatment in human myelomatosis. *Brit. J. Haemat.* 16:607, 1969.

Kyle, R. A., and Bayrd, E. D. Benign monoclonal gammopathy: A potentially malignant condition. *Amer. J. Med.* 40:426, 1966.

Kyle, R. A., Pierre, R. V., and Bayrd, E. D. Multiple myeloma and acute myelomonocytic leukemia: Report of four cases possibly related to Melphalan. *New Eng. J. Med.* 283:1121, 1970.

Martin, N. H. The immunoglobulins: A review. *J. Clin. Path.* 22:117, 1969.

Mattioli, C., and Tomasi, T. B. The human serum immunoglobulins. *D.M.*, April 1970.

McArthur, J. R., Athens, J. W., Wintrobe, M. M., and Cartwright, G. E. Melphalan and myeloma. *Ann. Intern. Med.* 72:711, 1970.

McCallister, B. D., Bayrd, E. D., Harrison, E. G., and McGuckin, W. F. Primary macroglobulinemia. *Amer. J. Med.* 43:394, 1967.

Metzger, H. Myeloma proteins and antibodies (editorial). *Amer. J. Med.* 47:837, 1969.

Moore, D. F., Migliore, P. J., Shullenberger, C. C., and Alexanian, R. Monoclonal macroglobulinemia in malignant lymphoma. *Ann. Intern. Med.* 72:43, 1970.

Ogawa, M., Kochwa, S., Smith, C., Ishizaka, K., and McIntyre, D. R. Clinical aspects of IgE myeloma. *New Eng. J. Med.* 281:1217, 1969.

Osserman, E. F. Plasma cell dyscrasias. Current clinical and biochemical concepts. *Amer. J. Med.* 44:256, 1968.

Putman, F. W. Immunoglobulin structure: Variability and homology. *Science* 163:633, 1969.

Seligman, M., Mihaesco, E., Hurez, D., Mihaesco, C., Preud'homme, J., and Rambaud, J. Immunochemical studies in four cases of alpha chain disease. *J. Clin. Invest.* 48:2374, 1969.

Snapper, I., and Kahn, A. I. Multiple myeloma. *Seminars Hemat.* 1:87, 1964.

Waldenström, J. *Diagnosis and Treatment of Multiple Myeloma.* New York: Grune & Stratton, 1970.

Williams, R. C., Brunning, R. D., and Wollheim, F. A. Light-chain disease. *Ann. Intern. Med.* 65:471, 1966.

Wochner, R. D., Strober, W., and Waldmann, T. A. The role of the kidney in the catabolism of Bence Jones proteins and immunoglobulin fragments. *J. Exp. Med.* 126:207, 1967.

Zawadzki, Z. A., Benedek, T. G., Ein, D., and Easton, J. M. Rheumatoid arthritis terminating in heavy chain disease. *Ann. Intern. Med.* 70:335, 1969.

Zawadzki, Z. A., and Edwards, G. A. M-components in immunoproliferative disorders. *Amer. J. Clin. Path.* 48:418, 1967.

30. THE CLASSIFICATION AND STAGING OF MALIGNANT LYMPHOMAS

John M. Bennett

THE MALIGNANT LYMPHOMAS are a group of chronic but progressive disorders of lymphatic tissue involving the lymphocytic or histiocytic series, or both, by a neoplastic proliferation of cells, producing architectural obliteration and organ invasion. In the past decade significant advances have been made in both the pathologic classification and the clinical staging of these diseases. Moreover since the histology, clinical features, and therapeutic response of Hodgkin's disease are considerably different from those of the other malignant lymphomas, it is useful to discuss this entity separately.

HODGKIN'S DISEASE

Hodgkin's disease constitutes 40% of all malignant lymphomas. Its incidence among the white population is comparable to that of acute leukemia. Males predominate by a ratio of approximately 4 to 3 and generally have a worse prognosis than females. Indeed, Hodgkin's disease is the leading cause of nonaccidental death of males between the ages of 15 and 35. The majority of cases occur in patients between the ages of 20 and 40 years, with less than 10% recognized under the age of 10 or over the age of 60 years.

The unique feature of Hodgkin's disease has been the recognition of the Reed-Sternberg cell, an abnormal reticulum cell with huge inclusion-like nucleoli and polyploidism, in association with an inflammatory cellular pro-

This work was supported in part by Grant Ca 11083 (ECOG) from the National Cancer Institute and by Grant RM 25-02 from the Rochester Cancer Regional Medical Program.

liferation. This cell is probably the end stage of the malignant reticulum cells that are recognized as an important feature of this disease (Fig. 30-1). It is of interest that recently the Reed-Sternberg cell has been identified by Lukes in conditions other than Hodgkin's disease. However, without the recognition of this cell and the insistence that it be present as a prerequisite for the diagnosis of Hodgkin's disease, nonneoplastic conditions such as postvaccination lymphadenitis and other reactive processes may be mistaken for Hodgkin's disease. Indeed the incidence of such mistaken diagnoses may approximate 15% if these criteria are not adhered to rigidly.

In 1944 Jackson and Parker, drawing on their vast experience at the Boston City Hospital, proposed a division into three pathologic types (Table 30-1). They suggested that those patients with a paragranuloma had a favorable prognosis, whereas those with a sarcoma had a very poor prognosis. Though this represented the first attempt to correlate pathology with the clinical response of a patient, it had very definite practical and predictive limitations because of the small numbers of patients that presented with either a paragranuloma type or sarcoma type of Hodgkin's disease. It was for this reason that Lukes and Butler proposed a new classification in 1964 (Table 30-1). The significant features of this classification, and of the revised one suggested at the Rye conference in 1966, were the

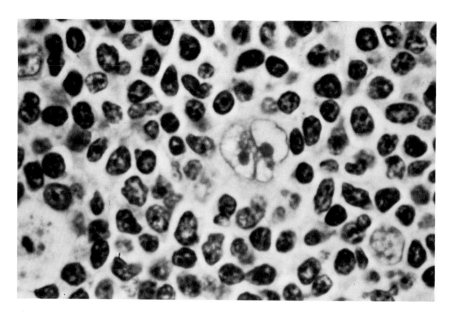

Figure 30-1. Reed-Sternberg cell among numerous lymphocytes. Note normal histiocyte in lower left. Hodgkin's disease, lymphocyte predominant type. (H & E; × 1200.)

Table 30-1.   Comparison of Histologic Classifications in Hodgkin's Disease

Parker-Jackson	Lukes-Butler (Rye modification)	R-S cells
(5%) Paragranuloma ──→	Lymphocyte predominance (5%)	Rare
(90%) Granuloma ──→	Nodular sclerosis (50%)	Occasional to moderate
	Mixed cellularity (40%)	
(5%) Sarcoma ──→	Lymphocyte depletion (5%)	Moderate to many

recognition of the nodular variety with collagen bands and atypical Reed-Sternberg cells, representing 50% of all cases with a preponderance in females, the majority occurring above the diaphragm (Fig. 30-2). Other important prognostic features are the presence of large numbers of normal-appearing lymphocytes and small numbers of Reed-Sternberg cells and malignant reticulum cells.

CLINICAL STAGING

The next important advance in the management of Hodgkin's disease was that of clinical staging. Although currently under review, the present acceptable anatomic classification is outlined in Table 30-2. Several retrospective analyses have indicated that patients with recognizable disease above the diaphragm, limited to one anatomic region (Stage I) or two or more anatomic regions (Stage II), have a significantly better prognosis than patients with disease above and below the diaphragm (Stage III) or with organ involvement (Stage IV). Moreover, when one includes the presence or absence of systemic symptoms, defined as documented fever (cyclical, intermittent, or Pel-Ebstein) seen in from 30 to 50% of patients, pruritus, night sweats, or weight loss equal to at least 10% of body weight, there may be as much as a threefold difference in survival figures in favor of those patients who present without symptoms.

Evaluation of Patient

The clinical and laboratory evaluation of a patient with biopsy-proved Hodgkin's disease should probably be carried out by a brief hospitalization. Clinical examination should include careful appraisal of the spleen size, in light of recent evidence by Kaplan's group that palpable spleens in untreated patients were histologically involved by Hodgkin's disease in 76% of cases, and 56% of these were associated with biopsy-proved liver in-

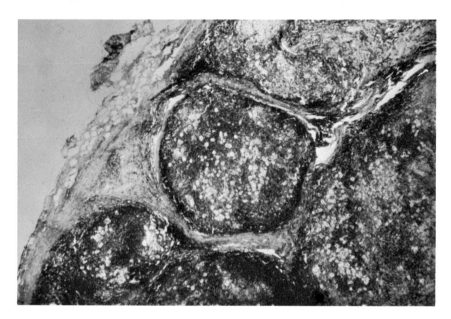

Figure 30-2. Large nodules separated by broad collagen bands. Pale areas are lacunae containing atypical Reed-Sternberg cells. Hodgkin's disease, nodular sclerosing type. (H & E; × 45.)

volvement. Lymphangiography represents a decided improvement over the intravenous pyelogram or an inferior vena cavagram. The demonstration of previously unsuspected retroperitoneal adenopathy may be as high as 30% of clinical Stage IIA and 90% of clinical Stage IIB. The use of this technique has enabled Kaplan and co-workers to unveil the probable mode of spread of this illness. Their concept that the disease begins in a single node or node group and spreads via contiguous involvement has decided implications for therapy.

Laboratory evaluation should include a complete blood count with platelet count, liver screening studies including a serum alkaline phosphatase, uric acid, serum calcium, and Coombs' test and serum iron test if anemia is present. Common hematologic findings, particularly in advanced disease, are neutrophilic leukocytosis, eosinophilia, and lymphopenia. The majority of patients with Stage I or Stage II disease have lymphocyte counts of greater than 2000 per cubic millimeter, whereas patients with Stage III or Stage IV disease have lymphocyte counts usually below 1500 per cubic millimeter. Of patients presenting with Hodgkin's disease initially, 15% have leukocytosis of greater than 15,000 per cubic millimeter. The usefulness of a bone marrow aspiration has been seriously questioned. Bone marrow biopsy using the closed biopsy technique may be of value in patients

Table 30-2.   Clinical Staging of Hodgkin's Disease

Stage	Location	Total (%)
I	Disease in one anatomic region or two contiguous regions on the same side of the diaphragm	10
II	Disease in more than two anatomic regions or two non-contiguous regions on the same side of the diaphragm	20
III	Disease on both sides of the diaphragm (excluding spleen)	60
IV	Disease in marrow, liver, bone, lung, G-I tract, skin, kidneys	10

Note: Subclassify as A or B in the absence or presence of fever, night sweats, and pruritus.

with symptoms in Stage III. With this technique a small number of patients may be advanced to Stage IV by the finding of Hodgkin's granuloma within the bone marrow specimen. Elevated leukocyte alkaline phosphatase activity has been correlated with active disease and may be useful in following the course of the patient during therapy.

The employment of a variety of skin tests including dinitrochlorobenzene (DNCB), tuberculin, histoplasmin, and mumps vaccine may demonstrate cutaneous anergy in 50% of patients, the vast majority being seen in Stages II, III, and IV. Lymphocyte transformation studies are altered significantly in these last three stages, the lowest percentage being in Stage IV. In one study no patients with anergy demonstrated by the preceding tests had both a normal lymphocyte count and a normal percentage of lymphocyte transformation.

The usefulness of combining pathologic classification with clinical staging can be seen in Table 30-3, which summarizes Keller's experience at the Stanford University Medical Center with these techniques. The principles of treatment and the various modalities of therapy will be discussed in the next chapter, but it is apparent from the table that with supravoltage radiotherapy today, a significant percentage of patients will survive 5 years when staged in this manner. Moreover, since the possibility of developing a new manifestation of disease after 5 years is less than 5%, the probability of a 95% cure rate in this population is within reach or already obtainable.

Since prognosis can be correlated statistically with both the histologic features and clinical staging at presentation in Hodgkin's disease, the importance of these procedures should be emphasized. Because, however, even in the best of hands lymphangiography may miss 20% of involved abdominal nodes, and also because clinical and laboratory assessment of liver involvement is often difficult, some centers are beginning clinical trials to evaluate the role of laparotomy, including open liver biopsy, abdominal

Table 30-3.   Survival Figures (%) for Hodgkin's Disease[a]

Pathological Findings %	Anatomic Stage		Symptoms		5-Year
	I–II	III–IV	A	B	Survival
Lymphocyte predominance (5)	90	10	100	0	85
Nodular sclerosis (50)	70	30	65	35	60
Mixed cellularity (40)	60	40	55	45	40
Lymphocyte depletion (5)	30	70	30	70	40 (2 years)

[a] Based on data from A. R. Keller et al., 1968.

node biopsy, splenectomy, and open wedge marrow biopsy, to improve the clinical staging of Hodgkin's disease. Whether or not these trials will alter survival statistics is hard to say at the present time, but it represents to some a logical extension of an attempt to be as accurate as possible in the staging procedure.

MALIGNANT LYMPHOMA (NON-HODGKIN'S TYPE)

The non-Hodgkin's lymphomas constitute a diverse group of primarily lymph node malignancies that range from the well-differentiated lymphocytic lymphomas to the poorly differentiated histiocytic or reticulum cell sarcomas. Although certain similarities exist between this group and Hodgkin's disease, there are several striking differences. First, a significant percentage of cases occur over the age of 50 in both males and females, in contrast to Hodgkin's disease. The disease presentation is more often extranodal than in Hodgkin's disease and is much less frequently localized at the onset. In contrast to Hodgkin's disease, leukemic transformation is frequent. The probability of cure in these disorders is of a much lower order of magnitude than in Hodgkin's disease. Multicentric origin is the rule rather than the exception.

At the present time, unlike the general acceptance of the new classification of Hodgkin's disease proposed by Lukes and Butler, there is no general agreement among pathologists on the classification of the non-Hodgkin's lymphomas. A classification that appears to be simple and to offer clinical usefulness is outlined in Table 30-4. This is a modification of the classification proposed by Lukes. There are several important features to be noted in examining this table. First, although the obliteration of lymph node architecture, infiltration of the capsule, and cellular atypia are all important criteria for establishing a diagnosis of lymphoma, primary importance is

Table 30-4. Classification of the Malignant Lymphomas

Cytology	Histology		Distribution		Peripheral Blood and Bone Marrow	Leukemia Terminology	5-Year Survival (%)
	Diffuse	Nodular	Irreg.	Systemic			
LYMPHOCYTIC							
Well differentiated	+++	+ᵃ	+	++++	++++	Chronic lymphocytic leukemia	25
Poorly differentiated	+	+++	++++	++	++	Leukemic lympho-sarcoma (sub-acute lymphocytic leukemia)	5–10
Stem cell	++++	?	+++	+++	+++	Acute lymphocytic leukemia (stem cell leukemia)	5–10
Burkitt's type	++++	?	++++	+	+ (rare)	—	15–20 (long-term)
HISTIOCYTIC							
Well differentiated	+	+++	+++	+	?	—	5–10
Poorly differentiated	+++	+	+	+++	+++	Acute histiocytic or monocytic leu-kemia (Schill-ing's)	Less than 5

ᵃ So-called nodular or giant follicle type may have longer survival.

given in this tabulation to the identification of specific cytologic types. A leukemia terminology is included to allow the clinician to identify with a more familiar cell type seen in the peripheral blood and also to indicate that often the diseases merge one into the other and are not easily separated.

The well-differentiated lymphocytic lymphoma consists of an abnormal proliferation of small to medium-sized lymphoid cells that often are indistinguishable from normal-appearing lymphocytes (Fig. 30-3). Air-dried imprints stained with a Romanowsky stain reveal a cell type identical to that seen in chronic lymphocytic leukemia (Fig. 30-4). The poorly differentiated lymphoma consists of a proliferation of medium-sized to large cells with an irregular nucleus, occasionally a small single nucleolus or at most two nucleoli, and a chromatin pattern that is finer and not as clumped as in the well-differentiated lymphomas. In addition, cells with amitotic cleavage planes (clefted lymphocytes) are observed frequently. Imprints reveal a more pleomorphic population of cells of the prolymphocyte type, although a moderate number of more differentiated cells with a fine to coarse chromatin pattern can be seen (Fig. 30-5). A nodular pattern in the distribution of lymphocytes in the lymph nodes is more common with this variety of tumor than with the well-differentiated lymphocytic lymphoma. The stem cell lymphoma (lymphoblastic lymphoma) is more commonly seen in children than adults and consists of a relatively uniform population of very poorly differentiated cells with fine chromatin, a single nucleolus or two

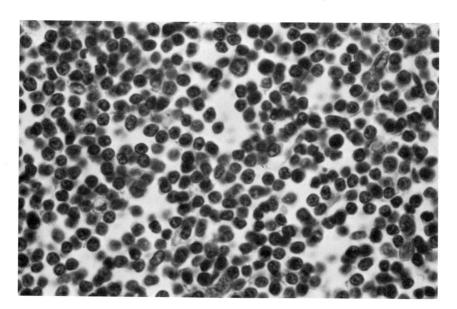

Figure 30-3. Numerous well-differentiated lymphocytes in spleen. Malignant lymphoma, well-differentiated type. (H & E; × 120.)

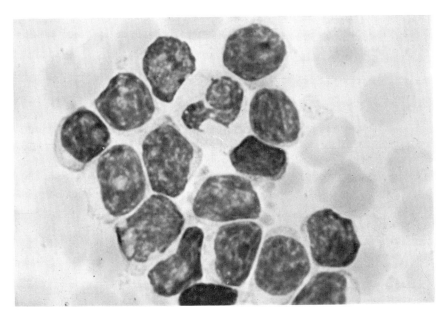

Figure 30-4. Small and medium-sized lymphocytes. Malignant lymphoma, well-differentiated type. (Wright's stained imprint; × 1500.)

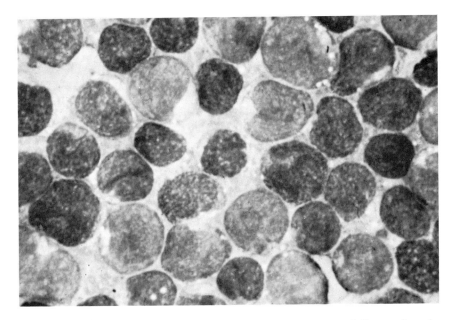

Figure 30-5. Note variability in nuclear contour and size. Malignant lymphoma, poorly differentiated type. (Wright's stained imprint; × 1500.)

nucleoli, and a moderate amount of cytoplasm that is slightly acidophilic. Imprint preparations reveal cells that are indistinguishable from those of acute lymphocytic leukemia.

BURKITT'S TUMOR

Burkitt's tumor is a malignant lymphoma consisting of primitive lympho-reticular cells often associated with benign-appearing histiocytes (macrophages), which give to the section under low power a "starry-sky" pattern (Fig. 30-6). This tumor, originally described in equatorial Africa and indeed the most prevalent childhood tumor in Uganda, often presents as a jaw swelling in males and as ovarian tumors in females. As discussed later, it has provoked considerable interest among epidemiologists, immunologists, and chemotherapists because of its many unique features. Air-dried imprints reveal a monotonous cell type with a very fine nuclear chromatin, several nucleoli, and intense basophilic cytoplasm, often with vacuoles (Fig. 30-7). Unlike the other forms of malignant lymphoma, Burkitt's tumor rarely presents with peripheral blood involvement, although terminally, with bone marrow invasion, a leukoerythroblastic picture may be seen.

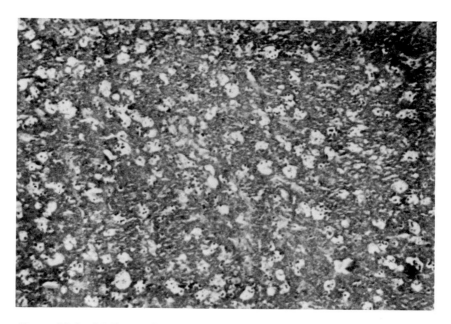

Figure 30-6. Malignant lymphoma, Burkitt's type. Note numerous histiocytes surrounded by cohesive tumor cells. (H & E; × 45.)

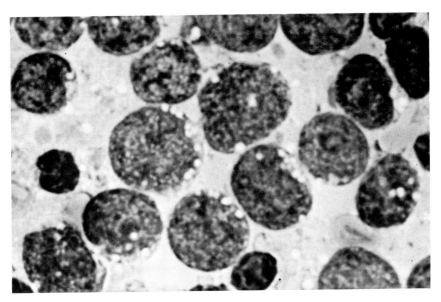

Figure 30-7.   Malignant lymphoma, Burkitt's type. Note vacuolated cytoplasm and large oval to round nuclei. (Wright's stained imprint; × 1500.)

HISTIOCYTIC LYMPHOMAS

The histiocytic lymphomas (reticulum cell sarcomas) include a number of cytologic variants and are more difficult to classify. The use of only two cytologic types is probably arbitrary and may well be modified in the future. However, the nucleus in both types tends to be very large with a finely reticulated chromatin pattern, and there is usually abundant acidophilic cytoplasm. The better differentiated types often contain phagocytic particles and may have fibril production associated with them, demonstrated by the use of a reticulin or silver stain. Imprints reveal very large nuclei with a fine stippled chromatin pattern, one or two very large nucleoli, and usually abundant basophilic cytoplasm in the undifferentiated cells (Fig. 30-8) and acidophilic cytoplasm in the differentiated variety. The monocytic leukemias (Schilling's type) are regarded in this classification as a systemic progression of the histiocytic lymphomas.

MALIGNANT LYMPHOMAS

In the evolution of the malignant lymphomas, leukemia is often interpreted as a natural evolution from irregular to systemic involvement. Note from Table 30-4 that the diffuse lymphomas more often are associated with leukemia than the nodular type. The so-called giant follicular lym-

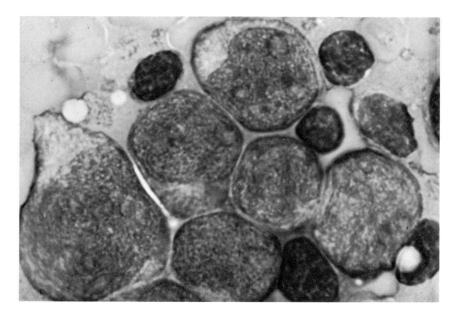

Figure 30-8. Malignant lymphoma, histiocytic type. Note large and pleomorphic cells. (Wright's stained imprint; × 1500.)

phoma, which has been considered to have a very favorable prognosis, has been reinterpreted by Rappaport and his co-workers as a nodular variety of either a well-differentiated or a poorly differentiated lymphocytic lymphoma. The prognosis, therefore, depends more on the cytologic type than on the pattern of disease. In addition, as high as 20% of such cases, on independent review, were considered to be examples of benign follicular hyperplasia in Firat's series.

Brief mention should be made of some of the other proliferative processes related to the malignant lymphomas that are more uncommon and again controversial in regard to classification. Mycosis fungoides is generally regarded as a neoplasm of skin or tissue reticulum cells which may evolve through a systemic form with marked lymph node enlargement and visceral involvement. On rare occasions cells may proliferate in the peripheral blood and can be recognized and differentiated from other abnormal lymphoid cells by their resemblance to monocytes and the markedly increased content of glycogen as demonstrated by a periodic acid–Schiff reaction. This latter condition has been referred to as the *Sézary syndrome.*

CLINICAL COURSE OF NON-HODGKIN'S LYMPHOMAS

The clinical picture of the non-Hodgkin's lymphomas is more variable than that seen during the initial presentation of Hodgkin's disease. This relates primarily to the more generalized involvement of both lymph node tissue and extranodal sites such as the tonsil, thyroid, or gastrointestinal tract. Systemic manifestations such as fever, sweats, and itching are much less common, though occasionally seen. Whereas the cellular immune defect predominates in patients with Hodgkin's disease, in the non-Hodgkin's group an acquired antibody deficiency syndrome is commonly present. A routine serum electrophoresis is often rewarding in revealing a pattern of hypogammaglobulinemia and, on rare occasions, hypergammaglobulinemia. Similarly hematologic manifestations, particularly Coombs'-positive hemolytic anemia, are recognized frequently in patients with lymphocytic lymphomas and in those with chronic lymphocytic leukemia. Increased susceptibility to infection of bacterial, viral, and fungal types can be seen in all the malignant lymphomas. The reasons for this are complex but include both the disturbances of immunoglobulin production and the reduction in granulocytic reserves secondary to both chemotherapy and marrow replacement. The physician, then, is confronted with the problem of evaluating fever, sweats, and chills in a setting in which the symptoms may also reflect the underlying disease as well as infection. An example of one uncommon pathogen in patients with Hodgkin's disease is the association of listeriosis, usually in the form of meningitis or septicemia or both. Within the viral group, infection with varicella zoster, either localized or generalized, probably reflects the altered immune state in this group of disorders and can be one of the disabling complications seen during treatment.

In patients with generalized disease and particularly with known bone involvement, hypercalcemia may develop. On rare occasions this may be found without the presence of bone involvement and may indicate that a humoral mechanism is playing a role. Again, hyperuricemia may result, particularly when there is a considerable amount of tumor present and after vigorous therapy has been instituted.

EPSTEIN-BARR VIRUS

Although the etiologic agent or agents responsible for the malignant lymphomas are presently unknown, evidence does favor at least a strong association for one form of the malignant lymphomas, namely Burkitt's tumor. From several cell-line cultures of the tumor cells of both African and non-African cases, isolates have been found of a herpes-like virus (HLV) originally detected by Epstein and his co-workers and designated as EB virus. Extremely high antibody levels against this virus have been found in patients with Burkitt's tumor, and what is most provocative are recent studies that have demonstrated these identical antibodies in virtually 100% of patients recovering from classic heterophil-positive infectious mononucleosis. It is possible that the high incidence in Equatorial Africa relates to the repeated stimulus of the reticuloendothelial system in African children due to malaria or other infectious agents, with release of a latent virus such as an EB virus coinciding with the development of the disease. As can be seen in Table 30-4 this tumor is also remarkable in the high initial rate of response to chemotherapy and the markedly prolonged remissions induced by a short course of drug therapy in approximately 20% of all cases.

AN APPROACH TO PATIENT EVALUATION

In the past decade it has become increasingly apparent that a multidisciplinary approach is required for developing a prognostic profile in the malignant lymphomas. This is true for both Hodgkin's disease and the non-Hodgkin's lymphomas. It appears, therefore, that to achieve the most accurate evaluation and to predict prognosis, one should have information relating to the cytologic type of malignant lymphoma, the histologic pattern, whether the disease is localized or generalized (i.e., anatomic staging), whether there is peripheral blood or bone marrow involvement, the presence or absence of symptoms, and an accurate picture of the immunologic status, of both the immediate and the delayed type. With such an approach to patient evaluation, the physician is in the best possible position to recommend the most ideal therapy, whether it be radiotherapy, chemotherapy, or a combination of both modalities.

REFERENCES

Bennett, J. M.   A successful safari. *New Eng. J. Med.* 280:328, 1969.
Bennett, J. M., Nathanson, L., and Rutenburg, A. M.   Significance of leukocyte alkaline phosphatase in Hodgkin's disease. *Arch. Intern. Med.* (Chicago) 121:338, 1968.
Brown, R. F., Haynes, H. A., Foley, H. G., Godwin, H. S., Berard, C. W., and Carbone, P. P.   Hodgkin's disease: Immunologic, clinical and histologic features of 50 untreated patients. *Ann. Intern. Med.* 67:291, 1967.
Firat, D., Stutzman, L., Studenski, E. R., and Pickren, J.   Giant follicular lymph node disease. *Amer. J. Med.* 39:252, 1965.
Glatstein, E., Guernsey, J. M., Rosenberg, S. A., and Kaplan, H. S.   The value of laparotomy and splenectomy in the staging of Hodgkin's disease. *Cancer* 24:709, 1969.
Histopathological definition of Burkitt's tumor. *Bull. W.H.O.* 40:601, 1969.
Jackson, H., and Parker, J.   Hodgkin's disease: II. Pathology. *New Eng. J. Med.* 231:35, 1944.
Keller, A. R., Kaplan, H. S., Lukes, R. J., and Rappaport, H.   Correlation of histopathology with other prognostic indicators in Hodgkin's disease. *Cancer* 22:487, 1968.
Lee, D. J.   Correlation between lymphangiography and clinical status of patients with lymphoma. *Cancer Chemother. Rep.* 52:205, 1968.

Lukes, R. J.   The Pathologic Picture of the Malignant Lymphomas. In C. J. D. Zarafonetis (Ed.), *Proceedings of the International Conference on Leukemia-Lymphoma*. Philadelphia: Lea & Febiger, 1968. Pp. 333–356.

Lukes, R. J., and Butler, J. J.   The pathology and nomenclature of Hodgkin's disease. *Cancer Res.* 26:1063, 1966.

Lukes, R. J., Tindle, B. H., and Parker, J. W.   Reed-Sternberg-like cells in infectious mononucleosis. *Lancet* 2:1003, 1969.

Rappaport, H., Winter, W. J., and Hicks, E. B.   Follicular lymphomas: A re-evaluation of its position in the scheme of malignant lymphomas based on a survey of 253 cases. *Cancer* 9:792, 1956.

Rosenberg, S.A., and Kaplan, H. S.   Evidence for an orderly progression in the spread of Hodgkin's disease. *Cancer Res.* 26:1225, 1966.

Simpson, J. S., Leddy, J. P., and Hare, J. D.   Listeriosis complicating lymphoma. *Amer. J. Med.* 43:39, 1967.

31. THERAPY OF THE MALIGNANT LYMPHOMAS AND CHRONIC LYMPHOCYTIC LEUKEMIA

Richard F. Bakemeier

AMONG THE major advances in the management of neoplastic disease within the past two decades have been the concept of curability of Hodgkin's disease and Burkitt's lymphoma when diagnosed in a relatively localized stage and the attainability of long remissions even in generalized malignant lymphomas. These advances, involving the use of extensive radiotherapy or chemotherapy or both, have created a challenging obligation for the clinician. The necessity is clear for accurate diagnosis of lymph node histo-pathology—a task often requiring the assistance of an experienced hemato-pathologist—before undertaking the thorough staging procedures described in the preceding chapter. The importance of accurate staging becomes strikingly apparent when one considers the degree of bone marrow suppression and decreased resistance to infections which may attend current techniques of radiotherapy and chemotherapy. The "go-for-broke" option now available in potentially curable malignant lymphomas, particularly with high-dose, extended-field radiotherapy, is rational only when virtually all neoplastic tissue can be encompassed in the treatment field, or when virtually all neoplastic cells are susceptible to the toxic effects of the therapeutic agent (or both).

Natural defenses, possibly immunologic, may also be available to eradicate a limited number of neoplastic cells. In reference to lymphoma, such defenses are suggested by the relatively improved prognosis of Hodgkin's disease patients with increased numbers of lymphocytes in involved lymph nodes. However, the "body burden" of neoplastic cells in clinically apparent malignant disease is generally considered to exceed the numbers which

The author is recipient of U.S. Public Health Service Research Career Development Award AM-14902.

can be handled by such mechanisms. Therefore cure or prolonged, disease-free remission can be the rational goal of therapy only when the choice and method of application of therapeutic agents permits (1) destruction of perhaps 99.99999% of all malignant cells, as judged by certain animal leukemia models, and concurrently (2) adequate preservation of normal tissues, perhaps augmented by transfusions of red blood cells, white blood cells, or platelets. It is obvious that many factors, including the age of the patient, any associated diseases which might affect life expectancy, and the natural history of the untreated or palliatively treated lymphoma must also be considered in deciding the extent and goals of therapy.

With these general preliminary considerations brought to the reader's attention, we shall turn to a discussion of the therapeutic approaches to lymphoma and chronic lymphocytic leukemia now available.

HODGKIN'S DISEASE

RADIOTHERAPY

The concept of curability of Hodgkin's disease, developed over the past decade through the work of Easson, Peters, Kaplan, Rubin, and others, depends on a primary role of radiotherapy in the treatment program. High doses of radiation—over 4000 rads to each involved area—have been demonstrated to be necessary to prevent local recurrences. The inclusion of adjacent, apparently uninvolved nodes in the treatment field has become generally accepted, although definitive cooperative studies are currently in progress to compare such *extended field treatment* to more localized irradiation to the involved nodes.

Hodgkin's disease at Stages I and II, as determined by thorough staging, can be expected to remit totally for over 2 years in about 70% of patients treated with a *mantle field* (outlined in Fig. 31-1) which treats simultaneously the cervical, supraclavicular, axillary, mediastinal, and hilar lymph nodes, or with an *inverted-Y field* (lower segment blackened in Fig. 31-2C), for disease above or below the diaphragm, respectively. Such results, reported from several large series by Peters, Kaplan and Rosenberg, Rubin, and others, justify the moderate side effects that occur from such extended field therapy, including dysphagia, cough, nausea, diarrhea, and skin changes, and the slight risk of severe complications such as pericarditis and spinal cord damage. Remissions of more than 3 years have better than a 90% chance of being complete cures. Considering histopathology as well as staging, the lymphocyte predominant and nodular sclerosing types of Hodgkin's disease have a somewhat better outlook than mixed cellularity or lymphocyte depletion types.

Such results still leave 30% of patients who initially have apparently

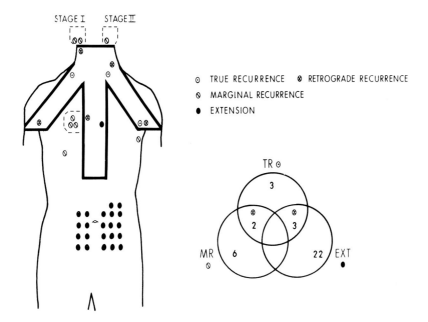

Figure 31-1. Patterns of recurrence of Hodgkin's disease after mantle field therapy. Stage I patients are indicated on the left side of the diagram and Stage II patients on the right. Extension below the diaphragm has been the predominant pattern of recurrence. (From P. Rubin et al., *Amer. J. Roentgen.* 105:814, 1969.)

localized disease with unsatisfactory long-term results. An analysis of such relapses at Rochester by Rubin, Haluska, and Poulter revealed that retroperitoneal lymph node extension, undetected by lymphangiography during initial staging, was the major reason for treatment failure. (Recent reports suggest up to 15 to 20% false-negative lymphangiograms with experienced radiologists.) Even the addition of laparotomy as a staging procedure may not detect such microscopic involvement, particularly in the upper para-aortic nodes. Data from laparotomies performed at Stanford University indicate that *left* supraclavicular node involvement should increase suspicion of para-aortic node involvement.

Therefore more extensive radiation fields are being investigated in Stage IIB as well as Stage III Hodgkin's disease by Kaplan, Rubin, Johnson, and others. Such therapy, termed *total lymphoid irradiation* (Kaplan), *segmental sequential irradiation* (SSI) (Rubin), or *total·nodal irradiation* (Johnson), delivers 3500 to 4500 rads sequentially to the areas blackened in Figure 31-2. For example, a patient with Stage IIB disease above the diaphragm would receive mantle irradiation over a 4- to 5-week period, followed by a rest period of 3 to 4 weeks. Then the remaining lymph node–

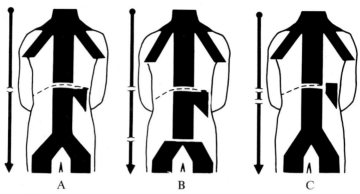

Figure 31-2. Segmental sequential irradiation fields. The "total lymphoid irra-diation" can be divided in various segments to improve tolerance. Pattern C has been followed at Rochester. Splenectomy reduces the size of the upper abdomi-nal fields and reduces lung and kidney irradiation. (From P. Rubin et al., *Amer. J. Roentgen.* 105:814, 1969.)

bearing areas below the diaphragm, and the spleen, if not removed at lapa-rotomy, would receive irradiation in either one or two fields. Such treatment therefore lasts 3 to 4 months and is usually attended by significant leukope-nia and thrombocytopenia (white cell count below 2000 per cubic milli-meter and platelet count below 30,000 per cubic millimeter in over half the patients in Rubin's series at Rochester). Life-threatening infections and bleeding have not been problems, however. Women of child-bearing age or younger present the additional problem of ovarian damage when subjected to the inverted-Y field. The ovaries can be surgically placed in the midline, menstrual function may continue after treatment, and one normal preg-nancy following such treatment has been reported by Kaplan. However, Rubin has calculated a gonadal dose of 400 to 500 rads with the equipment used at Rochester. The high genetic burden, which may not be manifest for several generations, has led us to allow sterilization of the unmoved ovaries to occur in those patients for whom SSI appears to offer hope for improved survival and who accept this sterilization.

It is yet rather early to state the effectiveness of this extensive radiation therapy, although Johnson's preliminary data from the National Institutes of Health indicate an increase in 2-year survival of Stage IB and IIB, from 35% with involved and adjacent nodes treated, to 70% with total nodal irradiation.

Stage III Hodgkin's disease presents a particular challenge to the physi-cians planning therapy. Radiotherapy designed for potential cure must in-clude the extensive fields described above to encompass the disease. Even then, especially with Stage IIIB patients, recurrence in treated nodes and extension to extranodal sites occur in up to two-thirds of patients within 2 years. Patients with systemic symptoms and either mixed cellularity or lymphocyte depletion histology are particularly liable to have extranodal relapse. Since tolerance of chemotherapy for recurrences is often poor up to a year following such radiation therapy, careful selection of patients, probably including prior laparotomy and splenectomy as criteria, is vital to avoid extensively damaging the bone marrow of a patient requiring chemotherapy for Stage IV disease within a year or less. Splenectomy is suggested because of the difficulty of identifying splenic involvement without careful sectioning of the spleen, because of the correlation of splenic involvement with liver involvement, and because subsequent irradiation to the area can be decreased. The additional potential benefit of better tolerance of myelosuppressive therapy after splenectomy has been suggested but not proved as yet except in patients with anemia, leukopenia, or thrombocytopenia related to hypersplenism. Accepted therapy for Stage III disease in many centers is either extensive radiation therapy *or* chemotherapy. Combinations of radiation therapy with chemotherapy are under study, but reports are still preliminary. Such a combined approach has the potential advantage of controlling or even eradicating microscopic disease in sites outside the radiation therapy fields.

CHEMOTHERAPY

The choice of chemotherapeutic agents for the treatment of Hodgkin's disease has broadened considerably in the past decade. Chemotherapy is generally accepted as the appropriate therapy for symptomatic, progressive Stage IV Hodgkin's disease and, in most centers, for many Stage III patients. Local irradiation remains the preferred therapy, even in Stage IV patients, for serious localized problems such as superior vena caval or spinal cord compression, painful local bone lesions, or painful local node enlargement without systemic symptoms. Kaplan has treated unilateral lung involvement by radiation therapy and hepatic involvement by both external irradiation and colloidal radioactive gold with some success, but these remain largely investigational approaches.

Single-drug therapy of widespread Hodgkin's disease effects a good objective response in about 70% of patients. However, combination chemotherapy has been demonstrated to give more prolonged remissions in over 80% of patients with disseminated disease who have not been previously treated, and its use may become more widespread (see below).

A study by Ezdinli and Stutzman indicates that either nitrogen mustard (0.4 mg per kilogram of body weight intravenously) or vinblastine (Velban, a periwinkle alkaloid) (0.15 to 0.2 mg per kilogram intravenously every 7 to 14 days) can produce a decrease in tumor size by one-third to two-thirds in 70 to 80% of patients, with a mean remission duration of about 3 months. Relief of fever, sweating, and pruritus and regression of enlarged nodes may occur within a few days to weeks. Cyclophosphamide and chlorambucil are alkylating agents which also are effective in Hodgkin's disease. Cyclophosphamide is particularly useful in combination regimens which include other myelosuppressive agents because of its relative platelet-sparing effect. Even after resistance to alkylating agents has developed, over 60% of patients demonstrate good responses to vinblastine.

Procarbazine (Matulane, formerly Natulan, a methylhydrazine derivative) is also effective in over half the patients resistant to irradiation, alkylating agents, and the periwinkle alkaloids. However, remissions are usually relatively short (median duration 16 weeks in Samuels' study). Dosage is usually begun at 50 mg daily and increased slowly, by 50 mg daily, to avoid excessive nausea. The customary maximum adult dosage is 300 mg per day, with reduced maintenance doses following clinical remission.

Corticosteroids, in adult doses of 20 to 40 mg of prednisone per day, may be useful in controlling systemic symptoms and hemolytic anemia in advanced cases of Hodgkin's disease. Larger doses (45 to 300 mg per day) have been demonstrated to produce objective regression of the disease in lymph nodes, liver, and spleen in two-thirds of advanced cases refractory to irradiation and alkylation. Although useful in the presence of marrow suppression, corticosteroids may cause serious infectious, peptic ulcer, and hyperglycemic complications.

BCNU [1,3,bis (β-chloroethyl)-1-nitrosourea] is a promising drug, currently used in investigative trials, which has been found effective in over half the patients with far-advanced Hodgkin's disease resistant to other therapy. Marrow suppression, which may have a delayed onset of 3 or 4 weeks after intravenous administration of 1 or 2 doses, constitutes the major toxicity.

Combinations of drugs having additive therapeutic benefit but differing in toxicity are being actively studied. One such combination, referred to as *MOPP* (nitrogen *m*ustard, vincristine (*O*ncovin), *p*rocarbazine, and *p*rednisone), has induced prolonged complete remissions in 81% of untreated Stage III and IV patients studied by DeVita and co-workers (Table 31-1) in an intermittent 6-month regimen (2 weeks of treatment alternating with 2 weeks of rest). Unmaintained remissions as long as 42 months, with a mean response duration over 24 months, are longer than one expects with the use of a single drug. Additional intermittent MOPP therapy beyond 6 months (e.g., two cycles every 3 months) may lead to even longer remissions. Bone marrow toxicity is usually not a serious limiting factor unless previous extensive radiation therapy has been given. However, the neurotoxicity of vincristine may be a problem, and in our experience the recurrent nausea and vomiting from nitrogen mustard eventually conditions some patients to have these symptoms *prior* to each cycle, particularly

Table 31-1. MOPP Regimen

Drug	Dosage (mg/m²)	Day					
		1 2	8	10 11	14	28	
Nitrogen mustard (HN₂)	6 (IV)	X	X			Rest period	
Vincristine	1.4 (IV)	X	X				
Procarbazine	100 (PO)	X X X X X X X X X X X X X X					
Prednisone (1st and 4th cycles only)	40 (PO)	X X X X X X X X X X X X X X					

NOTE: Repeat at minimum of 14-day intervals, omitting prednisone second, third, fifth, and sixth cycles. Additional cycles (e.g., two cycles at 3-month intervals) may prolong remissions.

when the therapy is continued past 6 months. One such patient at Rochester, whose pulmonary Hodgkin's disease has been controlled for 14 months by 12 courses of MOPP, with relapses during two 1-month intermissions, has had no serious toxicity but strikingly demonstrates this conditioned pretreatment vomiting. Other combinations useful in advanced Hodgkin's disease are cyclophosphamide-vinblastine-prednisone and cyclophosphamide-vincristine-prednisone, with or without procarbazine, the myelosuppressive agents being used in doses smaller than when used singly. Complete remissions may be induced in half or more of the patients, but the attendant increased risk of complications must be kept in mind.

In summary, combination regimens may produce prolonged remissions in the majority of patients presenting with good bone marrow function, and an initial 6- to 9-month course in patients not candidates for potentially curative radiation therapy may permit a longer treatment-free interval than single-drug therapy can. However, the latter is still standard therapy for palliative treatment and may provide equally long remissions in some patients, with fewer side effects than occur with combination chemotherapy.

At the risk of excessive generalization, and emphasizing that each patient's total clinical picture must be analyzed individually, I suggest the therapeutic approaches indicated in Table 31-2. The feasibility of these programs presupposes the availability of a skilled radiotherapist using appropriate supravoltage equipment in close cooperation with a hematologist, medical oncologist, or internist with chemotherapeutic experience. It is apparent that segmental sequential irradiation requires particular expertise and that referral to a center experienced in its application may be necessary to afford the patient optimum management.

Table 31-2.   Outline of Suggested Treatment of Hodgkin's Disease

Stage	Histology	Suggested Treatment
IA, IIA	LP, NS	Extended field irradiation
IA, IIA	MC, LD	Segmental sequential irradiation
IA, IIA	Left supracla-vicular nodes	Segmental sequential irradiation
IB, IIB, IIIA	LP, NS	Segmental sequential irradiation
IB, IIB, IIIA IIIB	MC, LD All histology	Segmental sequential irradiation preceded by combination chemotherapy (2 or 3 cycles suggested, possibly more after irradiation)
IVA or IVB	All histology	Initial therapy: 6–9 months combination chemotherapy With previous widespread irradiation, cautious use of combination or single agent (vinblastine, cyclophosphamide, procarbazine; HN_2 for most rapid response) Local irradiation for localized problems

MALIGNANT LYMPHOMA: LYMPHOCYTIC AND RETICULUM CELL TYPES

RADIOTHERAPY

Malignant lymphomas of the lymphocytic and reticulum cell types vary somewhat in their radiosensitivity, but in general they respond well. Enthusiasm for extended field irradiation or total lymphoid irradiation, as contrasted to therapy to involved sites alone, is tempered by the tendency of these lymphomas to be generalized when first diagnosed. Furthermore, the more advanced age of many of these patients, in contrast to those with Hodgkin's disease, and the increased incidence of associated diseases and decreased tolerance to therapy make long-term cure a less rational goal. Total-body irradiation to doses of 100 to 300 rads is currently under investigation for treating generalized disease, however.

Radiation therapy is used to treat symptomatic local sites, often in combination with chemotherapy if there are systemic symptoms. Mediastinal compression can be relieved by a rapid dose schedule of 400 rads × 3 and diuretics. This should be followed by daily doses of 150 to 200 rads to levels of 3000 to 4000 rads. Spinal cord compression, if detected within a few hours after onset, can be treated successfully without surgical decompression, using the same rapid dose schedule. Osseous involvement should be treated, if symptomatic, with doses of 2000 to 3000 rads. Even without visible mediastinal lymphadenopathy, irradiation to the mediastinum is often successful in controlling pleural effusions resulting from lymphatic obstruction. Gastrointestinal involvement, if part of generalized lymphoma and not amenable to surgical cure, should be treated with small, fractionated doses to avoid perforation from rapid tumor lysis.

Pretreatment with allopurinol to prevent hyperuricemia should be considered if large lymphoid masses are to be lysed by radiation therapy or chemotherapy.

CHEMOTHERAPY

Progressive, symptomatic disease too extensive for local or regional radiation therapy can be effectively controlled by several different chemotherapeutic agents, singly or in combination. Nitrogen mustard can produce rapid, dramatic relief of systemic symptoms. Chlorambucil is widely used as an oral agent (0.1 to 0.2 mg per kilogram per day). Cyclophosphamide has become the most commonly used alkylating agent for non-Hodgkin's lymphoma in our center, because of the ease of oral administration and the relative platelet-sparing effect. Doses of 50 to 150 mg per day by mouth are used for maintenance therapy. Induction of remission may be effectively produced with intermittent intravenous cyclophosphamide in doses of 15 mg per kilogram per week. An interesting recent report by Mendelson and co-workers describes the use of intravenous cyclophosphamide in larger doses (1500 mg per square meter of body surface, or about 35 mg per kilogram of body weight) every 3 weeks. Five of 17 patients with generalized lymphoma developed a complete response (no clinical, radiologic, or laboratory evidence of disease). Such intermittent regimens take advantage of the observations of Bruce and co-workers concerning the "cycle-active" nature of cyclophosphamide, i.e., greater toxicity for cells in the mitotic cycle than for resting cells. Many marrow stem cells may be relatively protected from this toxicity by being in the resting state. Bone marrow suppression from such intermittent regimens is not severe even with lymphomatous infiltration. Adequate hydration must be maintained to prevent hemorrhagic cystitis.

Vincristine (Oncovin), a periwinkle alkaloid, appears to produce objective responses in about one-third of patients with lymphocytic lymphoma and reticulum cell sarcoma. It may be used in cases resistant to alkylating agents, even when considerable bone marrow suppression is present, in doses of 20 to 30 μg per kilogram of body weight per week, intravenously.

Corticosteroids have a definite lympholytic effect in about three-fourths of patients with lymphocytic lymphomas and give tumor responses in some patients with reticulum cell sarcoma. They are particularly useful when there is bone marrow suppression or severe infiltration and in the presence of hemolytic anemia. The complications of prolonged corticosteroid therapy are well known, and alternate-day schedules should be considered to minimize these.

Combinations of agents, similar to those described for Hodgkin's disease (Table 31-1), have been widely tested in lymphocytic lymphoma and reticulum cell sarcoma in recent years. Reports such as that of Lowenbraun, DeVita, and Serpick indicate that these regimens may produce quite prolonged remissions (mean durations 11.7 and 30.6 months, respectively). The immunosuppressive nature of these regimens must be kept in mind, however, particularly since these patients often are already immunologically crippled by their disease. We have recently been fortunate in curing a patient of severe *Pneumocystis carinii* pneumonia which developed during treatment of his lymphocytic lymphoma with cyclophosphamide, vincristine, and prednisone. As stated before, the age of a patient, his tolerance for therapy, and the natural history of his disease, sometimes indolent even when untreated, should be considered in planning therapy. It may be that, whereas certain older patients may be in danger of overtreatment, younger patients with aggressive disease might benefit from more intensive, early radiation therapy, perhaps combined with chemotherapy, to limit the body burden of neoplastic cells.

In summary, in managing lymphocytic lymphomas and reticulum cell sarcoma, local irradiation is recommended for local symptomatic disease. Systemic symptoms—fever, sweats, weight loss, fatigue—or progressive symptomatic generalized nodal enlargement warrant systemic chemotherapy. Cyclophosphamide is a particularly useful agent. While daily oral maintenance is effective, convenient, and relatively economical, intermittent intravenous regimens, if feasible, offer the potential advantages of less immunosuppression and less marrow suppression.

BURKITT'S LYMPHOMA

Prolonged remissions or even cures following brief courses of cyclophosphamide or methotrexate in African patients with Burkitt's tumor have stimulated much interest and speculation concerning participation by a host antitumor response, possibly immunologic. For excellent discussions of this lymphoma the reader is directed to the paper by Cohen and associates and the Symposium in *Cancer*, 1968 (see references). About one-half of reported American patients with tumors histologically identical to Burkitt's tumor in Africans have shown prolonged remissions following large intravenous doses (40 to 50 mg per kilogram of body weight) of cyclophosphamide every 3 to 4 weeks for 6 courses. It should be noted that such intermittent therapy should minimize the otherwise considerable immuno-suppressive effects of cyclophosphamide.

CHRONIC LYMPHOCYTIC LEUKEMIA

Chronic lymphocytic leukemia (CLL) may vary in its clinical behavior from a *benign* form, which may be asymptomatic and stable, to an *aggressive* form, usually seen in younger patients (30 to 50 years) and character-ized by fatigue, weight loss, fever, progressive generalized lymphadenopa-thy and splenomegaly, anemia, thrombocytopenia, and susceptibility to infections.

The benign variety need not be treated unless symptoms develop that are attributable to the disease, although such symptoms may be very subtle and go unrecognized for considerable periods. The aggressive type can be effec-tively treated by chemotherapeutic agents. Local radiation therapy may re-duce a massively enlarged spleen or painfully enlarged nodes. Frequent blood counts should be obtained during splenic irradiation to avoid severe cytopenias. Johnson has recently studied the effects of total-body irradia-tion on CLL and has shown that 8 of 16 patients had complete disappear-ance of disease for a median duration of 19 months following doses in the neighborhood of 150 rads. This remains an investigational technique.

Chemotherapy employs alkylating agents and corticosteroids. Chloram-bucil (Leukeran) in doses of 0.1 to 0.2 mg per kilogram per day has been widely used. As the white blood count falls, the dose should be reduced. Maintenance therapy with chlorambucil (1 to 2 mg per day) may give pro-longed remission, although cyclophosphamide may have less long-term marrow toxicity than chlorambucil. As pointed out in Chapter 9, the onset of Coombs'-positive hemolytic anemia may occur in cases of CLL shortly after treatment with alkylating agents.

Corticosteroids may be used for their lympholytic effect in patients with progressive disease, particularly when bone marrow suppression is present, making alkylation therapy hazardous. Doses of 10 to 30 mg per day of prednisone will usually improve the patient symptomatically, but infectious complications may occur. Larger doses (100 to 150 mg per day) may pro-duce objective improvements in blood counts and lymph nodes, but these are usually short lived when the drug is stopped. Corticosteroids may effec-tively control acquired immune hemolytic anemia developing during the course of CLL.

An interesting experimental approach to CLL has been the administra-tion of antilymphocyte serum. Allogenic human immune plasma produced in volunteers causes a transient fall in peripheral lymphocytes and may cause a decrease in node size. Horse antisera are of limited usefulness because of the danger of anaphylactic reactions.

SUMMARY

Therapy of the malignant lymphomas has provided one of the brightest chapters in neoplastic disease management in the past 10 years. Effective control and even cure, especially of Hodgkin's disease, are now possible. Longer remissions may result from the careful use of combination chemotherapy, although the possible increase in complications must be weighed against the realistic goals of therapy. Further major advances await the more complete understanding of etiologic factors and the details of pathogenesis of these diseases.

REFERENCES

Bruce, W. R., Meeker, B. E., and Valeriote, F. A.   Comparison of the sensitivity of normal hematopoietic and transplanted lymphoma colony–forming cells to chemotherapeutic agents administered in vivo. *J. Nat. Cancer Inst.* 37:233, 1966.

Cohen, M. H., Bennett, J. M., Berard, C. W., Ziegler, J. L., Vogel, C. L., Sheargren, J. N., and Carbone, P. P.   Burkitt's tumor in the United States. *Cancer* 23:1259, 1969.

DeVita, V. T., Serpick, A. A., and Carbone, P. P.   Combination chemotherapy in the treatment of advanced Hodgkin's disease. *Ann. Intern. Med.* 73:881, 1970.

Ezdinli, E. Z., and Stutzman, L.   Vinblastine vs. nitrogen mustard therapy of Hodgkin's disease. *Cancer* 22:473, 1968.

Glatstein, E., Guernsey, J. M., Rosenberg, S. A., and Kaplan, H. S.   The value of laparotomy and splenectomy in the staging of Hodgkin's disease. *Cancer* 24:709, 1969.

Johnson, R. E.   Modern approaches to the radiotherapy of lymphoma. *Seminars Hemat.* 6:357, 1969.

Johnson, R. E., Thomas, L. B., and Chretien, P.   Correlation between clinico-histologic staging and extranodal relapse in Hodgkin's disease. *Cancer* 25:1071, 1970.

Kaplan, H. S.   On the natural history, treatment, and prognosis of Hodgkin's disease. *Harvey Lect.* 64:215, 1968–1969.

Lessner, H. E. (for the Southeastern Cancer Chemotherapy Cooperative Study Group).   BCNU [1,3,bis (β-chloroethyl)-1-nitrosourea]: Effects on advanced Hodgkin's disease and other neoplasia. *Cancer* 22:451, 1968.

Lowenbraun, S., DeVita, V. T., and Serpick, A. A.   Combination chemotherapy with nitrogen mustard, vincristine, procarbazine, and prednisone in lymphosarcoma and reticulum cell sarcoma. *Cancer* 25:1018, 1970.

Mendelson, D., Block, J. B., and Serpick, A. A.   Effect of large intermittent intravenous doses of cyclophosphamide in lymphoma. *Cancer* 25:715, 1970.

Rubin, P., Haluska, G., and Poulter, C. A.   The basis for segmental sequential irradiation in Hodgkin's disease: Clinical experience of patterns of recurrence. *Amer. J. Roentgen.* 105:814, 1969.

Samuels, M. L., Leary, W. V., Alexanian, R., Howe, C. D., and Frei, E., III. Clinical trials with N-isopropyl-α-(2-methylhydrazino)-P-toluamide hydrochloride in malignant lymphoma and other disseminated neoplasia. *Cancer* 20:1187, 1967.

Silver, R. T.   The treatment of chronic lymphocytic leukemia. *Seminars Hemat.* 6:344, 1969.

Third Symposium on Clinical Aspects of Acute Leukemia and Burkitt's Tumor. *Cancer* Vol. 21, No. 4, 1968.

Ultmann, J. E.   Current status: The management of lymphoma. *Seminars Hemat.* 7:441, 1970.

Ultmann, J. E., and Nixon, D. D.   The therapy of lymphoma. *Seminars Hemat.* 6:376, 1969.

APPENDIX
BIBLIOGRAPHY OF METHODOLOGY

I. ANEMIAS

A. GENERAL

Cartwright, G. E. *Diagnostic Laboratory Hematology* (4th ed.). New York: Grune & Stratton, 1968.

Dacie, J. V., and Lewis, S. M. *Practical Haematology* (4th ed.). New York: Grune & Stratton, 1968.

B. HEMOLYTIC

1. *Evaluation of Immune Hemolysis*

   Mollison, P. L. *Blood Transfusion in Clinical Medicine* (4th ed.). Philadelphia: Davis, 1967.

2. *Sugar Water Test*

   Hartmann, R. C., Jenkins, D. E., Jr., and Arnold, A. R. Diagnostic specificity of sucrose hemolysis test for paroxysmal nocturnal hemoglobinuria. *Blood* 35:462, 1970.

3. *Filterability*

   Jandl, J. H., Simmons, R. L., and Castle, W. B. Red cell filtration in the pathogenesis of certain hemolytic anemias. *Blood* 28:133, 1961.

   Teitel, P. Le test de la filterabilité erythrocytaire (TFE): Une méthode simple d'étude de certaines propriétés microrhéologiques des globules rouges. *Nouv. Rev. Franc. Hemat.* 7:195, 1967.

C. B_{12} AND FOLATE: ASSAY METHODOLOGY

Anderson, B. B. Investigations into the *Euglena* method for the assay of the vitamin B_{12} in serum. *J. Clin. Path.* 17:14, 1964.

Brozovic, M., Hoffbrand, A. V., Dimitriadou, A., and Mollin, D. L. The excretion of methylmalonic acid and succinic acid in vitamin B_{12} and folate deficiency. *Brit. J. Haemat.* 13:1021, 1967.

Herbert, V. Aseptic addition method for *Lactobacillus casei* assay of folate activity in human serum. *J. Clin. Path.* 19:12, 1966.

Hoffbrand, A. V., Newcombe, B. F. A., and Mollin, D. L. Method of assay of red cell folate activity and the value of the assay as a test for folate deficiency. *J. Clin. Path.* 19:17, 1966.

Klipstein, F. A.   The urinary excretion of orally administered tritium-labeled folic acid as a test of folic acid absorption. *Blood* 21:262, 1963.

Kohn, J., Mollin, D. L., and Rosenbach, L. M.   Conventional voltage electrophoresis for formiminoglutamic-acid determination in folic acid deficiency. *J. Clin. Path.* 14:345, 1961.

Lau, K. S., Gottlieb, C., Wasserman, L. R., and Herbert, V.   Measurement of serum vitamin B_{12} level using radioisotope dilution and coated charcoal. *Blood* 26:202, 1965.

McCurdy, P. R.   The detection of intestinal absorption of Co^{57}-tagged vitamin B_{12} by serum counting. *Ann. Intern. Med.* 62:97, 1965.

II. HEMOSTASIS

A. GENERAL

Biggs, R., and MacFarlane, R. G. (Eds.). *Human Blood Coagulation and Its Disorders* (3d ed.). Philadelphia: Davis, 1962.

Douglas, A. S.   *Anticoagulant Therapy.* Philadelphia: Davis, 1962.

Hardisty, R. M., and Ingram, G. I. C.   *Bleeding Disorders: Investigation and Management.* Philadelphia: Davis, 1965.

Hougie, C.   *Fundamentals of Blood Coagulation in Clinical Medicine.* New York: McGraw-Hill, 1963.

Quick, A. J.   *Hemorrhagic Diseases and Thrombosis* (2d ed.). Philadelphia: Lea & Febiger, 1966.

Tocantins, L. M., and Kazal, L. A. (Eds.). *Blood Coagulation, Hemorrhage and Thrombosis: Methods of Study.* New York: Grune & Stratton, 1964.

B. PLATELETS

Marcus, A. J.   Platelet function. *New Eng. J. Med.* 280:1213, 1276, 1330, 1969.

Salzman, E. W.   Measurement of platelet adhesiveness: Simple *in vitro* technique demonstrating abnormality in von Willebrand's disease. *J. Lab. Clin. Med.* 62:724, 1963.

Shulman, N. R.   Immunoreactions involving platelets: III. Quantitative aspects of platelet agglutination, inhibition of clot retraction and other reactions caused by the antibody of quinidine purpura. *J. Exp. Med.* 107:697, 1958.

Spaet, T. H., and Cintron, J.   Studies on platelet factor-3 availability. *Brit. J. Haemat.* 11:269, 1965.

Weiss, H. J., Aledort, L. M., and Kochwa, S.   The effects of salicylates on the hemostatic properties of platelets in man. *J. Clin. Invest.* 47:2169, 1968.

III. LEUKOCYTES

A. CYTOCHEMISTRY

Bennett, J. M., and Dutcher, T. F.   The cytochemistry of acute leukemia: Observations on glycogen and neutral fat in bone marrow aspirates. *Blood* 33:341, 1969.

Hayhoe, F. G. J.   Clinical and Cytological Recognition and Differentiation of the Leukemias. In C. Zarafonetis (Ed.), *Proceedings of the International Conference on Leukemia-Lymphoma.* Philadelphia: Lea & Febiger, 1968. P. 307.

Kaplow, L.   Simplified myeloperoxidase stain using benzidine dihydrochloride. *Blood* 26:215, 1965.

Rutenburg, A. M., Rosales, C. L., and Bennett, J. M.   An improved histochemical method for the demonstration of leukocyte alkaline phosphatase. *J. Lab. Clin. Med.* 65:698, 1965.

B. MURAMIDASE

Osserman, E. F., and Lawlor, D. P.   Serum and urinary lysozyme muramidase in monocytic and monomyelocytic leukemia. *J. Exp. Med.* 124:921, 1966.

Perillie, P. E., Kaplan, S. S., Lefkowitz, E., Rogaway, W., and Finch, S. C.   Studies of muramidase (lysozyme). *J.A.M.A.* 203:317, 1968.

C. NBT TEST

Baehner, R. L., and Nathan, D. G.   Quantitative nitroblue tetrazolium test in chronic granulomatous disease. *New Eng. J. Med.* 278:971, 1968.

D. IMMUNODIFFUSION AND IMMUNOELECTROPHORESIS

Ouchterlony, Ö.   Immunodiffusion and Immunoelectrophoresis. In D. M. Weir (Ed.), *Handbook of Experimental Immunology.* London: Blackwell, 1967. P. 655.

INDEX

INDEX